Teaching Psychiatry

Teaching Psychiatry

Putting Theory into Practice

Linda Gask
University of Manchester, Manchester, UK

Bulent Coskun
University of Kocaeli, Kocaeli, Turkey

David Baron
Keck School of Medicine, University of Southern California, Los Angeles, CA, USA

⊛WILEY-BLACKWELL

A John Wiley & Sons, Ltd., Publication

Library of Congress Cataloging-in-Publication Data

Teaching psychiatry : putting theory into practice / [edited by] Linda Gask, Bulent Coskun, David Baron
     p. ; cm.
   Includes bibliographical references and index.
   ISBN 978-0-470-68321-7 (cloth)
   1. Psychiatry–Study and teaching. I. Gask, Linda. II. Coskun, Bulent. III. Baron, David A.
   [DNLM: 1. Psychiatry–education. 2. Curriculum. 3. Psychotherapy–education. WM 18]
   RC459.T43 2011
   616.890076–dc22
                                                                                    2010035694

A catalogue record for this book is available from the British Library.

This book is published in the following electronic formats: ePDF: 978-0-470-97453-7; Wiley Online Library: 978-0-470-97454-4; ePub: 978-0-470-97493-3

Typeset in 10/12pt Bembo by Aptara Inc., New Delhi, India.
Printed and bound in Singapore by Markono Print Media Pte Ltd.

First Impression   2011

Contents

Contributors

Maarten Bak Department of Psychiatry and Neuropsychology, Maastricht University, PO Box 616, 6200 MD Maastricht, The Netherlands

David Baron Department of Psychiatry, Keck School of Medicine, University of Southern California, 2250 Alcazar St, CSC 2202, Los Angeles, CA 90033, USA

Sheldon Benjamin Department of Psychiatry, University of Massachusetts Medical School, 55 Lake Avenue North, Worcester, MA 01655, USA

Maria R. Corral Department of Psychiatry, University of British Columbia, St. Paul's Hospital, 1081 Burrard Street, Vancouver, BC V6Z1Y6, Canada

Bulent Coskun Department of Psychiatry, Kocaeli University Medical School, University of Kocaeli, Umuttepe Kampusu 41 380, Kocaeli, Turkey

Michael Curtis Standardized Patient Program, William Maul Measey Institute for Clinical Simulation and Patient Safety, Temple University School of Medicine, Room 361, Medicine Education and Research Building, 3500 N. Broad Street, Philadelphia, PA 19140-5104, USA

Rob van Diest Department of Psychiatry and Neuropsychology, Maastricht University, PO Box 616, 6200 MD Maastricht, The Netherlands

Nisha Dogra Greenwood Institute of Child Health, University of Leicester, Westcotes House, Westcotes Drive, Leicester LE3 0QU, UK

Mark Oliver Evans Gaskell House Psychotherapy Centre, Swinton Grove, Manchester M13 0EU, UK

Rodolfo Fahrer Department of Mental Health, School of Medicine, University of Buenos Aires, 2436 J. Salguero, Piso 8, Buenos Aires, Argentina

Glen O. Gabbard Department of Psychiatry and Behavioural Sciences, Baylor College of Medicine, 6655 Travis Street, Suite 500, Houston, TX 77030, USA

Linda Gask School of Community Based Medicine, University of Manchester, NPCRDC, 5th Floor Williamson Building, Oxford Road, Manchester M13 9LP, UK

David P. Goldberg Institute of Psychiatry, King's College, 16 De Crespigny Park, London SE5 8AF, UK

Rex Haigh Berkshire Healthcare NHS Foundation Trust, Fitzwilliam House, Skimped Hill Lane, Bracknell RG12 1LD, UK

Cyril Höschl Psychiatrické centrum Praha (Prague Psychiatric Centre affiliated with Charles University), Ústavní 91, 181 03 Prague 8 – Bohnice, Czech Republic

Niranjan Karnik Pritzker School of Medicine, The University of Chicago, 5841 S. Maryland, MC 3077, Chicago IL 60637, USA

Kath Lovell Emergence Community Interest Company, 59 Weltje Road, Hammersmith, London W6 9LS, UK

Brian Lunn School of Medical Sciences Education Development, The Medical School, Newcastle University, Royal Victoria Infirmary, Queen Victoria Road, Newcastle upon Tyne NE1 4LP, UK

Amanda B. Mackey Department of Psychiatry and Behavioral Sciences, University of Louisville School of Medicine, 501 E. Broadway Suite 340, Louisville, KY 40202, USA

Maria Margariti Eginition Hospital, Department of Psychiatry, University of Athens, Vasillissis Sofias Avenue 72-74, Athens 115 28, Greece

Adriana Mihai Psychiatric Department, University of Medicine and Pharmacy Tg Mures, 38 GH Marinescu Street, 540130TG Mures, Romania

Driss Moussaoui Ibn Rushd University Psychiatric Centre, Rue Tarik Ibn Ziad, Casablanca 20000, Morocco

Michael F. Myers Department of Psychiatry & Behavioral Sciences, SUNY Downstate Medical Center, 450 Clarkson Avenue, Brooklyn, NY 11203, USA

Allan Tasman Department of Psychiatry and Behavioral Sciences, University of Louisville School of Medicine, 401 E. Chestnut Street, Suite 600, Louisville, KY 40202, USA

Jon van Niekerk Rivington Unit, Royal Bolton Hospital, Greater Manchester West Mental Health Foundation Trust, Bolton BL4 0JR, UK

Raja Vellingiri Badrakalimuthu Cambridge and Peterborough NHS Foundation Trust, Ida Darwin Site, Fulbourn, Cambridge CB21 5EE, UK

Hugo de Waal East of England Deanery, Block 3, Ida Darwin Site, Fulbourn Hospital, Fulbourn, Cambridge CB21 5EE, UK

Foreword

This book aims to cover the history and future of medical education in psychiatry at every level of training from the undergraduate to medical student, to the resident and practitioner after graduation. This is a challenge that is very well met by the authors. The contributors represent educators from around the world and reference other dedicated educators over the centuries, from Hippocrates to the present. All this to make the point that we live in one world and that, perhaps more than ever with advanced communication and technology, we can and should learn from each other.

This text discusses effective ways for how to teach and learn, as psychiatric educators, including how to promote life-long learning. Some chapters focus on learning throughout one's psychiatric career, while others look at specific aspects of career development. For instance, Chapters 2 and 4 consider recruiting and teaching medical students about psychiatry – of great interest at a time when we need to attract quality graduates into our discipline. Importantly, this book is about educational methods and several chapters (5, 7, 8, 9, 10, 11, 14 and 18) review techniques for teaching residents, not just behavioural science, but interviewing skills, psychotherapy techniques and some introductory elements of clinical research. The skills imparted during psychiatric education are also required by primary care physicians, who treat many patients with comorbid 'physical' and psychiatric illnesses and often are the only available mental health providers. Other chapters (6, 10, 13 and 15) therefore present models for teaching interviewing and psychotherapy skills to primary care providers. Further, there is a comprehensive description of how one can learn life long through problem-based learning techniques (Chapter 6). These chapters also make the point that effective psychiatric teaching at all levels, including primary care, must include ward work, outpatient work and, particularly, community work, and highlight the various ways this can be done.

The use of technology in psychiatric education is addressed specifically in Chapter 16. This states that while technology can facilitate the educational process, it raises ethical issues that cannot be ignored. Ethical issues relevant to the whole educational process are described in Chapter 3, which notes that ever-expanding medical improvements create new social phenomena that must be addressed. It also highlights the need to become more global in our approach to education as we deal with regional variations in the delivery of psychiatric care. Chapter 12, Teaching Psychiatry Students About Cultural Diversity, takes ethical issues in another direction by describing the essence of culture and how cultural issues are intercalated into our everyday lives. It emphasizes that cultural diversity training, at any level of career development, involves the educational concepts of 'cultural expertise' and 'cultural sensibility'.

A strength of this book is that the multiple contributors do not just discuss what has been done and what needs to be done in the future, but consider the assessment and evaluation of the educational process as it proceeds. Chapter 17, Assessment in Psychiatric Education, features the key components of assessment, from formative to summative elements. It makes the point that assessment of the process of learning shapes the teaching and learning that will follow.

Throughout the book, excellent tables and 'boxes' provide the reader with take-home information that they can adapt to their own situation. Each of the 19 chapters can stand alone in giving the reader both a general curriculum, as well as specific tools to teach.

In closing, in the final chapter, the authors remind us that: 'The word "doctor" comes from the ancient term "docere". The translation of this word is not "to diagnose" or "to treat", but rather "to teach". When we stop and think about what we do as physicians, and particularly as psychiatrists, it is clear that we work to help our patients maintain health or treat disease. *Teaching* them how to maintain emotional homeostasis and better deal with life stress is an important component of every treatment strategy and clinical intervention.' Finally, we are presented with examples of how to teach our patients, their families, our students and ourselves.

This text provides a global perspective on teaching psychiatry, at every level, from a process point of view. It is not a 'what to teach' manual as much as it is a 'how to teach'. I believe it is a valuable addition to the psychiatry education literature geared for the teacher as well as useful to their students who want to better learn how to teach in their turn.

Michele T. Pato

Professor and Associate Chair of Education
Department of Psychiatry and the Behavioral Sciences
Keck School of Medicine, University of Southern California

1

Overview: The Need for Improvements in Psychiatric Education

Linda Gask[1], David Baron[2] and Bulent Coskun[3]

[1]School of Community Based Medicine, University of Manchester, Manchester, UK
[2]Department of Psychiatry, Keck School of Medicine, University of Southern California, Los Angeles, CA, USA
[3]Department of Psychiatry, Kocaeli University Medical School, Kocaeli, Turkey

Education includes more than the cognitive transmission of knowledge. Learning requires an affective and psychomotor component as well. Psychiatrists are uniquely qualified to appreciate, and apply, core tenets of the educational process.

This book developed out of recognition amongst the co-editors of a need for more attention within our profession to both the art and the science of teaching psychiatry. As past Chair (Gask) and present Chair (Coskun) and Co-Chairs (Gask and Baron) of the Section of Education of the World Psychiatric Association, we have debated the developments in teaching over the last decade, and have noted that our own speciality has sometimes seemed rather slow to adopt some of the newer educational technologies, using 'technology' in the broadest sense of the word to mean the methods and tools that can be brought to bear to solve a particular problem in society. In many parts of the world, psychiatric teaching is still delivered using a combination of the formal lecture programme, combined with the apprenticeship hands–on experience in the hospital and out-patient clinic often with limited supervision. As two young colleagues of one of the editors wrote in the *Psychiatric Bulletin* many years ago when reflecting on the experience of the trainee:

> No-one except you and the patient really know what happens when you take him for an interview. You learn from your own mistakes behind the closed door.
> —Adams and Cook [1]

Teaching Psychiatry: Putting Theory into Practice   Edited by Linda Gask, Bulent Coskun and David Baron
© 2011 John Wiley & Sons, Ltd

A view that will still be familiar to many of those starting psychiatry today.

However, at the same time we recognized that our own decisions to enter the profession were not always so much governed by the now quite traditional methods that were used in our teaching, but the qualities of an individual and often charismatic teacher who inspired enthusiasm for finding out about what sometimes seems like a quite difficult and nebulous subject to many students. In the chapter which follows this brief introduction, Cyril Höschl and Jon van Niekerk explicitly address the important role that education has to play in addressing the 'recruitment crisis' in psychiatry and the negative attitudes that medical students have been found to possess towards our speciality. This is followed by a discussion by Driss Moussaoui of the need to specifically address ethical issues in the teaching of psychiatry. In Chapter 4, a comprehensive overview of the development of an undergraduate curricula is presented by Nisha Dogra, Cyril Höschl and Driss Moussaoui using a model developed by the Royal College of Psychiatrists in the United Kingdom (UK) as an example. In a companion chapter, Amanda Mackey and Allan Tasman specifically examine the design of the residency curriculum; an up-to-date overview of methods in assessment is provided in a later chapter by Brian Lunn, Maria Corrall and Adriana Mihai.

How to teach 'behavioural sciences' in ways that seem to be relevant and interesting to undergraduate students (some of us remember this being addressed in a particularly uninspiring way in dusty lecture theatres) is covered by one of the co-editors, Bulent Coskun. Problem-Based Learning is one of the newer 'technologies' to arrive in medical education, and how this can be used in both undergraduate and postgraduate or residency education is addressed by an international group of authors: Badrakalimuthu, van Diest, Bak and de Waal. Those seeking a more literal use of the term 'technology' will find the chapter by Sheldon Benjamin and Maria Margariti extremely enlightening.

The art and skills of listening and talking with patients is central to our professional lives and we make no apologies for our emphasis on acquisition of both basic interviewing skills (Gask) and more complex skills in conducting psychotherapy (in chapters by both Glen Gabbard from the United States of America (USA) and Mark Evans from the United Kingdom), in addition to specific chapters dealing with innovative techniques, such as the Standardized Patients (Michael Curtis and Dave Baron), and with imaginative involvement of real users of our services (from Rex Haigh and Kathleen Lovell).

Looking beyond the teaching of psychiatrists, we have also addressed the other important roles that teachers of psychiatrists have to play, specifically in training in primary care (Gask, Coskun and Fahrer), where the vast majority of people with mental health problems receive care. Many psychiatrists will be involved in teaching in this setting, but we also need to consider how to teach psychiatrists to be educators within the community (Baron and Coskun) and, finally, how we can help our students to acquire the skills to carry out a research project of their own (addressed by David Goldberg).

We set out to try and get an international team of authors to work with us in producing this book and, through this collaboration, we believe new international alliances have been forged. From our correspondence with the writing teams this does indeed seem to be the case but it has not always been easy. As one of the authors commented in his e-mail correspondence with us, it was a little ironic that the vagaries of new technology (failure in e-mail) made it difficult for him to deliver to us as early as he had hoped a chapter which addressed use of new technologies in medicine.

It is our hope that readers will find this compendium of knowledge about how, what, where and, above all, why to teach psychiatry. We need to inspire ourselves before we can inspire our students, whoever they may be. Quality education is our best recruiting tool, shaper of public health policy sensitive to the needs of our patients, the keystone of the research process and the most important component of clinical care. We must all teach wisely. Our profession depends on it.

Reference

1. Adams, G. and Cook, M. (1984) Beginning psychiatry. *Bulletin of the Royal College of Psychiatrists*, **8**, 53–54.

2

Recruitment of Psychiatrists: the Key Role of Education

Cyril Höschl[1] and Jon van Niekerk[2]

[1]Prague Psychiatric Centre affiliated with Charles University, Prague, Czech Republic
[2]Rivington Unit, Royal Bolton Hospital, Greater Manchester West Mental Health Foundation Trust, Bolton, UK

2.1   Introduction

The image of psychiatry as a modern medical specialty that deals with a vast range of mental disorders, some of which are very common in the general population, and that delivers a variety of therapeutic interventions, some of which are among the most effective that medicine has at its disposal, is currently unfamiliar to the general public in most countries of the world.

—Mario Maj, President, World Psychiatric Association

The case to make for recruiting more psychiatrists is an easy one. The reports of a 'Recruitment crisis' in the developed world need to be put into context, however. The World Health Organization (WHO) recommends that there should be approximately one psychiatrist per 10 000 population, but most countries fall far below this level [1]. The WHO Mental Health Atlas 2005 showed that one fifth of the more than 100 countries supplying figures spent less than 1% of their health budget on mental health. This despite estimates that one third of global disease burden is caused by brain diseases and that more than three quarters of the costs of brain diseases are attributed to mental disorders [2]. The survey of 192 countries did show a slight increase in the total number of psychiatrists, from 3.96 to 4.15 per 100 000 people worldwide, since 2001; however, distribution across regions ranged from 9.8 in Europe to just 0.04 in Africa. In 47.6% of countries covering 46.5% of the world's population, there is less than one psychiatrist per 100 000 population. The trend is set for this disparity to increase. Recruitment in developing nations is also undermined by medical immigration of potential psychiatrists to developed nations.

Teaching Psychiatry: Putting Theory into Practice   Edited by Linda Gask, Bulent Coskun and David Baron
© 2011 John Wiley & Sons, Ltd

In 1994, only 3.2% of US medical school graduates chose psychiatry, the lowest proportion since 1929 [5]. This longstanding shortage of psychiatrists may be due to a number of factors, including a low rate of recruitment into psychiatry, a high rate of failure to complete training, failure to practise after completion of training and poor retention of psychiatrists [4]. It is recognized that much needed reform in mental health care will be seriously hampered if recruitment problems persist. On the other hand, careful thought needs to be given on how reforms impact on the way psychiatrists work, otherwise these radical reforms in mental health care may put off medically orientated potential adepts for a psychiatric career ('We did not study medicine to become social workers'). In response to the recruitment problems, the World Psychiatric Association (WPA) made a commitment to enhance the image of psychiatry as a dynamic speciality to the general public, mental health professionals and policy makers [3]. The WPA recognized that the negative image of psychiatry has an effect on those suffering from mental illness and their families being motivated to access services and on medical students not choosing psychiatry as a career option.

The authors reviewed all recruitment-related English language publications since 1959 and found that recruitment has been cyclical, with success from 1940 to 1969 and from 1985 to 1988, decline from 1970 to 1984 and from 1989 to 1994. The first success began with (i) public recognition of a dramatic shortage of psychiatrists to serve in the military and treat casualties and (ii) the fervour of the community mental health movement, which focused more on prevention of mental illness; massive resources were provided for psychiatry during this period. The declines were associated with (i) the failure of the community mental health movement to fulfil its promise, (ii) psychiatry becoming more biologically orientated and medically conventional and (iii) the effects of managed care and increased competition for patients. The psychiatry departments that have high recruitment rates are in public-supported schools or give considerable priority and resources for medical student psychiatric education.

In the United Kingdom it has been recognized for many years that there are insufficient local graduates interested in pursuing a career in psychiatry [6]. The annual figure in the United Kingdom has been consistent at around 4–5% of graduate doctors choosing psychiatry [7]. The recruitment shortfall has been hailed as catastrophic at times with overseas trainees filling the gap. There are ethical implications of recruiting foreign medical doctors from countries where psychiatrists are already scarce. Psychiatry is a culturally sensitive speciality and overseas trainees sometimes struggle with the cultural nuances and communication difficulties that exist. This has been shown by the difference between the success of United Kingdom graduate trainees and non-UK graduates at the final clinical exams.

Evidence of negative attitudes toward psychiatry by medical students is an international phenomenon and has been observed in other countries, including France [8], Australia [9], Saudi Arabia [10], Korea [11] and China [12], and by French and Norwegian medical students [13] and Dutch medical students [14].

In this chapter what has worked in the past and how to implement effective educational strategies to improve recruitment are explored and innovative developments are looked at.

2.2 Stigma

If we regard medicine as a microcosm of general society, then we would expect the impact of stigma to be highlighted in those specialities that deal with the disenfranchised. This seems to be true for geriatric medicine [15], HIV medicine [16] and psychiatry [6]. Educating the general public with anti-stigma campaigns needs to continue to address this. The media should be made aware of the importance of how they portray the mentally unwell and psychiatrists should put themselves forward to correct misunderstandings. Indeed, some should be trained to deal with the media effectively. There is an onus on governments to promote education and dispel myths about mental illness on a public health level and this should start early [17]. Dealing with stigma in the general population falls outside the scope of this chapter, but it is important that psychiatrists are engaged and involved in these campaigns.

In a qualitative research paper Dogra asserts that medical schools in general still stigmatize psychiatrists and psychiatry as a subject [18]. A pragmatic way for this to be addressed may be through the involvement of psychiatrists in all aspects of medical school life. In a scoping group commissioned by the Royal College of Psychiatrists, the authors proposed that psychiatrists need to be all over the curriculum 'like a rash'. An example is the integrated curriculum of the Third Faculty of Medicine of Charles University at Prague, where, besides neurobehavioural sciences, psychiatrists can participate in subjects as diverse as 'Needs of the patient', 'Structure and function of human body', 'Theoretical foundations of clinical medicine', 'Introduction to Clinical Practise', 'Pain', 'Clinical and pathological foundations of medicine', 'Dyspnoea and Chest Pain', and so on. (www.lf3.cuni.cz).

The evidence that students and non-mental health staff hold negative views is strong [19, 20]. An extensive survey [21, 22] has revealed similar findings. Nearly half the patients felt that they were discriminated against by their general practitioners. They viewed the physicians as insensitive, dismissive and overly reliant on drugs for treatment. Psychiatrists and other health care professionals were also reported as sometimes discriminating negatively towards people with mental health problems. There is evidence that some health professionals also keep quiet about a family member or a colleague with a mental disorder, just like the rest of the public [23]. Psychiatrists feel undervalued in their speciality and this can have an added

---

Box 2.1   How Education can Play a Role in Reducing Stigmatization of Mental Illness

1. Communication skills should be taught effectively (culturally informed).

2. Competence in examining mental state should be seen as of equal importance to that given to physical examination.

3. Respect for the uniqueness of the individual is sustained (not diagnostic label).

4. The knowledge that the doctor–patient encounter can be a powerful instrument for favourable or unfavourable change in the patient's condition.

5. Develop insight into their temperaments such that they can guard against any tendency to reinforce patients' fears.

6. Programmes should consider using input from people with mental illnesses.

negative impact on how medical students perceive the speciality. According to a survey of more than 5000 members of the American Psychiatric Association, most psychiatrists (80%) felt that their profession was very important, but 45% 'felt that other medical specialists perceived psychiatry as a less-than-moderately important speciality' [24].

The Royal College of Psychiatrists published a report dealing with stigmatization and made several recommendations on how education can play a role in reducing stigmatization of mental illness [25]. The recommendations attempt to ensure that those competencies that are essential to recognize and manage mental health problems become generic to all doctors (Box 2.1).

2.3 The Selection Process: Getting to Know the Target Audience

For every man there exists a bait which he cannot resist swallowing.
—Friedrich Nietzsche

The way medical students are selected has a profound effect on the recruitment of psychiatrists. This group of students for whom scientific achievement is favoured over the humanity studies creates a position where most medical students find psychiatry as interesting but uncharted territory. Psychiatrists should influence selection of more psychologically minded medical students, so that tomorrow's doctors have the necessary skills to treat patients in a holistic way, whether they choose psychiatry as a career or not. The psychologically minded medical student will be more open to choosing psychiatry as a career option. An interesting finding of several studies, however, is the precocity of the commitment to the discipline shown by those who do choose psychiatry as a career before entering medical school [26]. The trend for medical students to change their career choice during their training does not seem to affect psychiatry as much as other subspecialities. This has clear implications for early recruitment to the speciality of those who are interested in psychiatry even before they enter psychiatry clerkships or even enter medical school. Weintraub argues starting recruitment of those interested in psychiatry before their psychiatric placements [27].

Eagle and Marcos found that psychiatry attracted students from a lower social class, from cities, more often single and politically liberal [28]. Walton [29–32] found that medical students that choose psychiatry consisted of a group who were more reflective and responsive to abstract ideas. They found complexity intriguing and could tolerate ambiguity. Pasnay found non-authoritarian attitudes, open-mindedness, greater interest in theoretical issues and social welfare amongst these students [33].

There are indications that female students have more positive attitudes towards psychiatry [34] and are more likely to opt for psychiatry as a career choice [35]. Neglecting male students may have significant implications for the numbers of doctors likely to be active in the psychiatric workforce over the longer term. Identifying students that are interested in psychiatry early and fostering and supporting this interest should be developed by medical departments. Nielsen and Eaton found that the group of students whose interest in psychiatry was stronger than average was more impressed by psychiatry's comprehensiveness, the recent biological advances in psychiatry and the efficacy of treatments [36].

> **Box 2.2   Characteristics of Medical Students Interested in Psychiatry (or our Target Audience)**
>
> More reflective
>
> Liberal views
>
> Responsive to abstract ideas
>
> More open minded
>
> Less authoritarian.

In a comprehensive study Scher found that those intending to undertake a residency in psychiatry were more likely than their peers to rate more positively the efficacy of psychiatric treatments, the gratification from psychiatric work, the adequacy of psychiatric conceptual models and the quality of the psychiatric teaching [37]. They also appreciated the holistic approach psychiatry takes to patients, the opportunity to get to know patients in depth, the breadth of the field and its interactions with other disciplines and its recent neuroscientific advances.

Lee found that the factors that made the speciality more attractive to those who were interested in psychiatry were the perceived amount of intellectual challenge of the discipline, the number of novel and unique problems, emphasis on treating the whole person, the range of practice options in psychiatry, the psychiatric clerkship, biological advances in psychiatry,

> **Box 2.3   Positive Views about Psychiatry Expressed by Students Showing more Interest in Psychiatry**
>
> 1. Psychiatry's comprehensiveness as a speciality
>
> 2. Recent biological (neuroscientific) advances
>
> 3. The efficacy of psychiatric treatment
>
> 4. Gratification from psychiatric work
>
> 5. Adequacy of psychiatric conceptual models
>
> 6. The quality of the psychiatric teaching and placements
>
> 7. The holistic approach of psychiatry
>
> 8. The opportunity to get to know patients well.

the possibility of a return to a humanities or social science background, the experience with the psychiatric faculty, the opportunity for long-term relationships with patients and the emotional experience of working with psychiatric patients [38]. Characteristics of students showing an interest in psychiatry are shown in Boxes 2.2 and 2.3.

2.4 Undergraduate Teaching Programmes

It will come as a ray of hope to educators that there is evidence that recruitment into psychiatry is correlated with the quality of undergraduate medical school teaching programmes [5, 39]. However, there needs to be a commitment to major resources to teaching as well for this to be most effective. In the United States of America (USA) medical schools with the strongest academic departments have shown the best recruitment [40, 41]. Sierles showed that two of the three most important factors were the academic rank of the psychiatry teaching director and whether they had won an award for their teaching abilities. This shows the importance of clear leadership within departments and the importance of charisma. The relative academic prestige of the psychiatric department within the medical school was the second most important factor. This clearly shows that if educators enhance their programmes, they will see an increase in recruitment.

A limiting factor exists where universities have to put pressure on academics to produce research to promote the department's national standing. Educational research is not normally valued as highly as this. This results in education and training being less of a priority for academic departments. The importance of providing high quality psychiatric teaching programmes needs to be made and recruiting highly motivated educational directors is crucial. Sierles and Taylor found that psychiatric departments that have high medical student recruitment rates prioritize and resource medical education sufficiently for quality teaching to be delivered [5]. Langsley concluded that high quality programmes for teaching medical students psychiatry are characterized by a well rounded faculty who are psychologically informed, a greater commitment to medical student education than to resident training, varied teaching methods, enthusiastic student response and systematic evaluation that produces change in subsequent years [42]. The latter indicates that students feel heard and valued.

A lack of consistency in the curriculum of medical schools has been reported in both Japan [43] and Australia [44], with significant variations in the content and the amount of time devoted to the subject. Both of these studies emphasized the need to make the teaching relevant for future clinical practice. Oakley makes the case to focus on scenarios which students will commonly encounter in their initial years of employment and that psychiatry should be better integrated into the overall curriculum, with the opportunity for teaching in different settings [45]. The World Psychiatric Association (2001) published a core curriculum in psychiatry (Chapter 4), and also provided a justification for the need for all future doctors to know about psychiatric problems.

There should be a healthy balance between having a student responsive curriculum and the necessity of teaching the fundamentals and principles of a speciality [45]. Previous studies looking at priorities of medical students and psychiatrists have shown that there was agreement between the groups that basic psychiatric skills needed by most doctors were more important than specialized psychiatric knowledge [46]. If core psychiatric skills were viewed as being as indispensable as physical examination skills, the incentive to learn these well would be inculcated.

2.5 Clinical Undergraduate Placements: 'What Made You Choose Psychiatry?'

The answer to this question is different for everyone, but most cite a charismatic teacher or an interesting patient drawing them in. It has been shown that clinical placements can have a positive impact on recruitment into psychiatry. The subjective experience of the speciality by the medical student is highly correlated with their future choice of a career in psychiatry [7]. This may explain the extensive literature that exists on attitudes towards psychiatry, psychiatry as a career choice and promoting psychiatry [47–51]. Encouragement from more senior doctors during a psychiatric attachment increases the number of students wanting to pursue psychiatry [52].

The setting of teaching and how interactive and purposeful it is can make all the difference. El-Sayeh argues that modern teaching in ward rounds and clinics needs to be active and goal-directed [53]. Here students play a useful role in the clinical team and are given specific tasks. Murdoch Eaton and Cottrell [54] also advise several tips for teaching on psychiatric ward rounds, including: regular ward rounds dedicated to teaching, students having a specific role within the ward round, students following a specific patient from admission to discharge, allocating specific tasks during the ward round and allowing time for feedback and adequate supervision.

The need for clinical psychiatrists to be actively involved in psychiatric education (especially clinical teaching) has been highlighted [18]. Student non-attendance and professional attitudes need to be addressed to give the message that psychiatrists value the subject as important [53].

General practice is a useful setting for learning psychiatry, but requires collaboration between psychiatry and primary care departments. It has been found in the United Kingdom that integrating general practice sessions into a hospital psychiatric attachment demonstrated benefits of increasing breadth of experience, understanding the patients' experience, learning about mental illness from a primary care physicians' perspective, 'normalization' of mental illness and increased empathy [55]. A total of 90% of patients with mental health problems and up to 50% of those with serious mental illness use primary care services exclusively [56, 57].

Mowbray found that 65% of junior doctors chose psychiatry after graduation [58]. The limited 4–11 week placements do not adequately prepare the young doctor to recognize mental health problems or equip them in managing complex cases within secondary and primary care [59]. In the United Kingdom only 5% of the total Foundation Posts are allocated to psychiatry, despite the speciality being the third biggest hospital-based speciality. The fact that so few junior doctors rub shoulders with psychiatrists during these formative years will continue to hamper recruitment factors. Kelly *et al.* noted that much needed to be done to improve the status of the psychosocial aspects of medical care for students and their clinical teachers [60]. A survey of newly qualified doctors showed that they rarely asked questions on psychological state when admitting patients to hospital and often believed they lacked the skills to assess and treat common psychiatric problems, such as depression, anxiety and alcohol misuse [61]. There has been a view of moving more towards an integrative curriculum for those newly qualified doctors to enhance their knowledge of psychiatry and develop more psychologically minded doctors.

2.6   Innovative Ways of Recruiting into Psychiatry

2.6.1   Psychiatry Interest Group University Societies

The establishment of student-led psychiatric societies affiliated with medical schools has been discussed for some time in the United States. As part of the a new recruitment drive, the Royal College of Psychiatrists' Psychiatric Trainees' Committee (PTC) took a lead on establishing psychiatry interest group societies. The aims of these societies are to promote psychiatry as a career option for medical students and raise the profile of mental health amongst all would-be clinicians. The students are usually supported by their local psychiatry schools and academic departments but an important feature of the more successful ones are that they are student-led. This is a key requirement for the creative ideas of the students to come to the fore. One of the authors (van Niekerk) has been involved in setting up such a society at the University of Manchester in the United Kingdom and the surprising result was a society that was popular with students and created stimulating debate.

A description of how to set up such a society is given on the Royal College of Psychiatrists' Web site. The successes of these societies are being replicated across the United Kingdom and this has dispelled a number of myths about the lack of interest in psychiatry as a subject. The Royal College of Psychiatrists has also established a Student Associate membership with certain benefits to students and foundation doctors. As associates they receive a free online subscription to the College's Journal, a free annual conference and e-newsletter. The Royal College of Psychiatrists also sponsors free attendance at its annual international congress and has created specific days designed to cater for them. Student Associate membership is also open to Foundation Doctors free of charge.

2.6.2   Clinical Case Discussion (Balint) Group Development for Foundation Doctors

Medical training has drastically changed over the last decade. A high turnover of patients in hospital settings and the reduction in junior doctor training hours has important psychological consequences and impact on the doctor–patient relationship. To develop psychologically minded junior doctors in the twenty-first century the case is being made that we need to intervene early in their careers. One way of addressing this is to create Clinical Case Discussion (Balint style) groups. There is good evidence that these groups lead to increased job satisfaction and 'increase doctors' competence in patient encounters and enables them to endure in their job and find joy and challenge in their relationships with patients' [62].

2.6.3　Engaging Before Medical School Entry

Although it seems to be too early to recruit future psychiatrists, even from secondary schools, a lot can be done there to change public attitudes toward psychiatry, to diminish the stigma and to correct common prejudices about psychiatry. One way is to organize meetings, debates and encounters of secondary school students with psychiatrists. The personal problems of students and general questions about mental health can be one part of the content and indirect education about psychiatry, about major mental diseases, their management and prevention the other part.

One of authors (Hoschl) experienced a chain of student–guest meetings at secondary schools in the Czech Republic in which he repeatedly realized that this age group may be optimal to form a compact opinion and attitude towards a discipline. The motivation of students aged 16–19 to learn is high, as is their enthusiasm and authenticity. Their questions are usually sincere. At the same time, the secondary school students are flexible, open to change and sensitive to charismatic personalities.

2.7　Conclusion

The key learning points from this chapter are summarized in Box 2.4.

Box 2.4　Key Learning Points

- Recruitment shortfall of psychiatrists in the most developing nations is far more acute than in developed countries.

- Relying on doctors from developing countries to fill recruitment gaps in developed countries has ethical implications.

- Creating a self-sufficient workforce is crucial for both the developing and developed nations to serve their respective communities.

- Communication skills should be taught effectively (culturally informed).

- Competence in examining mental state should be seen as of equal importance to that given to physical examination.

- Stigma in the general population translates into the medical profession.

- Patients experience stigma within hospital and primary care settings.

- Psychiatry remains stigmatized within the medical profession.

- Emphasizing the importance of psychiatric assessment will raise the importance of mental health care.

- Psychiatrists need to be involved in the development of the undergraduate curriculum of medical students.

- Medical students are on the whole selected on their science grades.

- Psychiatrists should be involved in the selection of medical students and be visible and engaged throughout the curriculum.

- Once psychiatry is chosen as a career option, students tend to stick with that decision more than with other specialities.

- Early recruitment is justified – even before medical school.

- Psychiatrists should emphasise that psychiatry lends itself to more reflective practice and allows abstract thought.

- Designing of teaching programmes should be done with the target audience in mind.

- Quality of teaching programmes correlates with increased interest in psychiatry.

- Adequate resources need to be made available–time and funding.

- Psychiatric departments need enthusiastic leaders with exceptional teaching abilities.

- The curriculum needs to prepare the newly qualified doctor to recognize, diagnose and manage common psychiatric presentations.

- Well-rounded courses need to be psychologically informed.

- Systematic evaluation and feedback is crucial.

- Core psychiatric skills need to be viewed as essential for the newly qualified doctor.

- The undergraduate subjective experience of the speciality correlates highly with the final choice of career.

- Encouragement from senior doctors remains vital.

- Modern teaching demands participatory and goal-directed teaching in ward rounds and clinics.

- Sessions within primary care need to be incorporated.

- Innovative ways of making psychiatry more accessible should be explored – student societies.

Recruitment into psychiatry needs a whole systems approach and there are no easy answers. Despite the stigma that psychiatry carries within the medical profession there are examples of recruitment excellence from across the globe where the enthusiasm and charisma of psychiatric teachers are making a real difference in terms of recruitment. The impact of psychiatrists as engaging educators and role models remains crucial. We need to make sure that psychiatry remains a priority within medical schools and that these departments are well funded and produce good academic output. The speciality lends itself to creative teaching and should have good feedback mechanisms to remain relevant to teachers and students. How we present the speciality as a dynamic and fascination subject is important and we need to be visible and engaging with the undergraduate and postgraduate curricula. The speciality needs to be careful not to alienate those they seek to attract by attempting to dress the speciality up as something that it is not. The recent trend to focus more on the biological and neuroradiological advances needs to be balanced by psychological informed curricula. It is vital that we keep our target audience in mind. These liberal, open minded, abstract loving medical students are often put off by a limiting view of the speciality where complex problems are supposed to be fixed by medication. We need to be brave enough to try different approaches and nurture interest shown at undergraduate level. The recent emergence and interest shown in student societies shows how complex issues in mental health can be explored in a creative and inspiring fashion. Ultimately it will be our patients that benefit from a coordinated and well resourced recruitment plan.

References

1. World Psychiatric Association and World Federation for Medical Education (2001) Core Curriculum in Psychiatry for Medical Students, http://www.wpanet.org/detail.php?section_id=8&content_id=111 (accessed 17 December 2009).
2. Andlin-Sobocki, B., Jonsson, H., Wittchen, U. et al. (2005) Cost of disorders of the brain in Europe. European Journal of Neurology, 12, 1–27.
3. Maj, M. (2009) The WPA Action Plan is in progress. World Psychiatry, 8 (2), 65–66.
4. Moloney, J. and MacDonald J. (2000) Psychiatric training in New Zealand. Australian and New Zealand Journal of Psychiatry, 34, 146–153.
5. Sierles, F.S. and Taylor, M.A. (1995) Decline of U.S. medical student career choice of psychiatry and what to do about it. American Journal of Psychiatry, 152, 1416–1426.
6. Brockington, I.F. and Mumford, D.B. (2002) Recruitment into psychiatry. British Journal of Psychiatry, 180, 307–312.
7. Goldacre, M., Turner, G., Fazel, S. et al. (2005) Career choices for psychiatry: national surveys of graduates of 1974–2000 from UK medical schools. British Journal of Psychiatry, 186, 158–164.
8. Samuel-Lajeunesse, B. and Ichou, P. (1985) French medical students' opinion of psychiatry. American Journal of Psychiatry, 142, 1462–1466.
9. Yellowlees, P., Vizard, T. and Eden, J. (1990) Australian medical students' attitudes towards specialities and specialists. Medical Journal of Australia, 152, 587–592.
10. Soufi, H.E. and Raoof, A.M. (1992) Attitude of medical students towards psychiatry. Medical Education 26, 38–41
11. Koh, K.B. (1990) Medical students' attitudes toward psychiatry in a Korean medical college. Yonsei Medical Journal, 31, 60–64
12. Pan, P.C., Lee, W.H. and Lieh-Mak, F.F. (1990) Psychiatry as compared to other career choices: a survey of medical students in Hong Kong. Medical Education, 24, 251–257.

13. Roupret, M., Hupertan, V. and Chartier-Kastler E. (2005) The choice of a medical career in a population of 600 second-cycle French medical students preparing the national-ranking exam. *Presse Médicale*, **34**, 786–790.

14. Tijdink, J.K., Soethout, M.B.M., Koerselman, G.F., *et al.* (2007) Teaching undergraduate psychiatry in primary care: the impact on student learning and attitudes. *Medical Education*, **41**, 100–108.

15. British Geriatrics Society (2006) Report to Health Select Committee on Medical Workforce Issues.

16. American Academy of HIV Medicine (2009) Averting a Crisis in HIV Care: A Joint Statement of the American Academy of HIV Medicine (AAHIVM) and the HIV Medicine Association (HIVMA) On the HIV Medical Workforce.

17. Jorm, A.F. (2000) Mental health literacy: Public knowledge and beliefs about mental disorders. *The British Journal of Psychiatry*, **177**, 396–401.

18. Dogra, N., Edwards, R., Karim, K. *et al.* (2008) Current issues in undergraduate psychiatry education: the findings of a qualitative study. *Advances in Health Sciences Education*, **13**, 309–323.

19. Jorm, A.F., Korten, A.E., Jacomb, J.A. *et al.* (1997) Helpfulness of interventions for mental disorders: beliefs of health professionals compared with the general public. *British Journal of Psychiatry*, **171**, 233-237.

20. Mental Health Foundation (2000) Pull Yourself Together, Mental Health Foundation, London.

21. Chadda, D. (2000) Discrimination rife against mental health patients. *British Medical Journal*, **320**, 1163.

22. Lefley, H.P. (1987) Impact of mental illness in families of mental health professionals. *Journal of Nervous and Mental Disorders*, **175**, 613–619.

23. Phelan, J.C., Bromet, E.J. and Link, B.G. (1998) Psychiatric illness and family stigma. *Schizophrenia Bulletin*, **24**, 115–126.

24. Berman, I., Merson, A., Berman, S.M. *et al.* (1996) Psychiatrists' attitudes towards psychiatry. *Academic Medicine*, **71**, 110–111.

25. Royal College of Psychiatrists (2001) Mental Illness: Stigmatization and Discrimination within the Medical Profession, Royal College of Psychiatrists, London.

26. Babbott, D., Baldwin, D.C., Jolly, P. *et al.* (1988) The stability of early specialty preferences among US medical graduates in 1983. *Journal of the American Medical Association*, **259**, 1970–1975.

27. Weintraub, W., Plaut, S.M. and Weintraub, E. (1994) Recruitment into psychiatry: increasing the pool of applicants. *Canadian Journal of Psychiatry*, **44**, 473–477.

28. Eagle, P.F. and Marcos, L.R. (1980) Factors in medical students' choice of psychiatry. *American Journal of Psychiatry*, **137**, 423–427.

29. Walton, H.J., Drewery, J. and Carstairs, G.M. (1963) Interest of graduating medical students in social and emotional aspects of illness. *British Medical Journal*, **2**, 588–592.

30. Walton, H.J., Drewery, J. and Philip, A.E. (1964) Typical medical students. *British Medical Journal*, **2**, 744–748.

31. Walton, H.J. (1966) Differences between physically-minded and psychologically-minded medical practitioners. *British Journal of Psychiatry*, **112**, 1097–1102.

32. Walton, H.J. (1969) Personality correlates of a career interest in psychiatry. *British Journal of Psychiatry*, **115**, 211–219.

33. Pasnau, R.O. and Bayley, S.J. (1971) Personality changes in the first year psychiatric residency training. *American Journal of Psychiatry*, **128**, 79–84.

34. Alexander, D.A. and Eagles, J.M. (1986) Attitudes of men and women medical students to psychiatry. *Medical Education*, **20**, 449–455.

35. Shelley, R.K. and Webb, M.G.T. (1986) Does clinical clerkship alter students' attitudes to a career choice of psychiatry? *Medical Education*, **20**, 330–334.

36. Nielsen, A.C. and Eaton, J.S. (1981) Medical students' attitudes about psychiatry: implications for psychiatric recruitment. *Archives of General Psychiatry*, **38**, 1144–1154.

37. Scher, M.E., Carline, J.D. and Murray, J. (1983) Specialization in psychiatry: what determines the medical student's choice pro or con. *Comprehensive Psychiatry*, **24**, 459–468.

38. Lee, E.K., Kaltreider, N. and Crouch, J. (1995) Pilot study of current factors influencing the choice of psychiatry as a specialty. *American Journal of Psychiatry*, **152**, 1066–1069.

39. Stoudemire, A. (2000). Quo vadis, psychiatry? Problems and potential for the future of medical student education in psychiatry. *Psychosomatics*, **41**, 204–209.

40. Nielsen, A.C. (1979) The magnitude of declining psychiatric career choice. *Journal of Medical Education*, **54**, 632–637.

41. Sierles, F.S. (1982) Medical school factors and career choice of psychiatry. *American Journal of Psychiatry*, **139**, 1040–1042.

42. Langsley, D.G., Freedman, A.M., Haas, M. *et al.* (1977) Medical student education in psychiatry. *American Journal of Psychiatry*, **134**, 15–20.

43. Yamauchi, T. (1998) Education of psychiatry in Japan. *Psychiatry and Clinical Neurosciences*, **52**, S256–S258.

44. O'Connor, D.W., Clarke, D.M. and Presnell, I. (1999) How is psychiatry taught to Australian and New Zealand medical students. *Australian and New Zealand Journal of Psychiatry*, **33**, 47–52.

45. Oakley, C. and Oyebode, F. (2008) Medical students' views about an undergraduate curriculum in psychiatry before and after clinical placements. *BMC Medical Education*, **8**, 26.

46. Chatham-Showalter, P.E., Silberman, E.K. and Hales, R.E. (1993) Learning priorities of staff, residents, and students for a third year psychiatric clerkship. *Academic Psychiatry*, **17**, 21–25.

47. Abramowitz, M.Z. and Bentov-Gofrit, D. (2005) The attitudes of Israeli medical students toward residency in psychiatry. *Academic Psychiatry*, **29**, 92–95.

48. Baxter, H., Singh, S.P., Standen, P. *et al.* (2001) The attitudes of 'tomorrow's doctors' towards mental illness and psychiatry: changes during the final undergraduate year. *Medical Education*, **35**, 381–383.

49. Malhi, G.S., Parker, G.B., Parker, K. *et al.* (2003) Attitudes towards psychiatry among students entering medical school. *Acta Psychiatrica Scandinavia*, **107**, 424–429.

50. Pailhez, G., Bulbena, A., Coll, J. *et al.* (2005) Attitudes and views on psychiatry: a comparison between Spanish and U.S. medical students. *Academic Psychiatry*, **29**, 82–91.

51. Tharyan, P., John, T., Tharyan, A. *et al.* (2001) Attitudes of 'tomorrow's doctors' towards psychiatry and mental illness. *The National Medical Journal of India*, **14**, 355–359.

52. Maidment, R., Livingston, G., Katona, C. *et al.* (2004) Change in attitudes to psychiatry and intention to pursue psychiatry as a career in newly qualified doctors: a follow-up of two cohorts of medical students. *Medical Teacher*, **26**, 565–569.

53. El-Sayeh, H.G., Budd, S., Ealler, R. *et al.* (2006) How to win the hearts and minds of students in psychiatry. *Advances in Psychiatric Treatment*, **12**, 182–192.

54. Murdoch Eaton, D. and Cottrell, D. (1998) Maximising the effectiveness of undergraduate teaching in the clinical setting. *Archives of Diseases in Childhood*, **79**, 365–367.

55. Walters, K., Raven, P., Rosenthal, J., *et al.* (2007) Teaching undergraduate psychiatry in primary care: the impact on student learning and attitudes. *Medical Education*, **41**, 100–108.

56. Department of Health (1999) National Service Framework for Mental Health: Modern Standards and Service Models, Department of Health, London.

57. Kendrick, T., Burns, T., Garland, C. *et al.* (2000) Are specialist mental health services being targeted on the most needy patients? The effects of setting up special services in general practice. *British Journal of General Practice*, **50**, 121–126.

58. Mowbray, R.M., Davies, B. and Biddle N. (1990) Psychiatry as a career choice. *Australian and New Zealand Journal of Psychiatry*, **24**, 57–64.

59. Karim, K., Edwards, R., Dogra, N. *et al.* (2009) A survey of the teaching and assessment of undergraduate psychiatry in the medical schools of the United Kingdom and Ireland. *Medical Teacher*, **31**, 1024–1029.

60. Kelly, B., Raphael, B. and Byrne, G. (1991) The evaluation of teaching in undergraduate psychiatric education: students' attitudes to psychiatry and the evaluation of clinical competency. *Medical Teacher*, **13**, 77–87.
61. Williams, C., Milton, J., Strickland, P., *et al.* (1997) Impact of medical school teaching on preregistration house officers' confidence in assessing and managing common psychological morbidity: three centre study. *British Medical Journal*, **315**, 917–918.
62. Kjeldman, D. and Holmstrom, I. (2008) Balint groups as a means to increase job satisfaction and prevent burnout among general practitioners. *Annals of Family Medicine*, **6**, 138–145.

3

Ethical Issues in Teaching Psychiatry

Driss Moussaoui

Ibn Rushd University Psychiatric Centre, Casablanca, Morocco

3.1   Introduction

Ethics in psychiatry is a branch of medical ethics [1] that is part of the larger domain of ethics, which has been a chapter of philosophy for thousands of years. Psychiatry is probably the oldest medical speciality. The ancestors of physicians were sorcerers and shamans, using both physical treatments (herbal medicines) and magical invocations within ceremonies that could be partly considered as group psychotherapy with individual impacts. It is no surprise that psychiatric disorders were mentioned in the earliest medical documents we know of, such as the Ebers papyrus (depression, the illness of uterus) or Hippocratic works (melancholia, hypochondriasis) [2].

From the very beginning, law (Hammurabi code) and ethics were at the heart of the medical profession, and the Hippocratic Oath is still sworn by medical students before becoming medical doctors everywhere in the world. In this oath, essential ethical issues, such as confidentiality and prioritizing the interests of the patient, were already there, 2500 years ago. Very early, doctors and society understood that the asymmetrical relationship between the doctor and the patient needed clear guidelines in order to protect the patient from the power of the sorcerer/doctor.

It is a fact that the more power medicine has, the more ethical guidelines and regulations it should have. The problem is that technological advances in all branches of medicine are so rapid, inducing tremendous changes in the way diagnosis and treatment are conducted, that ethical thinking is lagging behind. In psychiatry, many ethical issues are posed; one of the most important is the fact that it is the only medical speciality that can deprive a person from liberty, letting aside the judicial system. This is why it is essential for all doctors, especially

Teaching Psychiatry: Putting Theory into Practice   Edited by Linda Gask, Bulent Coskun and David Baron
© 2011 John Wiley & Sons, Ltd

psychiatry, to learn how to solve the multiple ethical dilemmas each patient might bring to the table.

As a matter of fact, psychiatry is probably the most complex branch of medicine. Psyche is indeed the most sophisticated production of the brain, that is the most complex 'machinery' we know of in the universe. Psychopathology adds to the complexity of normal psyche. If we add to it the social and cultural aspects which impact on mental life of people, it is no surprise that the daily work of every psychiatrist is full of unexpected situations, and sometimes difficult to resolve ethical dilemmas.

More than in any other period in human history, human rights, democracy and ethics have become part of the public discourse, because expectations in this field are rising everywhere in the world. High sensitivity to these issues has put increasing pressure on doctors, adding to the other one: doctors need to demonstrate that they have the best technical abilities, along with the newest knowledge and technologies. This double pressure creates mounting suspicion between patients and doctors, the latter thinking first and before everything else to protect themselves from lawsuits. In some cases, information collected on the Internet may add to confusion in controversial domains in medicine. This is why it is more difficult than before to be a good doctor; for that, he/she has to find the way, despite increasing pressures, to build up with the patient the best possible alliance, through empathy and good science.

All this taken into account, one of the most important fields to teach medical students and postgraduates is definitely ethics. This represents a powerful tool, not only to make the right decisions, but also to improve the doctor–patient relationship and, hence, the medical management of each case. This teaching necessitates the capacity of the teacher to show the way, the capacity of the student to receive and contribute to this learning/teaching process, and the capacity of the institution to absorb the necessary changes and adaptations to evolve towards a more ethical environment.

3.2 Medical Power, Ethics and Doctor–Patient Relationship

One of the main objectives in teaching medical ethics is how to deal with the medical power, which is based on knowledge and know-how. The first part is less of a power now because information is readily available on the Internet and because it is more and more shared with the public via the media. Often, patients come to doctors with their diagnosis in hand and are knowledgeable enough to discuss the treatment with the doctor. I have personally seen this even in illiterate patients, who have heard about depression or schizophrenia on television or radio stations. This is another reason why users and families need to be accepted as partners by doctors, who should help them complete their knowledge. The more they know about the illness and treatment, the better.

The only effective medical power remaining in the hands of the doctor is experience. Having treated hundreds or thousands of cases, having had the experience with this or that treatment, makes a difference.

The sick person needs to imbue the doctor, perceived as healthy and powerful, with an aura of medical power that makes him worthy of trust and confidence. This is the origin of the dissymmetrical relationship between the doctor and the patient. The danger for the doctor is to be seized by the vertigo of the power lent to him by the patient; the error would be to use it for other purposes than the strict interest of the patient. The doctor must reduce the distance constructed by the perception of the patient, in order to make him/her available to work with the patient and the family as partners. Compassion and empathy are excellent tools to reduce this distance. Unfortunately, this is not what characterizes exactly the relationship between doctors and patients in most parts of the world. One of the revolutions to initiate in mentalities and behaviours is to bring more humane and human rights relationships, especially in low and middle income countries. Should we be reminded that 80% of the patients of the world belong to these countries?

Ethics is not only principles; it is mostly action. This is why, in this field, the teacher is before anything else a role model. Saying that all doctors must serve their patients is important (some say 'their servant'); doing it in daily practice is of essence. Ethics is not merely words. The discourse is only the path towards ethics, and in no way replaces it. From the ethics point of view, deadly danger comes from speaking good words and doing wrong things. This hypocrisy may contaminate quickly the vast majority of students, who then learn how best to lie to patients, to their families and to the community through beautiful discourses. There is no better way to kill the confidence of patients in doctors than doing this; confidence remains the indispensable ingredient of every doctor–patient relationship.

3.3 The Teacher

An excellent way of teaching dissymmetrical relationships is to take the teacher–student relationship as an example. I used to tell my students: 'I am your servant as we should all be servants of the patients. Let's list my duties towards you and see if I do it the right way'. It is very important that the teacher puts the power he/she has in question. For example, when it comes to small ethical flaws we all might have suffered from in our daily practice, it is crucial that the teacher starts with his own experiences. The students follow then much more easily. Instead of a vertical relationship between the teacher and the student, the ideal position is that they work in partnership with the leading position of the teacher. In many ways, the doctor–patient relationship follows the one built between the teacher and the student.

A difficult situation might arise when one or more senior doctors or teachers behave in an unethical way. In this case, the teacher has to reassert the principles of ethical conduct with the students, and try to solve institutionally the misconduct of the colleague.

Another aspect that might create a problem in the teacher–student relationship is the boundaries that must exist between the two. Some teachers might open part of their private life to one or to all students. In no way this should lead to exploitation of the students by the teacher, especially in the sexual domain, and this is because of their dissymmetrical relationship.

3.4 The Student

Each student must do their best to actively participate to their learning and teaching in ethics, especially by reading the proposed literature as well as ethical guidelines and by participating in the various discussions during the teaching. The student must also bring personal case-vignettes of difficult situations from the ethical point of view when asked to do so. Also, the student has the responsibility to try his best to adapt clinical practice to what he learned. For example, the student must discuss with more senior doctors and with other students encountered cases that pose ethical dilemmas.

The student has to be informed from the beginning that the main objective of teaching ethics is to create a psychological system that analyses through one question: 'What is good, what is bad in what I say, in what I do, in the way I behave, in the decision I am taking?'; this system should function in a permanent way. In case of great difficulty, especially when we have nobody to consult with and we have to take a quick decision, another question can bring some light in the darkness of the dilemma: 'Where does the interest of the patient lie?'

The psychological integration of such a continuous system of ethical analysis of the patient–doctor relationship and of the decisions taken is a necessity for the prevention of unethical behaviours and choices.

It is also important that the students discuss amongst themselves litigious cases from the ethical point of view, as they do when they have technical problems. There is a need to teach the students that the most experienced person in medical ethics might find themselves in a difficult situation and have to ask for advice and guidance from others. Whenever possible, collective decision is better in difficult cases than an individual one.

3.5   The Institution

There are two ways of teaching ethics in psychiatry: through specific sessions with lectures and workshops, but also in the daily practice of the student or the psychiatrist. From the institutional point of view, it is important to have a good ethical environment. Amongst important tools of this environment, an ethics committee is to be created if it does not exist. Most of the psychiatric institutions in the world do not have such a committee. One of its missions is to promote research and education in medical ethics in general and in psychiatry in particular. It should also organize debates on ethics about new situations in medical practice, especially because of the introduction of new technologies (e.g. psychosurgery in obsessive compulsive disorder (OCD), brain stimulation). Debates could be organized between colleagues who disagree on the way to manage ethical dilemmas dealing with psychiatric or mental health issues, for example terminating or not a pregnancy, feeding against one's will a hunger striker for political reasons, how absolute is medical confidentiality?, or access to mental health care for those in socially precarious conditions. This form of teaching represents a component of the continuing ethical education (CEE) for doctors of the institution. Another mission of the ethics committee is to train trainers in ethics.

A different exercise could be initiated: teaching ethics in psychiatry to medical students and residents with other members of the team (nurses, social workers, clinical psychologists) or even with specialists of human sciences (e.g. sociologists, anthropologists, historians). One of the issues that may arise in such cases is the communication difficulties and division of the medical power between various components of the medical team. The teacher then has to focus the discussion on the sometimes complex relationship between the treating member of the team, the other members, and the patient.

The ethical value of a team is essential for the good functioning of each doctor. In many low to middle income countries, scarcity of resources tends to push some health workers with low salaries to ask for money from families of patients, corrupting the entire environment of the institution. Such detrimental behaviours must be fought through clear guidelines and procedures, including administrative and judicial sanctions. It is important also to have institutional discussions about such unethical behaviours.

3.6 Teaching Ethics in Psychiatry

Teaching of ethics could be part of general teaching of medical ethics, or could be specific to students working in psychiatry. It could be through a systematized teaching leading to an academic recognition (certificate, diploma) or it could be done regularly in a psychiatric hospital or unit with no connection to university.

The teacher should use simple words, metaphors and avoid philosophical jargon, in order to allow better understanding by the majority of students and to allow a wider participation in discussions. The teacher can use all kinds of references to explain his positions: films, literature, or recent political or sport events.

Teaching ethics is first of all asking questions and debating about clinical cases. Xenophon wrote: 'Questioning is teaching' and this is the best path for a good teaching of ethics. The doctor has to deal with uncertainty in technical aspects (diagnosis, prognosis and treatment) and should be able to cope with it. The same applies to ethical issues. There is often no ideal solution for ethical dilemmas, only the least bad that is finally chosen after long discussion and analysis [3].

The **curriculum** of the teaching of ethics in psychiatry should contain at least four parts:

- It should start with a historical perspective of psychiatry: history of the creation of asylums in the sixteenth and seventeenth centuries in Europe and the Americas, the highly symbolic act of Philippe Pinel and Jean–Baptiste Pussin when they removed the chains of the mental patients in Bicêtre Hospital in Paris, the political abuse of psychiatry in the ex-Soviet Union and in South Africa in the 1960s and 1970s.

- The second part could be the explanation of the Madrid Declaration of the World Psychiatric Association [4] and the distribution of the electronic content of the various codes of ethics and guidelines by national and international non- governmental organizations (NGOs) [5]. Examples given by the teacher will illustrate the various assertions of the Madrid Declaration. Other hand-outs and Web site addresses should be given to the students.

- The third part can deal with the main ethical questions that psychiatry has to deal with, such as:

  - validity of informed consent in research on patients with severe mental disorders,

  - hospitalization against the will of the patient with various degrees of dangerous behaviours,

  - access to medication in needy psychotic patients,

- stigmatization of mental patients, including by some psychiatrists,

- relationship to the pharmaceutical industry,

- the situation of human rights in psychiatric institutions,

- human rights of mental patients in prison.

- The fourth and most important part, and which should last at least half of the time of teaching, will comprise case-vignettes. They could be in a written form, videotaped, through presentation of actual patients, or oral report by the teacher or the students. Very few are ready to accept spontaneously the idea that ethical flaws might have occurred in their daily practice in a recurrent way. This is why the teacher should be the first to present cases with ethical difficulties. The students follow easily then. It is important to convey to them that having an ethical problem is a not a curse, because it happens to everybody, all the time. I tell my students: 'the most ethical person, a saint, is visited by the devil ten times each day'.

Analysis must take into account not only the clinical and therapeutic aspects, but also the psychosocial ones. It is necessary then to widen the debate. Like politics, ethics deals with power. The first tries to conquer it and to maintain its grip on it; the second tries to analyse it, to manage it and to control it when it goes the wrong way. It is important to convey the message that there is only one real power in medicine: the recognition of the patient that he has been well served by the doctor. This is not merely a narcissistic benefit for the latter; it is a moral credit which can help building confidence of future patients in that doctor, because of a good reputation.

The student must also learn that no research can be conducted without the green light of the ethics committee, even when it is a simple epidemiological study. On the same note, no teaching with patients can be done without their expressed agreement, and no written clinical material will be used without being sure that the identity of the patient is preserved in the teaching group. If necessary, a case-vignette can be invented, or biographical data of a patient can be altered.

Another important message to convey to the students is the necessity of continuing ethical education (CEE). Reading textbooks and articles on ethics in psychiatry [6–9], as well as philosophical magazines (there is, for example, a simple one for the francophone public 'Philosophie Magazine') on a regular basis may be very helpful. Attending meetings organized by the ethics committee is another way of progressing in the field.

The **evaluation** of the teaching/learning process is an important moment. The ideal outcome of teaching ethics is when the student is able to take the right ethical decisions in an autonomous way, far from the guidance of the teacher. A small part of the evaluation may address the memorizing of important concepts. Most of the evaluation could be through the attendance and actual participation of the student during the teaching. Examination could be done through the discussion of written or videotaped case-vignettes containing ethical dilemmas.

Another interesting aspect of evaluation could be to ask students to conduct research studies on various aspects of the life of patients and of the institution. Examples of such research are: criteria of putting a patient in a seclusion room, how much information is given to the patient about prescribed medication, how much a person with schizophrenia is able to understand a proposed clinical trial before giving informed consent, how to present a diagnosis of Alzheimer's disease and to whom.

3.7 Conclusions

In a more and more complex world, teaching ethics in psychiatry is a necessity. This is not only because it is a moral obligation, but because it helps and protects the patient and the psychiatrist. One of the best ways of teaching ethics to undergraduates in a medical school is to teach philosophy within a corpus of human sciences. This helps acquiring critical thinking and understanding the frustration of uncertainties, which are amongst the most important attitudes the student should have to become a good doctor. This helps also to ask the correct questions when it comes to ethical issues.

It should be clear that theoretical education and training in ethics is not enough. Vigilance must accompany each moment of the medical practice. Collaboration with the patient, with the medical team and other colleagues is necessary to track down ethical problems, under their various masks, in order to find the most satisfactory solutions. There is also the necessity of improving one's thinking on various social phenomena that impact on medical practice. Thinking global is part of ethics at large and helps improve the ethical thinking of the student. The teaching needs also to be reinforced by CEE courses in ethics.

All this is time and energy consuming, but we cannot afford not to invest permanently in ethics. The opposite would put psychiatry and medicine at risk of dangerous moral weakness. Maintaining and improving the value of psychiatrists, doctors and medicine at large are at the price of this life long effort.

References

1. World Medical Association (2005) *Medical Ethics Manual*, Ferney-Voltaire.
2. Hippocrates (1998) *The Works*, Diachronic Publications, Athens.
3. Carmi, A., Moussaoui, D. and Arboleda-Florez, J. (2005) Teaching ethics in psychiatry: case-vignettes, UNESCO Chair in Bioethics, Haifa, and World Psychiatric Association of Psychiatry Committee on Ethics.
4. World Psychiatric Association (2008) Declaration of Madrid and guidelines, http://www.wpanet.org/detail.php?section_id=5&category_id=9&content_id=48 (accessed 22 July 2010).
5. Moussaoui, D. and Murthy, S. (2005) Declarations and codes of ethics related to psychiatry and mental health (CD-Rom), World Health Organization EMRO and World Psychiatric Association.
6. American Psychiatric Association (2001) Opinions of the Ethics Committee on the Principles of Medical Ethics with Annotations Especially Applicable to Psychiatry, American Psychiatric Association, Washington, DC.
7. Woolbridge, K. and Fulford, B. (2004) *Whose Values?* The Sainsbury Centre for Mental Health, London.
8. Fulford, B., Thornton, T., and Graham, G. (2006) *Oxford Textbook of Philosophy and Psychiatry*, Oxford University Press.
9. Okasha, A., Arboleda-Florez, J. and Sartorius, N. (2000) *Ethics, Culture and Psychiatry, International Perspectives*, American Psychiatric Press, Washington, DC.

4

Developing a Medical Student Curriculum in Psychiatry

Nisha Dogra[1], Cyril Höschl[2] and Driss Moussaoui[3]

[1]*Greenwood Institute of Child Health, University of Leicester, Leicester, UK*
[2]*Prague Psychiatric Centre affiliated with Charles University, Prague, Czech Republic*
[3]*Ibn Rushd University Psychiatric Centre, Casablanca, Morocco*

4.1 Introduction

The aim of this chapter is to highlight necessary changes in medical curricula to reflect the needs and challenges of contemporary psychiatry. Psychiatry as a medical discipline on one hand shares the fate of other medical disciplines, on the other hand as a profession dealing also with *mental health* it overlaps with non-medical domains, such as social care, well-being, consumers' protection, human rights, gender issues, ethics and so on. Psychiatry as a medical discipline investigates the brain and its relationship to human experience and behaviour. On the other hand, *social* psychiatry is concerned with social influences on human mental health. It can provide partial social explanations for psychiatric phenomena. Students need to be aware of both these aspects. Psychiatry also faces challenges in the guise of the anti-psychiatry movements.

In Europe, and to some extent worldwide, psychiatry made its contributions in eighteenth and nineteenth century medicine, mainly in Germany (e.g. W. Griessinger, E. Kraepelin, E. Bleuler), France (J.-É. Esquirol, J.-P. Falret, Ph. Pinel, B. Morel) and the United Kingdom (W. Tuke). Since the twentieth century psychiatry has developed on a more global level, and more increasingly under the influence of North American research progress in the neurosciences and related disciplines. These common denominators, as well as common challenges of a globalized world, justify to some extent our contemporary attempts to find a common way forward.

Teaching Psychiatry: Putting Theory into Practice   Edited by Linda Gask, Bulent Coskun and David Baron
© 2011 John Wiley & Sons, Ltd

Quite recently, reflecting increasing emphasis on human rights, ethics and public health, attention has been increasingly paid not only to illness as such but also to mental health, and, therefore, to quality of life and well-being. This development raises new needs and challenges for the discipline. We need to ensure it remains within medicine and this may need re-conceptualization of psychiatry and re-definition of its position amongst other medical disciplines. On one hand, psychiatry is fighting stigma, on the other hand it needs to find a new place in taking care of human beings in their complexity. The medical curriculum is a good place to begin [1].

Last, but not least, we see a declining interest of medical students in choosing psychiatry as a specialization. Besides the low rate of recruitment into psychiatry, a shortage of psychiatrists may be also due to a high rate of failure to complete training, failure to practise after completion of training and poor retention of psychiatrists. There is a danger that much needed reform in mental health care will be seriously hampered if recruitment problems persist (see Chapter 2 for more discussion of recruitment). Again, the undergraduate medical curriculum is the appropriate place to start in order to attempt to increase students' motivation and interest in psychiatry.

4.1.1 Defining a Curriculum

For the purpose of this chapter, a *curriculum* is the set of courses, and their content, offered at a school or university. A *core curriculum* is a curriculum, or course of study, which is deemed central and usually made mandatory for all students of a school. Historically, curriculum (from the Latin word for race-course) was understood as an idea, the course of deeds and experiences through which children become the adults they should be (John Franklin Bobbitt in 'The Curriculum', the first textbook published on the subject in 1918 [2]).

Curriculum usually has two meanings [3]. Firstly, the range of courses from which students choose what subject matters to study and, secondly, a specific learning programme. In the latter case, the curriculum describes the teaching, learning and assessment materials needed and/or available for a given course of study. So the curriculum is a superior set to syllabuses or modules.

In this chapter, while talking about curriculum, we have in mind first of all a core curriculum at a medical school. If we refer to *education,* we usually talk about a broader system of gaining knowledge, skills and attitudes. It may include also residency programmes, postgraduate education, continuing medical education and public education in large.

4.1.2 Devising and Implementing a Curriculum

There is a big difference between devising a curriculum and implementing it. For example, most accreditation bodies require a certain minimum amount of hours of teaching to recognize a university grade in medicine. A school outlines the proportion of different subjects and forms (lectures, practices, workshops etc.). This structure can be quite uniform across a region or country but still lead to huge differences in the content, in the practice, in the student experience, outcomes and the overall atmosphere and culture of a school.

4.1.3 Historical Background of Development of a Core Curriculum in Psychiatry for Undergraduates

It has been known for decades that the majority of mental patients are first seen by general practitioners (GPs) and that 30–40% of the patients seen by GPs suffer from mental disorders, mostly depression and anxiety disorders [4]. On the other hand, it is well documented that the presence of mental disorders is associated with significant worsening in health-related quality of life, and that impairment associated with mental disorders is greater than that associated with physical illness in patients seen by GPs [5]. It was therefore felt in the early 1990s by the World Psychiatric Association (WPA) that it was necessary to address the quality of undergraduate teaching in psychiatry and to sensitize future GPs and non-psychiatric specialists to psychiatry and mental health. Additionally, it is arguable that there is a need for **all** doctors to have a working understanding of mental health issues, as patients with mental health disorders and problems may present to any health care professional. Being able to undertake a mental state examination should be part of every doctor's basic skill set. This is supported by the fact that patients with mental health problems may receive care for their physical health problems that is not as good because doctors may not address their biases or fail to involve the patients in decisions about their care (on false assumptions of what decisions the patient may or may not be able to make).

In 1994, The WPA (president: F. Lieh Mak) decided with the World Federation of Medical Education (WFME) (president: H. Walton) to devise a core curriculum for undergraduates in psychiatry [6]. It was the second time after neurology, all medical specialities included, that such collaboration between the WFME and a major medical speciality took place. The WPA Section on Education in Psychiatry undertook this task.

The project was designed by one of the authors (Moussaoui) and A. Freedman within a committee chaired by M. Gelder. The first step was to conduct a survey in medical schools about the existing curricula for undergraduates in psychiatry. Out of a list of 1305 medical schools provided by the WFME, the questionnaire was sent to 500 faculties of medicine. Responses came from 124 departments of psychiatry belonging to 40 different countries; only 113 responses were usable. Seventy seven departments were from high income countries and 44 from low to middle income countries.

Almost half (47.8%) of these departments had a national curriculum for undergraduates in psychiatry, and more than half (53%) were dissatisfied with their teaching. There was no relationship between the availability of a national core curriculum and satisfaction with the teaching of psychiatry to undergraduates. The most frequently taught topics were: mental state assessment, psychopathology, personality disorders, affective disorders, schizophrenic disorders, alcoholism and drug dependence, psychosexual disorders, organic psychosis, psychiatric aspects of medical disorders and psychosomatic medicine, mental handicap and treatment in psychiatry.

The mean duration of theoretical teaching of psychiatry was 46.4 ± 24 hours. Most of it was lectures (34.9%) or lectures and discussions (24.8%). Rotations or practical training varied from 1 to 32 weeks (mean: 6.2 ± 4 weeks). The teaching was done through clinical cases (70%), presentation of patients (79%), writing case reports by medical students (56.9%). Only 46.9% of the responders mentioned that undergraduates were involved in emergency rooms by being on duty. Another interesting finding was that only 10% of all departments used audiovisual means to teach psychiatry to undergraduates in 1994.

The learning was assessed through the following means: written examination (68.8%), student participation (62.3%), checklist (20.2%), oral examination (20.2%), multiple choice questions (0.9%) and evaluation by objectives (0.9%).

The suggested topics for inclusion in the core curriculum were psychiatric disorders (63.5%), especially depression (25.4%), substance abuse (22.2%), anxiety disorders (22.2%) and organic mental syndrome (19%), as well as psychopharmacology (39.7%), psychotherapy (28.6%), interviewing skills (28.6%) and patient–doctor relationship (17.5%). There was no expectation that curricula would be different between high and low to middle income countries.

The main outcomes were that there was a need to sensitize other specialities to the importance of psychiatric teaching, to stress the importance of mental health in the community, to improve teaching of behavioural sciences and psychotherapy, and to emphasize the importance of an internationally coordinated education for undergraduates in psychiatry.

The majority of departments of psychiatry (86.7%) were also in charge of the teaching behavioural sciences to undergraduates (Chapter 5).

This kind of survey concerning curricula for undergraduates in psychiatry, to our knowledge, has not been replicated. It is unclear whether the results of a similar survey would be fundamentally different today, 16 years after the first one. A survey of teaching undergraduate psychiatry in United Kingdom and Irish medical schools in 2005 found that the content of programmes remain highly variable with a range of teaching and assessment methods applied [7]; this is discussed further below in the example described. The variation of time allocated for the clinical discipline also varied between two and twelve weeks, which is perhaps somewhat surprising given that all UK schools are expected to deliver the curriculum as outlined by the General Medical Council (GMC) in *Tomorrow's Doctors* [8].

The use of the Internet as a major source of medical information and teaching has certainly led to changes in teaching methods (Chapter 16). Audiovisual teaching is also probably more used than before. There has also been a greater emphasis on teaching those who teach medical students how to teach more effectively. It is also likely that GPs more frequently diagnosis and treat depression [9]. However, the main concerns of the profession are probably still the same today.

4.2   The Evidence and Context

When devising a curriculum, the responsible authorities should first of all respect general rules regarding the educational system in a country (e.g. presence of colleges) and the accreditation criteria (total amount of teaching hours – usually not less than 5000 per the whole study, and the proportion of different teaching settings). In this respect it is important to ask whether the retention of knowledge is proportional to the amount of a teaching burden [10]. It seems that the relationship between self-education and the amount of teaching activities in the curriculum is bell shaped (Figure 4.1).

Several studies have shown that problem-based learners retain knowledge much better than students receiving conventional teaching [11]. Problem-based learning (PBL) (Chapter 6) leads to better recall of information for three reasons: (i) mobilization of previous knowledge stimulates learners to constructs explanatory models, and this facilitates the processing and comprehension of new information; (ii) new information is better understood if learners are

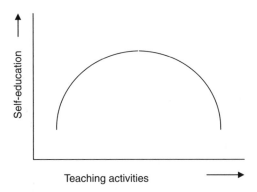

Figure 4.1 Correlation between self-education and the amount of teaching activities in the curriculum.

stimulated to elaborate on it (elaboration in PBL can take several forms, such as discussion); and (iii) learning in context makes information more accessible for later use [12].

There are basically two models of learning: one based on active problem solving and the second based on learning in terms of conditioning (Table 4.1). The latter corresponds with traditional European curricula while the former represents problem-based learning. However, problem-based learning is highly dependent on student motivation and the skills of their facilitators. There is some evidence that when the psychosocial sciences are not highlighted, students using problem-based learning may pay minimal attention to these components [13].

4.2.1 Socio-Political Considerations

Medical curricula in Europe, particularly in traditional countries and in Central and Eastern Europe (CEE), share the tradition and transformation of the university training under the strong German influence, modified in CEE by decades of the communist educational system. This tradition is characterized mainly by the classical educational formats (plenary lectures and practices), by the split of a discipline into 'general' (psychopathology) and

Table 4.1 A comparison of models of learning.

Learning		
Model:	Constructivist	Behaviouristic
Principle:	Active formation	Stimulus → Reaction
Theoretical background:	Piaget and others	Skinner, Pavlov and so on.
Learned behaviour:	Problem solving	Avoidance behaviour
Condition:	Previous experience	Inherited patterns
External influence:	Support and 'scaffolding'	Reward and punishment
Environment:	Democratic	Restrictive

'special' (diseases) parts, and by a predominant medical approach based on the Kraepelinian nosological system. In recent decades, however, a more problem orientated, integrated and interactive style of medical training has also penetrated into this part of Europe. It was reflected by the introduction of new medical curricula with diversified teaching, meaning that psychiatry could be taught in many different modules, such as applied neuroscience, medical ethics, patient orientated approach and modern educational formats including electives in psychotherapy, biological psychiatry, psychopathology, assessment techniques and methodology. Psychiatry would also be a relevant component of modules on specific presentations such as pain, dyspnoea, basic medical problems and the broader medical context. Neurobehavioural sciences are now more integrated and clinical rotation is more practically orientated (that is problem orientated). Examples of such curricula can be found at the University of Dundee in the United Kingdom (the so called *Dundee model*, based on outcome – Figure 4.2) [14].

The Maastricht, Limburg (the so called *Limburg model*) is characterized by the training in communication skills and a significant proportion of self-study assignments with emphasis on review sessions (see also Chapter 6). The Linköping curriculum (characterized by the so called *Srimman*, that is the *common thread*) has at its core contact with patients; from the

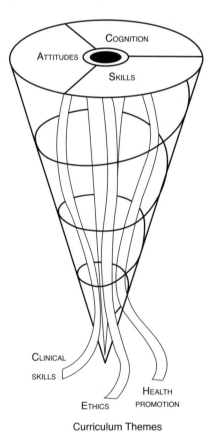

Curriculum Themes

Figure 4.2   The Dundee curriculum.

time they begin training medical students are exposed to patient contact and this remains constant throughout their undergraduate experience. This is also the case for CEE at the Third Faculty of Medicine of Charles University in Prague [15, 16] and some other schools. The key does appear for psychiatrists to remain integral to the teaching programme wherever it appears in the curriculum. There is evidence that medical students value teaching that is taught by clinicians and relates their learning to practice [17].

4.3   Developing the Curriculum

4.3.1   The Process of Devising a Curriculum

To paraphrase Citrad John, a Czech immunologist:

> Students are mainly interested in theoretical aspects of their learning for its application to their future roles as clinical doctors.

Although medicine had significantly changed during twentieth century, undergraduate medical curricula in many European countries had not reflected this. In particular, the medical curricula had not been responsive to the clinical (practical) needs of the undergraduate student. Moreover, the traditional curricula did not motivate students to learn the theory, as the theory and practice are often artificially separated and there might be few links made to highlight the relevance of the theory to practice. Plenary lectures used to prevail as a form of education, although this has changed and continues to do so, but are dependent on appropriate resources. Lectures remain an important part of delivery but perhaps now are more thoughtfully used.

In some countries, the medical curriculum became a matter of bitter criticism from students. Therefore, attempts to launch new curricula occurred in different parts of Europe (see above). Their main objectives usually were:

1. To adjust the medical curricula to the 'state of art' of contemporary medicine.

2. To support more individual contact of students with both teachers and patients.

3. To increase the motivation of students to study the theory by demonstrating its relevance to practice, and also to encourage students to conduct research.

4. To support active training forms and the acquisition of skills.

5. To gain the skills in data processing and its interpretation.

6. To support critical thinking and the ability to discuss.

7. To evaluate long-term feedback from students and incorporate their perspectives into curriculum development.

Any change of a system of education, including the introduction of a new curriculum, is a social and political process dependent on the strength of authority, charismatic leadership and external circumstances [18]. In the worst case, leadership may be delegated to someone else and diluted in different committees and thereby provides little direction. On the other hand, it may have its source in an authority of a strong personality. A successful leader supports leadership, hires managers and leaders who induce reliability, understands obstacles, plans how to tackle them and strategically avoids islands of resistance. Effective communication means problem anticipation, recognition and description, necessity of change, and buy-in of the new vision. The goal is that others will identify themselves with the new curriculum (or with the change) and take full responsibility for it because they have a vested interest to do so. It inevitably needs constant communication and interaction face-to-face (not just written circulars or e-mail messages). To a leader some of this may feel redundant but even those committed to change can be dissuaded if the direction becomes altered or lacks focus. The centralization of a system is the basic condition of its function. It enables both its quality control and the balance between orders, recommendations and instructions. In addition, curricular problems are much easier solved from the top. Centralized leadership also enables the participation of different stakeholders and their burden to be balanced better. Appropriation of a central fund for a new curriculum is absolutely essential. Without that it is not possible to administer a new curriculum. A central budget enables power to be removed from individual departments, which is essential when introducing teaching activities that cut across the old institutional structure. Central budgeting also emphasizes institutional responsibility for a curriculum. A system of incentives, rewards, prizes and recognition must be introduced to support the implementation of a new curriculum.

A major problem is the image projected by psychiatry in the general population, and particularly amongst the medical students. This may be due to the complexity of the bio-psycho-social model in psychiatry, which makes it both fascinating as a concept to medical students but means that it also perceived as too difficult a speciality to be implemented. This is why it is essential to develop sophisticated educational mechanisms for the best possible teaching of psychiatry to undergraduates, if we do not want to see psychiatry and psychiatrists to become an 'endangered species' [19].

4.4 Developing a Core Curriculum: Example from the UK

A survey of UK medical schools regarding their teaching of undergraduate psychiatry, [7] found that some aspects of the curriculum were consistent across the medical schools while other areas showing great variability. The course content was broadly similar but the assessment, length of experience and course structure differed. The authors concluded that there are significant differences in how psychiatry is taught to undergraduate students in the United Kingdom and Ireland, and it is unclear if this variation has any effect on the levels of competency achieved. A qualitative study of key personnel involved in the education of psychiatry at undergraduate level found that educators identified several problems and potential solutions. The fact that teaching was not valued much either by universities or the National Health Service was seen as a significant issue. The research was reviewed in the context of the evidence that psychiatric departments that have high recruitment rates prioritize and resource medical education sufficiently for quality teaching to be delivered [20]. This built on work by Langsley *et al.* [21] who concluded that high quality programmes for teaching medical students psychiatry are characterized by a well rounded faculty, a psychodynamic orientation, a greater commitment to medical student education than to resident training, varied teaching methods, enthusiastic student response and systematic evaluation that produces change in subsequent years.

The above research played a part in the Royal College of Psychiatrists establishment of a scoping group to review undergraduate psychiatry education as a means of trying to address some of the issues raised; one of which was the benefits or otherwise of having a core curriculum and how this might help improve the quality of teaching [22].

Until recently the *ad hoc* nature of medical curricula has resulted in curricula of which the objectives bear little relationship to what is actually delivered to students, how students learn and how students are assessed, and this is probably true for other countries as well as the United Kingdom. The intervention of medical educationalists has perhaps enabled the relationship between these four components to become more coherent. In the United Kingdom, since 1993 the GMC has produced *Tomorrow's Doctors* (now on version three) [23]. By publishing *Tomorrow's Doctors,* the GMC set the framework within which it expected medical education in the United Kingdom to develop. Although the GMC and the Quality Assurance Agency (QAA) regularly visit medical schools to monitor standards of medical education, medical schools remain free to develop curricula as they see fit. The criteria used by the QAA are similar to those used for other university courses and cover six aspects: (1) curriculum design, content and organization; (2) teaching, learning and assessment; (3) student progression and achievement; (4) student support and guidance; (5) learning resources; and (6) quality management and enhancement [24]. The GMC choses not to develop a national curriculum, as diversity within medical education was, and is, considered important for innovation [25].

Medical schools in the United Kingdom have had to review what is most important for students to know and how might they best learn it rather than subjects being taught because they have always been taught. The newer medical schools curricula (for example the Peninsula Medical School and the University of East Anglia Medical School) have been in a position to develop courses with less historical baggage than perhaps the more traditional schools. They have also been in a position to engage with educationalists from the outset. The drive behind *Tomorrow's Doctors* was a desire to overhaul medical school curricula. There was a great emphasis on a shift from a heavily content-laden taught curriculum to teaching students key facts and other skills, which are transferable, for example attitudes towards life-long learning. There was also an emphasis on moving away from formal didactic teaching and working towards self-directed student learning. This was, in part, an acknowledgement of the growing evidence that curricula could not continue to expand at the same rate as medical knowledge [26–28].

4.4.1   Development of the College Core Curriculum

The development of this Core Curriculum was carried out by a subgroup within the Royal College of Psychiatrists' Scoping Group on Undergraduate Education in Psychiatry [22]. The subgroup met over a year and produced a draft core curriculum, which was then reviewed by members of the wider Scoping Group. It was modified and then sent for consultation, specifically to the educational leads for psychiatry in each medical school, to key academic General Practitioners with expertise in teaching on mental health issues and to key members of the Royal College of Psychiatrists. In addition, members of the College were invited to comment via the College e-bulletin. The Core Curriculum subgroup then integrated many of the comments received into the final version, which went before the Education Training Committee of the Royal College of Psychiatrists as part of the final project report. The final version is reproduced below. Medical students were consulted through their membership of the Scoping Group and also through discussion with students undertaking their clinical placements with those working on the document. Unfortunately, funding was not available to allow any detailed consultation with users or carers or medical students. However, use was made of some research which had been undertaken with service users on their views of the contents of an undergraduate programme [29]. It may be helpful to be aware that most of the comments received related to specialist interest but the document on the whole was well received. Three United Kingdom medical schools are using the document in its entirety as they review their undergraduate programmes.

In formulating this 'Core Curriculum', those involved recognized that there are variations between medical schools in the amount of time allocated to, and integration between, 'core' theoretical and clinical teaching within psychiatry (usually in the third or fourth year of the undergraduate programme) and what is taught on related topics, often in other years in the 'preclinical components' of the course, such as psychology, sociology, psychopharmacology and communication skills. There was also an acknowledgement that the document could not be too lengthy to be unusable. The variation in curricula was also relevant to consider, as some schools have considerable 'vertical integration' of aspects of psychiatry throughout the curriculum. In other schools psychiatry may be less well integrated across the curriculum and appear mainly in one clinical block. The purpose of the core curriculum proposed is to outline the 'core' aspects of knowledge, skills and attitudes related specifically to psychiatry that medical students require for basic competence and to meet the standards of '*Tomorrow's Doctors*'. That is, these learning outcomes should be the minimum requirement of UK medical schools. There was a recognition that being prescriptive was unlikely to be useful. This learning then becomes the scaffolding for further learning. The philosophy of the Scoping Group was that all doctors need to be able to safely and comprehensively undertake a full assessment of patients' health. Students must be able to assess mental health as well as physical health and be aware of the importance of social circumstances [22].

The core curriculum presented here is relevant for all doctors and can easily be supplemented by other components, such as student selected components or elective to meet the needs of those with a greater interest in psychiatry. Those devising the core curriculum accepted that the areas of knowledge, skills and attitudes are linked and that there may be overlap. However, in developing curricula it is helpful to think about the three domains to ensure comprehensive cover.

The learning outcomes are described in the following section; the eight appendices that formed the document are also included. Six appendices give greater detail regarding what might reasonably be included within the knowledge, skills and attitudes required. The final two appendices provide brief statements regarding delivery and assessment of the curriculum, again suggesting what may be an ideal approach.

4.4.2   The Royal College of Psychiatrists Core Curriculum (UK)

Specific to teaching in clinical psychiatry, the principal **aims** of the undergraduate medical course should be:

- To provide students with knowledge of the main psychiatric disorders, the principles underlying modern psychiatric theory, commonly used treatments and a basis on which to continue to develop this knowledge.

- To assist students to develop the necessary skills to apply this knowledge in clinical situations.

- To encourage students to develop the appropriate attitudes necessary to respond empathically to psychological distress in all medical settings.

The **Learning Outcomes** are:

4.4.2.1   *Knowledge*

On completion of undergraduate training the successful student will be able to:

1. Describe the prevalence and clinical presentation of common psychiatric conditions and how these may differ according to age and developmental stage.

2. Summarize the major categories of psychiatric disorders, for example using ICD-10 (International Classification of Diseases, version 10).

3. Explain the biological, psychological and socio-cultural factors which may predispose to, precipitate or maintain psychiatric illness and describe multifactorial aetiology.

4. Describe the current, common psychological and physical treatments for psychiatric conditions, including the indications for their use, their method of action and any unwanted effects.

5. State the doctor's duties and the patient's rights under the appropriate mental health legislation and mental capacity legislation.

6. Describe what may constitute risk to self (suicide, self harm and/or neglect, engaging in high risk behaviour) and risk to and from others (including knowledge of child, adults with learning disabilities and elder protection requirements).

7. Describe how to assess and manage psychiatric emergencies, which may occur in psychiatric, general medical or other settings. In particular, be able to describe the elements of a risk assessment and the management of behavioural disturbance.

8. Describe the basic range of services and professionals involved in the care of people with mental illness and the role of self help, service user and carer groups in providing support to them. As part of this students should be able to describe when psychiatrists should intervene and when other clinicians should retain responsibility.

4.4.2.2 Skills

On completion of the course the successful student will be able to:

1. Take a full psychiatric history, assess the mental state (including a cognitive assessment) and write up a case. This includes being able to describe symptoms and mental state features, aetiological factors, differential diagnoses, a plan of management and assessment of prognosis.

2. Screen empathically for common mental health problems in non-psychiatric settings and recognize where medically unexplained physical symptoms may have psychological origins.

3. Evaluate and describe patients presenting with abnormal fears/anxieties, pathological mood states and problematic, challenging or unusual behaviours.

4. Summarize and present a psychiatric case in an organized and coherent way to another professional and be able to discuss management with doctors or other staff involved in a patient's care.

5. Recognize the differences between mental health problems and the range of normal responses to stress and life events.

6. Evaluate information about family relationships and their impact on an individual patient, which may involve gaining information from other sources.

7. Assess a patient's potential risk to themselves and others, at any stage of their illness and, in particular, be able to assess a patient following an episode of deliberate self harm.

8. Evaluate the impact of psychiatric illness on the individual and their family and those around them.

9. Find, appraise and apply information and evidence gained from in depth reading relating to a specific clinical case.

10. Discuss with patients and relatives the nature of their illness, management options and prognosis.

4.4.2.3 *Attitudes*

On completion of the course the successful student will be able to:

1. Use an empathic interviewing style, which is suitable for eliciting information from disturbed and distressed patients.

2. Recognize the importance of the development of a therapeutic relationship with patients, including the need for their active involvement in decisions about their care.

3. Demonstrate sensitivity to the concerns of patients and their families about the stigmatization of psychiatric illness.

4. Recognize the importance of multidisciplinary teamwork in the field of mental illness in psychiatric, community and general medical settings, primary care settings and some non-medical settings.

5. Demonstrate awareness of capacity, consent and confidentiality issues as they apply in psychiatry.

6. Reflect on their own attitudes to patients with mental health problems and how these might influence their approach to such patients.

7. Reflect on how working in mental health settings may impact upon their own health and that of colleagues.

Further information to clarify these learning outcomes is provided in the form of appendices and these are included at the end of the chapter.

4.5 Implementing the Curriculum

We should keep in mind that a new curriculum is a continuing dynamic process which inevitably needs to take into account the development plan of a school; many other factors will also need to be considered. Any problem has to be solved at various levels and diverse approaches may be needed. The main goal of the process would be an institutionalization of a school development. Such a process includes redefinition of roles, establishment of task forces to tackle specific challenges, definition of responsibility of individual members of academic community and, therefore, foundation of principles of a new culture. Hand in hand with the implementation of a new curriculum it is necessary to make a plan of outcome evaluation. A good change of curriculum has a chance to succeed if it minimizes the number of people losing a job, a position or a power and maximizes the number of those who keep the position or profit. A new curriculum is also likely to be more successfully implemented if staff are invested in the changes and have been involved in the development through meaningful consultation. This needs a directed and clear leadership which is able to make decisions when needed.

A new curriculum is likely to fail because of the following factors:

1. Ineffective leadership, which may result for several reasons and includes: an autocratic curriculum leader, a leader who is inefficient in coping with problems, unable to delegate and create several other leaders, has no charisma, cannot articulate his/her positions and visions, and is insufficient in motivation of others. It may also happen that newly appointed staff do not support changes and undermine the implementation of a new curriculum.

2. Ineffective communication. Some institutions are rather hierarchically structured, some are based rather on representation; some are rather formal in communication, and some are less formal. Bad communicators do not pay enough attention to faculty opposition and to concerns.

3. Insufficient centralization, which may be accompanied by the lack of support from individual departments and laboratories for interdisciplinary conception of teaching programmes. If a curriculum does not have support from different parts of a school or have central support and also lacks a clear infrastructure, then the curriculum may be unmanaged. This means that there is no central overview and individual departments end up doing what suits them as opposed to what might be required.

4. Lack of resources.

5. Resistance to change and an opposition based on different philosophy. Increasing demands on publications and research ('publish or perish') can further jeopardise the capacity for teaching, which is usually underestimated at evaluation processes. Faculty loses the motivation for a new curriculum because of a lack of sufficient reward. All of this can lead back to regression to the mean and to a failure of the whole plan.

4.6 Summary

As we have shown in this chapter, curriculum development is a complex area that is probably more influenced by socio-cultural and political aspects than by educational needs. Developing a coherent curriculum is only part of the challenge, as it is meaningless unless it is successfully implemented. We have suggested how curriculum planners may want to develop curricula in psychiatry and given an example of one such curriculum that could be modified for local use. We have also highlighted the potential pitfalls that may arise and need to be overcome if a curriculum is to be a dynamic entity that is responsive to changing needs. Keeping those who ultimately deliver the education involved in the development of curricula may be an important component, as it is at the point of delivery that success can be judged. Whilst the process is no doubt complex, it can be managed if the approach to it is systematic and focused.

Appendices for the Core Curriculum in the UK

These outline in more detail specific aspects of the knowledge and skills that are referred to above and also to wider areas of knowledge and skills that should ideally be taught across the curriculum.

Appendix 4.A – Brain function

This will include aspects of neuroanatomy, physiology and psychology:

- Physiology of neuronal function.

- Mechanisms underlying attention, perception, executive function, memory and learning.

- Mechanisms relevant to the experience of emotion.

- Mechanisms related to psychological function.

- Human development and life cycle.

Appendix 4.B – Sociological Issues

- The meaning of 'illness' to individuals and society.

- Awareness that different models of illness (and the competing claims made for each of the models promoted by various groups) are important to the understanding of psychiatric illness, its symptoms and associated behaviours. The following models should be considered: biopsychosocial, multi-axial, medical, developmental and attributional as they relate to mental health problems.

- Ethics and the values that underpin core ethical principles.

- The law and mental health and issues relating to 'capacity'.

- Relevance of family, culture and society and the individual's relationship with these.

- Importance of life events.

- Stigma.

- Understanding of the public health importance of mental health nationally and internationally in terms of personal economic and social functioning, including a knowledge of prevalence, disability, chronicity, carer burden, cultural attitudes and differences, suicide and service provision.

Appendix 4.C – Psychiatric Disorders and Related Topics

Knowledge of the following is a minimum:

- Simple classification of psychiatric disorders.

- Anxiety disorders.

- Mood disorders.

- Psychosis and specifically schizophrenia.

- Substance misuse, especially alcohol and cannabis (acute and chronic effects).

- Delirium.

- Dementia.

- Somatoform disorders.

- Acute reactions to stress and PTSD.

- Eating disorders.

- Disorders of personality.

- Effects of organic brain disease.

- Patients who self harm.

- Major disorders in childhood and differences in assessment.

- Differences in presentation in older people.

- Problems of those with learning disability.

- Comorbidity.

The degree to which a student may have clinical exposure to individual disorders will depend on the time allocated within the curriculum and the nature of the clinical experience available. It will not always be the case that exposure takes place in the setting of the psychiatric clinical attachment.

Appendix 4.D – Psychopharmacology

- Function of the main neurotransmitter systems in the CNS.

- Basic neurochemical theories of depression, schizophrenia and dementia.

- Mechanism of action and clinical pharmacology of commonly used psychotropic drugs:

  Anxiolytics

  Antidepressants

  Antipsychotics

  Mood stabilizers

  Drugs for dementia.

Mechanism of action of common psychoactive drugs used recreationally such as:

  Alcohol

  Cannabis

  Stimulants.

Appendix 4.E – Psychological Treatments

In understanding psychological treatments, students should have an understanding of the principles of psychological management of common psychiatric disorders, especially those that are likely to be seen in primary care such as depression and anxiety.

Approaches to common conditions include cognitive behavioural therapy, counselling and motivational interviewing.

Recognition of the importance of lifestyle on mental health and its impact on treatments, including: sleep hygiene, nutrition, social interaction, physical activity, education, occupation and family and community involvement.

Appendix 4.F – Communication Skills

The following aspects of interview skills are important but often difficult for undergraduate students to fully attain. Observation and feedback on assessments is recommended:

- Active listening.

- Empathic communication and building rapport.

- Understanding non-verbal communication.

- Skills in opening, containing and closing an interview.

Appendix 4.G – Delivery of the Curriculum

Delivery of the curriculum will depend on local resources, support and history and should involve a variety of different teaching methods. During the clinical attachment it is important to ensure that contact time with consultants is effectively used, as sometimes there may be very little of this. It is also important that consultant psychiatrists are a visible component of the student experience. Students need any teaching to be made relevant to practice [16] and there are benefits from seeing senior clinicians interested in their educational experience (especially for recruitment to psychiatry). Attention needs to be paid to consideration of which learning outcomes are expected to be achieved in different parts of the attachment. It is also important to ensure that where observation is used as a learning experience it is of little value without any adequate follow up. A ward round or clinic in which observation alone is used is unlikely to successfully help in meeting the learning outcomes outlined. Teaching should, where possible and appropriate, be delivered in the clinical settings where patients are present and include professionals involved in their care.

Appendix 4.H – Assessment

'Assessment drives learning' is a frequently quoted aphorism. It should also be recognized that assessment confers value to a course. For psychiatry to receive recognition as a valuable element of undergraduate medicine, assessment has to be robust and included in the terminal assessment of the whole undergraduate medical course.

Two elements are key to assessment of undergraduate students in psychiatry. These are formative and summative assessment:

- Formative assessment provides information for students about where they are in their learning process and what they need to do to reach their learning objectives. Ideally students should be directly observed interviewing patients and feedback should be given on their clinical skills. Additionally, through case presentations, students' progress in attaining required knowledge outcomes can be assessed. Further, by employing a continuing process of assessment, attitudes can be assessed and, if required, challenged.

- Summative assessment needs to be related directly to the specified learning outcomes for each medical school's course. It should be at the end-point of a student's learning in psychiatry. Each assessment should include components that address knowledge, skills and attitudes. For each of these areas differing assessment methods are indicated and assessors need to be clear about what objectives they are assessing in each component.

Clinical skills may be assessed using real patients or role players in a variety of objectively driven examination formats. It is important that the complexity of the cases is appropriate for the students' level of experience. Direct observation of students is the best means to assess clinical skills. The use of clinical cases for students at the end of their courses should allow them to demonstrate higher level skills, such as synthesis of multiple sources and types of information and clinical application of knowledge.

Acknowledgments

The contributions of Stephen Cooper, Brian Lunn and Barry Wright who were members of the subgroup that led the development of the core curriculum for the Royal College of Psychiatrists is gratefully acknowledged, as is the input of all those who fed back at the point of consultation.

References

1. Höschl, C. (2009) European psychiatry: needs, challenges and structures. *Eur Arch Psychiatry Clin Neurosci*, **259** (Suppl 2), S119–S122.
2. Bobbitt, J.F. (1918) *The Curriculum*, Houghton Mifflin, Boston.
3. Kelly, A.V. (2009) *The Curriculum: Theory and Practice*, 6th edn Sage Publications Ltd.
4. Wilkinson, M.J.B. and Barczak, P. (1988) Psychiatric screening in general practice: comparison of the General Health Questionnaire and the Hospital Anxiety Depression Scale. *Journal of the Royal College of General Practitioners*, **38**, 311–313.
5. Berardi, D., Berti Ceroni, G., Leggieri, G. *et al.* (1999) Mental, physical and functional status in primary care attenders. *The International Journal of Psychiatry in Medicine*, **29**, 113–148.
6. World Psychiatric Association and World Federation for Medical Education (1995) Core curriculum in psychiatry for medical students.
7. Karim, K., Edwards, R., Dogra, N. *et al.* (2009) A survey of the Teaching and Assessment of Undergraduate Psychiatry in the Medical Schools of the United Kingdom and Ireland. Undergraduate psychiatry: what's going on? *Medical Teacher*, **31** (11), 1024–1029.
8. General Medical Council (2009) Tomorrow's Doctors – Outcomes and Standards For Undergraduate Medical Education, General Medical Council, London. http://www.gmc-uk.org/TomorrowsDoctors_2009.pdf_27494211.pdf (accessed 1 March 2010).
9. Verhaak, P.F.M., Schellevis, F.G., Nuijen, J. and Volkers, A.C. (2006) Patients with a psychiatric disorder in general practice: determinants of general practitioners'psychological diagnosis. *General Hospital Psychiatry*, **28**, 125–132.
10. David, T.J., Dolmans, D.H., Patel, L. and Van Der Vleuten, C.P. (1998) Problem-based learning as an alternative to lecture-based continuing medical education. *J R Soc Med*, **91**, 626–630.
11. Norman, G.R. and Schmidt, H.G. (1992) The psychological basis of problem-based learning: a review of the evidence. *Acad Med*, **67**, 557–565.
12. Schmidt, H.G. (1993) Foundations of problem-based learning: some explanatory notes. *Med Educ*, **27**, 422–432.
13. Turbes, S., Krebs, E., and Axtell, S. (2002) The hidden curriculum in multicultural medical education. *Academic Medicine*, **77**, 209–216.
14. Höschl, C. (2000) A critical appraisal of medical education. *Psychiatrie*, **4** (2) 134–137. A report from the conference held in Linköping, Sweden, 29 August–1 September1999.
15. Höschl, C. (2007) Pathways of integrated medical curriculum. *Surg Radiol Anat.*, **29**, 423.
16. Höschl, C. and Kozeny J. (1997) Predicting academic performance of medical students: The first three years. *American Journal of Psychiatry*, **154**, 87–92
17. Dogra, N. (2004) The learning and teaching of cultural diversity in undergraduate medical education in the UK. PhD, University of Leicester.
18. van Mook, W.N., de Grave, W.S., van Luijk, S.J., *et al.* (2009) Training and learning professionalism in the medical school curriculum: current considerations. *Eur J Intern Med*, **20**, e96–e100. Epub 24 January 2009.

19. Katschnig, H. (2010) Are psychiatrists and endangered species? Observations on internal and external challenges to the profession. *World Psychiatry*, **9**, 21–28.

20. Sierles, F.S. and Taylor, M.A. (1995) Decline of U.S. medical student career choice of psychiatry and what to do about it. *American Journal of Psychiatry*, **152**, 1416–1426.

21. Langsley, D.G., Freedman, A.M., Haas, M. and Grubbs, J.H. (1977) Medical student education in psychiatry. *American Journal of Psychiatry*, **134** (Suppl), 15–20.

22. Dogra, N. (2009) *Report of the Royal College of Psychiatrists' Scoping Group on Undergraduate Education in Psychiatry.* http://www.rcpsych.ac.uk/pdf/Final%20Education%20in%20Psychiatry%20Scoping%20group%20report%20May%202009.pdf (accessed 29 December 2009).

23. General Medical Council (1993) Tomorrow's Doctors, General Medical Council, London.

24. Quality Assurance Agency (2001) [Online]. Available: www.qaa.ac.uk (accessed 22 July 2010).

25. Plomin, J. (2001) Tomorrow's doctors could lack medical expertise. *TheGuardian*, **19** June 2001.

26. Lowry, S. (1993) *Medical Education*, British Medical Association Publishing, London.

27. Richards, P. and Stockhill, S. (1997) *The New Learning Medicine*, 14th edn, BMJ Publishing Group, London.

28. Sinclair, S. (1997) *Making Doctors: An Institutional Apprenticeship*, Berg, Oxford.

29. Dogra, N., Cavendish, S., Anderson, J. and Edwards, R. (2009) Service user perspectives on the content of the undergraduate curriculum in psychiatry. *Psychiatric Bulletin*, **33**, 260–264.

5

Teaching Behavioural Sciences

Bulent Coskun

Department of Psychiatry, Kocaeli University Medical School, Kocaeli, Turkey

5.1   Introduction

> Never before have the challenges for behavioural sciences been more exciting or more urgent.
>
> —Rimer [1]

Different aspects of teaching Behavioural Sciences are considered in this chapter, with the main focus on how to teach, rather than what to teach. The titles, content, methods, teachers and even the recipients of these courses may differ between medical schools; but the importance of behavioural aspects of medical education continues to grow regardless of the dominance of biomedicine. Barriers, challenges and some recommendations for future teaching of behavioural sciences will also be considered using examples from different countries. A circular framework for different approaches to teaching behavioural sciences is presented and discussed.

It is worth considering the question of who should be the recipients of behavioural sciences teaching. Usually, the expected target is the medical student. But throughout the literature it is observed that physicians after graduation, mainly family physicians, International Medical Graduates (IMG) and also a wider group of professionals, as suggested in Chur-Hansen's article, may be expected to attend such courses [2].

5.2   Background

In the comprehensive document produced by the World Psychiatric Association and World Federation for Medical Education, the term 'behavioural science teaching' refers to three separate issues [3]. Firstly, to the scientific basis of psychiatry, which is the responsibility of the psychiatry department. Secondly, to what is sometimes called medical psychology,

Teaching Psychiatry: Putting Theory into Practice   Edited by Linda Gask, Bulent Coskun and David Baron
© 2011 John Wiley & Sons, Ltd

namely training in sensitivity, interviewing and communication skills, and in recognizing the role of family and other social factors in illness. The third use of the term refers to the scientific disciplines that are used to understand behaviour, including not only psychology and sociology but also aspects of genetics, biochemistry and physiology that underlie the origins of complex behaviour.

Another definition provided by Buyck *et al.* is: '. . .the interdisciplinary field concerned with development and integration of behavioural and biomedical science, knowledge and techniques relevant to the understanding of physical health and illness and the application of this knowledge and these techniques to prevention, diagnosis, treatment and rehabilitation' [4]. Benbassat *et al.* state that they use behavioural sciences 'as an all-inclusive term for a wide spectrum of diverse topics (e.g. interviewing skills, medical ethics, introductory courses in sociology, psychology and anthropology) that are not part of the biomedical programmes or clinical clerkships' [5].

Several different names are given to this course and a wide spectrum of topics has been listed in the curricula [5, 6]. Besides behavioural sciences, 'medical psychology' and 'social medicine' are also frequently used, depending on who is teaching the course. However, in addition to these more commonly used terms, programmes with similar aims and content are provided in courses called: 'Medical Professional Development' in Thailand; 'Medical Personal and Professional Development' at the University of Adelaide in Australia [2]; 'Medical Humanities and Behavioural Sciences (MHBS)' then 'Patient Centred Medicine (PCM)' in Ohio, USA [7]; 'Behavioural medicine' in Hungary [8]; 'Neurobehavioural sciences' in the third Faculty of Medicine at Charles University in Prague, Czech Republic (C. Höschl, Personal Communication, January 2010).; and, in addition, to behavioural sciences as 'a preparation programme for being a physician' in Kocaeli University Turkey. There is also a concept Biological Psychology, which is not taken into consideration in this chapter, as it focuses on psychology rather than medicine [9].

In a review of medical programmes in the United Kingdom, it was found that there was a behavioural science component in almost all of them. However, the extent and scope of teaching on social and behavioural sciences varied considerably [6]. It was also concluded that multidisciplinary teaching was often the key approach and, consequently, boundaries within and around social and behavioural sciences were often unclear; this has been noted elsewhere [5, 10].

5.3   History of Teaching Behavioural and Social Aspects of Medicine

Some authors date recognition of the importance of teaching socially orientated aspects of medical practice to the Flexner report of 1910 [11]. However, these ideas can be traced back almost 1000 years to the age of Avicenna [12, 13] and even to the age of Hippocrates [15].

For a long period, it was assumed that medical students, simply by their expressed wish to help other people, would recognize the importance of this topic [14]. Similarly, communication between doctors and patients was regarded as a simple task that did not need to be taught [15].

Then, as the importance of problems in doctor–patient relationships began to emerge in the literature, relevant professionals (mainly psychologists) were invited to give lectures to medical students. Also, awareness of the sociological dimensions of health and disease, especially for communicable diseases, raised the need for some sociological teaching for medical students, but this was still provided in lecture format. From the 1940s and 1950s steps were taken to organize special courses and develop specific departments to teach these topics in medical schools. But still the course on behavioural sciences was considered to be 'nice to know' rather than 'need to know' [6]. However, it is worth noting that in Brazil, during the late nineteenth century, psychology courses were taught at the medical schools. Psychology training was considered as part of Medicine and Law until 1962, when the Brazilian government recognized psychology training in separate schools [16].

In the 1940s at Yale University in the Unites States, the Institute of Human Relations was located in the Medical Centre and the departments of Psychiatry and Psychology worked collaboratively with input from representatives of several other behavioural science disciplines, including sociology and anthropology. It was advocated that medical schools should have divisions of social sciences along with natural sciences and clinical divisions [17]. For a considerable period, teaching psychology and the behavioural sciences was typically viewed as 'Western' and, more specifically, 'American' [2], however many countries across the world in fact included these courses in their medical curricula.

The social structures of the countries have also been found to have an impact on the choice of the medical school to teach behavioural sciences. For example, repression of social sciences such as sociology, psychology or anthropology was reported during Hungary's years of socialism. Training in these professions was revived in the 1980s and departments of behavioural sciences in Hungarian medical schools were founded after the collapse of socialism in the 1990s [8].

Another example may be provided from China. In a report on how to develop medical psychology in China in 1959, it was stated that:

> ...How to guarantee that the people could have healthy physique to resist the attack of illness and to eliminate the distress of fatigue has become the very important task which medicine and its related sciences have to tackle. In this sense medical psychology is to use the knowledge of the psychology of dialectic materialism to assist medicine in the prevention and care of illness, as well as in accomplishing the task of protecting the people's health. ...
> —Tsan [18]

In this quotation two points come forward: firstly, the preventive or protective function of medicine; and, secondly, the emphasis given to politics, which becomes evident with the words 'psychology of dialectic materialism'.

5.4   Rationale of Teaching Behavioural Sciences

Wedding quotes an interesting view of the rationale of teaching Behavioural Sciences from John Carr: [10]

> Before you change attitudes and behaviors around AIDS, you need to know how attitudes develop and change. Before you can change decisions about risky behaviors, you need to know how judgments and decisions are made. Before you address memory decline in the elderly, you need to know the basics of learning and memory and how that changes with age. And before you address the complexity of the interactions among genetics, the brain, and, say, schizophrenia, you need to know the basics of cognition, emotion, culture, behavioural and cognitive neuroscience, and behavioural genetics.

A similar message can be found in Kevin Mack's article, where he refers to the epidemiologists increasingly pointing to behavioural interventions as some of medicine's most powerful tools for reversing dangerous health trends in the United States. Thus he suggests 'to describe and promote curricular models that offer opportunities for the integration of behavioural sciences into the "rest" of medical education' [19].

In the key recommendations for 'Tomorrow's doctors', the General Medical Council states that:

> Tomorrow's doctors should know about, understand and be able to apply and integrate the clinical, basic, behavioural and social sciences on which medical practice is based.

With these recommendations behavioural sciences moved to the 'need to know' category [11].

As may be seen from the examples cited above, many authors agree on the necessity of having behavioural science education during medical education. As Benbassat states briefly: 'Courses in the behavioural sciences differ in contents, methods and settings of instruction; however, they all share the common interest of integrating key humanistic and social science principles into the medical curriculum' [5].

5.5   Who Teaches Behavioural Sciences?

Depending on the recruitment capacity of the medical school, behavioural sciences courses are provided by teachers representing different disciplines. Amongst the various social science specialists, psychologists traditionally dominate the arena, followed by sociologists, anthropologists and nurses. But in some places where there are limited resources, medical teachers, mainly psychiatrists, undertake the responsibility of teaching behavioural sciences. Ideally, a team of behavioural sciences experts should collaborate in the preparation, implementation and assessment of the behavioural sciences course [5].

Whatever the original background of the teacher they should be able to incorporate different perspectives. To attract and retain the attention of the medical students and involve them with the course, the teaching should have practical components drawn from real clinical experiences rather than only theoretical lectures. This means the teachers of behavioural sciences should have an active place in a clinical department if not at a special department or an institute for behavioural sciences, and should be able to enrich themselves with real cases. Even a teacher from a clinical department with strict adherence to their original discipline might have real difficulty in being an effective teacher. Flexibility of approach is essential. However, in a study carried out with teachers of behavioural sciences, it was found that some teachers felt isolated from disciplinary support and marginalized within medical schools [6].

5.6   Who Decides What and How to Teach?

It might be considered that 'what is taught' and 'how it is taught' are governed by the decision making procedures regarding the curriculum – the negotiations amongst teachers and the administrators. One cannot put aside the overall teaching policy and the resources and limitations of medical schools. This is inevitable, but the process may be overt or hidden

[20]. The policy of the university and the medical school, and the views of administrators, Deans or older and/or influential teachers, have considerable impact. Usually, the hidden agenda of the institution is rationalized to fit into the fashionable terminology of the 'mission and vision' of the school or university. Not infrequently there may be diverse views about the priorities. Sometimes personal relationships, frustrations or different dynamics between the administrators and the staff or amongst decision makers – mostly not related to the curriculum issues – may also affect the planning of the program (see Chapter 4 for further discussion of these issues).

Other factors which may influence the process of the development and implementation of the behavioural sciences curriculum may be the background of the people involved in the planning (psychiatrists, psychologists, sociologists, anthropologists or members of any other discipline present might prefer to have the topics they know best or think will be most helpful to appear in the curriculum). The special interest areas of course teachers may be crucial (sometimes some courses continue in a medical school until the teacher of that course is retired or moved to another place) [5]. Additionally, there may be special skills needed to 'translate behavioural sciences to medics' (as stated by one of the participants of a survey by Litva and Peters 20]. Cost of recruiting and availability of staff may be a factor (limited resources may be devoted to 'more medical' issues) [2], as are the overall political system [4, 8, 18] and the target population of the courses (usually, but not always, it is medical students). Finally, there is, as ever, the struggle for space in the curriculum, the expectations of the public, the media, the students and not forgetting the previous graduates!

A few innovative examples from different settings and medical schools are given in Box 5.1.

Sometimes the target population may not be the medical student. It has been shown that international medical graduates undergoing residency training in the United States benefit from a preparatory course on behavioural sciences. An interview study carried out with ten residents revealed that there were important differences in conceptualizing behavioural sciences and psychiatry in general in the home countries of the residents with what they were witnessing in United States. The tendency was to request a course on behavioural sciences in an early phase of their residency. The main differences were regarding physician–patient relationships, the meanings attributed to the roles of a physician, a patient and other health personnel [21].

Teaching of physician–patient relationships (including interviewing skills or communication skills) should not be in the monopoly of behavioural sciences or psychiatry courses. Different teachers from other medical specialities can provide ideal physician models for the medical students. For example, observing a surgeon talking about the risks of an operation while paying special attention to the anxiety and fears of the patient, the respectful attitude of the anatomist to the cadaver, and the sensitivity and the understanding attitude of the gynaecologist before genital examination of a patient with culturally rooted fears would be much more effective than the discussion of these issues at a lecture or even at a small group discussion with problem-based learning techniques or simulated patients. It would be much more effective to use all of these approaches.

A holistic approach should have continuity and complement both with the messages provided in different years from behavioural sciences teachers and also from other faculty members of the medical school from different disciplines.

Box 5.1   Some Examples of Innovative Methods for Teaching Behavioural Sciences

Use of auxiliary tools or activities during the course
Books, stories, poems (sometimes from artists who are physicians themselves) Other examples of art, drawings, paintings, photographs (again sometimes products of physician artists wherever available). Films, videos, clips from cinema, TV films, serials and documentaries [11, 32].

Inviting guests to the class or session of a course
Inviting physicians from general practice, other faculty members from other departments, previous graduates of the same school. Inviting interesting and/or well known people related to the topic under discussion.

Organizing visits to different settings
Other medical practice settings: health centres in the community, outpatient or inpatient units of other hospitals (general or psychiatry hospitals), health units of workplaces, consultation liaison units, institutions for the elderly, the children to be visited [26].

Visits to some art events with oral or written discussions afterwards (cinemas, theatres or exhibitions). These visits may provide the opportunity to observe human communication in different settings. It is always possible to make links with health and mental health issues.

Involvement of the students in modest research projects
Students may be encouraged to get involved with ongoing research projects or they may be asked to plan, implement and report some studies in topics which may help them to be sensitized to social and environmental issues [32].

Senior students and residents may also be encouraged to contribute to small group discussions with first year medical students.

Collaboration with other departments and relevant committees
As part of the patient–doctor course, first year medical students worked with diabetic patients who were selected by their primary care physicians. In preparation for their patient interactions, students were taught basic communication concepts and the role of the relationship in improving patient outcomes; continuity issues were addressed as students learned to collaboratively develop behavioural-change plans with their patients and then followed their patients' progress over the course of the year [30].

Together with anatomy department, first year medical students are invited to discuss their thoughts and feelings about the cadaver, their first 'patient', before entering dissection sessions [32].

5.7   When is the Proper Time to Teach Behavioural Sciences?

Thoughts on the proper time to teach behavioural sciences during medical training vary considerably. Some prefer to focus on early years; others suggest integration of behavioural sciences into the 'rest' the of medical education [19].

It may take years for a curriculum to stabilize in terms of time allocation and content. Actually it can be said that stability is not wanted. Continuous development is needed. Davis and Harden have cautiously suggested that that the success of their curriculum may be a potential danger [22]. They say there may be less incentive to change and there may be resistance to revising the curriculum. 'However,' they say, 'a curriculum is, a dynamic process that needs to respond to circumstances: the changes in society, medical practice and educational thinking'.

In practice, curricula are almost never the same for a long period due to several reasons: continuing developments on different aspects of the topic; inevitable changes regarding the preferences; changing teachers and costs of the course; duplications and conjoined teaching with other departments and, of course, the struggle for space and time. There may need to be considerable negotiation. The extent of teaching of communication skills occurring during other parts of the medical curriculum may also influence the process. In places where there are no special Behavioural Sciences Departments, Departments of Psychiatry may be in charge of planning teaching courses on behavioural sciences. Depending on the resources of the department and the medical school, some support may be needed from other faculties, which then brings in another important issue for proper timing of the imported teacher (out of his or her original department).

Usually behavioural sciences courses are placed in the early years of the training, particularly the first year [2, 6, 16]. In some cases these first year courses are supported with second and third year courses. Behavioural science topics may also be considered within the remit of general mental health or psychiatry training together with teaching psychiatric problems, their diagnosis and treatments [6].

In an example from Ohio State University, the course was shifted from a one year to a two year schedule, and from an all-day to a 90 minute, one session per week format. Teaching methods shifted from 80% lectures to 35% lectures, and teaching in small groups from 20 to 65% [7].

Russell *et al.* report several approaches which they gathered from medical schools in United Kingdom [6]. The authors state that it was generally felt that a 'spiral' curriculum is the best approach to achieving the attitudinal learning outcomes of the social and behavioural sciences in undergraduate medical education. They also underline that opinions differ, with 'continuous drip feeding of social and behavioural sciences' on one side and 'short and blocks of more intensive teaching' on the other. Benbassat *et al.* (2003) similarly discuss how integration of the course in the curriculum may be horizontal or vertical [5].

5.8 Methods of Teaching Behavioural Sciences

It is possible to look into the methods of teaching behavioural sciences from different perspectives taking into consideration different dimensions. As presented in Figure 5.1 six dimensions have been extracted from the literature to review various approaches of teaching behavioural sciences on a circular framework.

Although the list is composed of six single dimensions, there is no doubt that almost all may be considered to be interrelated with each other and that a dynamic balance would be present amongst these dimensions.

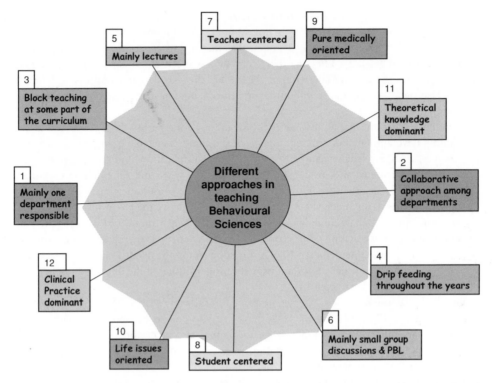

Figure 5.1 A circular framework for viewing different approaches to teaching Behavioural Sciences.

Before listing and discussing these six dimensions it would be right to say that other dimensions may also be added to this framework, or some dimensions may be omitted or replaced by others depending on the needs and the realities of the setting.

For any particular medical school, the present situation may be mapped out and future targets planned using this figure. It would not be fair to say there is one ideal profile for all. But each medical school may work on its own plan depending on the needs and realities of the institution.

5.8.1 Responsibility of the Course (1–2)

The first dimension is represented by the dimension, 'Mainly one department being responsible' of teaching behavioural sciences on one side, and 'Collaborative approach amongst departments' on the other side. In some places, due to lack of representatives from different disciplines, the course may be carried out through one department, on some occasions only by psychiatrists. At the other end of the scale, different disciplines from different departments may collaborate, starting from the planning of the course to the implementation and the assessment procedures (at horizontal or vertical levels). In some cases there may be a special department in charge of behavioural sciences but that department may act as a coordinator for the collaboration of teaching activities with support from different disciplines and departments. In the latter case, that medical school might be placed somewhere near the midpoint of the dimension on responsibility for the course [5, 6, 8, 9, 11, 17, 22].

5.8.2 Timing and Period of Teaching (3–4)

Some programmes are known to be provided as a block for a semester or a year, others may be disseminated throughout the years as a 'drip feed'. As stated earlier, usually behavioural sciences education starts in the first year of the training. The methods may change at the same school during the years depending on the preferences of the teachers, administrators and the resources of the institution [2, 5–7, 19, 22, 23].

5.8.3 Type of Teaching (5–6)

In this dimension it is possible to place classical lecturing on one side and relatively newer approaches of small group discussions and/or an extensively used specific example of innovative teaching such as problem-based learning (Chapter 6) on the other side. Many places use a combination of these methods depending mostly on the availability of teachers [2, 3, 7, 17, 19].

5.8.4 Having the Teacher or the Student at the Centre of the Teaching Process (7–8)

Teaching has traditionally been prepared according to the wisdom and perspective of the teachers. Teachers are generally believed to be capable of and without question responsible for deciding what is best to teach the students, being the focus of 'authority'. But in some places this view has been seriously challenged and the view expressed that students might better be brought into the centre of the teaching process – as Benbassat referred to it 'learner centred teaching'. This dimension may also be considered to be drawn between two points, one representing authority and only one unquestionable truth, the other point representing the attitude which encourages mastery of problem solving and seeking for evidence, questioning and challenging information, including what is presented by the instructor. The latter approach would certainly promote autonomy of the learner and bring him or her to the centre of the teaching or learning process (for more discussion of these issues see Chapter 6). If the teacher can manage to be a model in encouraging the student to be more active in the process, this may serve as an excellent example for the student in future relationships with patients [5, 15, 17, 21, 24, 25].

5.8.5   The Focus of the Teaching (9–10)

There may be several factors related to this dimension. Here we can draw the line between focusing on mainly medical issues at one extreme and daily life issues at the other. It could possibly be considered to focus on psychological, social, anthropological or some other aspects of knowledge and skills to be acquired by the candidate physicians. The term 'medically orientated' was preferred to mean that whatever the content may be the aim would be to equip the student with knowledge and skills for future role of being a physician. On the other hand, it has recently been a tendency to encourage medical students to get involved with social issues not necessarily directly related with being a physician, such as dealing with various aspects of arts, literature, poems, drawings, cinema and so on. Most of these topics, either elective or not, are considered to be under the umbrella of behavioural sciences or professional development, or human sciences and the humanities. A balance between the two ends may easily be constructed by harmonizing real life issues in health and disease topics through the use of art and technology during the course. Some innovative approaches are described elsewhere [2, 6, 10, 17, 24, 26–31].

5.8.6   Theory and Practice (11–12)

It is accepted that these two aspects complement each other but again it is recognized that it may be difficult to achieve harmony because of the issues discussed earlier. Even if the administration and the teachers may wish to increase practical exercises, the time allocated for such activities, ratio of the number of students and teachers, financial or physical limitations may act as barriers [5, 24].

5.9   Difficulties/Barriers and Recommendations Regarding Teaching Behavioural Sciences

Some of the difficulties have already been mentioned above while discussing other aspects of teaching behavioural sciences (definition, rationale, content, teaching time and methods), and it is evident that almost all are interrelated. Barriers or challenges and recommendations for overcoming them are listed in Table 5.1.

5.10   Conclusion

In this chapter, after an introduction on definition, historical development and rationale of teaching behavioural sciences, we have focused on a range of different methods of teaching behavioural sciences. A model for reviewing dimensions of teaching on a circular framework is presented which it is hoped will be of value. Various examples from different countries have been presented and discussed.

Table 5.1 Barriers and Challenges on Teaching Behavioural Sciences and Recommendations for Future.

	Barriers and challenges (areas of concern)	Recommendations (topics or activities for consideration)
Administrative issues	Overall health policy. Philosophy, principles and hidden agenda of the medical school and the university. Attitudes of the Dean and the Committee responsible for curriculum development, implementation and assessment. Financial capacity affecting recruitment policy, physical conditions, technological structure.	Collaboration in building up the curriculum and agreement on continuous development and use of feedback. Emphasis on giving priority to humane aspect of teaching medical students.
Characteristics and attitudes of the teachers	Being members of different disciplines with various backgrounds, interests, expectations, capacities for interpersonal relationships and ability to act as role models. Also with different beliefs, attitudes and skills on medical education. Different salaries, different levels of support from the associations of their own disciplines.	Collaboration of theoretical background with clinical skills (mainly on interviewing skills and respecting attitude). Organizing enrichment courses for faculty members on improving communication skills and dealing with 'difficult situations in physician–patient relationships'.
Characteristics and attitudes of the students	Motivations, expectations and stereotypes regarding medical education and psychosocial aspects of health and disease. Early experiences with diseases and model physicians. Facing differences amongst the principles taught at behavioural sciences and implementation at the clinical settings.	Encouragement about raising awareness on personal motivations, strengths and weaknesses. Gaining capacity for personal development, learning how to learn and the ability to give and take feedback assertively. Provision of role models open to discussion for development of caring and respecting physicians with the ability of critical thinking and problem solving skills.
Characteristics of the content and the method	Methods of making decisions about the curriculum. Different approaches to priorities about the content, implementation and assessment of the curriculum.	Collaboration of different approaches in synchonizing theory and skills with learning centred approach rather than teaching. Supplying the environment for learning by doing and contributing.
Interactions between the above	Level of recognition and transparency about the hidden agendas. Level of collaboration amongst behavioural sciences and other teachers. Attitudes of various disciplines towards each other and towards tomorrow's doctors.	Spiral development with contribution from all parties, administrators, behavioural sciences teachers, other faculty members, including the views of the students and also the consumers of the health services. Organization of joint teaching programmes with contributions from different disciplines.

References

1. Rimer, B.K. (1997) Toward an improved behavioural medicine. *Ann Behav Med*, **19**, 6–10.
2. Chur-Hansen, A., Carr, J.E., Bundy, C. *et al.* (2008) An international perspective on behavioural science education in medical schools. *J Clin Psychol Med Settings*, **15**, 45–53.
3. World Psychiatric Association and World Federation for Medical Education. http://www.wpanet. org/detail.php?section_id=8&content_id=109.
4. Buyck, D., Floyd, M., Tudiver, F. *et al.* (2005) Behavioural Medicine in Russian family medicine. *Patient Educ Couns*, **59**, 205–211
5. Benbassat, J., Baumal, R., Borkan, J.M. *et al.* (2003) Overcoming barriers to teaching the behavioural and social sciences to medical students. *Acad Med*, **78**, 372–380.
6. Russell, A., van Teijlingen, E., Lambert, H. *et al.* (2004) Social and behavioural science education in UK medical schools: current practice and future directions. *Medical Education*, **38**, 409–417.
7. Post, D.M., Stone, L.C., Knutson, D.J. *et al.* (2008) Enhancing behavioural science education at the Ohio State University College of Medicine. *Acad Med*, **83**, 28–36.
8. Piko, B.F. and Kopp, M.S. (2002) Behavioural medicine in Hungary: past, present, and future. *Behavioural Medicine*, **28**, 72–78.
9. Hoschl, C. (January 2010) Personal Communication.
10. Biological psychology, New World Encyclopedia. http://www.newworldencyclopedia.org/entry/ Biological_psychology (accessed January 2009)
11. Wedding, D. (2008) Innovative methods for making behavioural science relevant to medical education. *J Clin Psychol Med Settings*, **15**, 89–91.
12. Peters, S. and Livia, A. (2006) Relevant behavioural and social science for medical undergraduates: a comparison of specialist and non-specialist educators. *Medical Education*, **40**, 1020–1026.
13. Shoja, M.M. and Tubbs, R.S. Images in Psychiatry The Disorder of Love in the Canon of Avicenna (A.D. 980–1037). http://www.newworldencyclopedia.org/entry/ Biological_psychology (accessed January 2010).
14. Mohit, A. (2001) Mental health and psychiatry in the Middle East: historical development. *Eastern Mediterranean Health Journal*, **7**, 336–347.
15. Ramsden, E.L. (1976) Learning model for BS in Med Ed. *Public Health Reports*, **91**, 281–284.
16. Baumal, R. and Benbassat, J. (2008) Current trends in the educational approach for teaching interviewing skills to medical students. *IMAJ*, **10**, 552–555.
17. Hutz, C.S., Gomes, W. and McCarthy, S. (2006) Teaching of Psychology in Brazil. *International Journal of Psychology*, **41**, 10–16.
18. Straus, R. (1999) Medical sociology: A personal fifty year perspective. *Journal of Health and Social Behavior*, **40**, 103–110.
19. Tsan, T. (1959) How to develop medical psychology in China. http://www.stormingmedia. us/12/1203/A120373.html (accessed January 2010).
20. Mack, K. (2005) Innovations in the teaching of behavioural sciences in the preclinical curriculum. *Academic Psychiatry*, **29**, 471–473.
21. Litva, A. and Peters, S. (2008) Exploring barriers to teaching behavioural and social sciences in medical education. *Medical Education*, **42**, 309–314.
22. Russell Searight, H. and Gafford, J. (2006) Behavioural science education and the international medical graduate. *Acad Med*, **81**, 164–170.
23. Davis, M.H. and Harden, R.M. (2003) Planning and implementing an undergraduate medical curriculum: the lessons learned. *Medical Teacher*, **25**, 596–608.
24. Brownstein, E.J., Singer, P., Dornbush, R.L. *et al.* (1979) New concepts in the teaching of behavioural science in the preclinical curriculum. *Journal of Medical Education*, **54**, 423–425.

25. Kelly, B., Raphael, B. and Byrne, G. (1991) The evaluation of teaching in undergraduate psychiatric education: students' attitudes to psychiatry and the evaluation of clinical competency. *Medical Teacher*, **13**, 77–87

26. Benbassat, J. and Baumal, R. (2008) *A proposal for overcoming problems in teaching interviewing skills to medical students*, Advances in Health Sciences Education Theory and Practice, http://www.springerlink.com/content/v5288673322.315/fulltext.html (Published online 24 January 2008).

27. Levenkron, J.C., Greenland, P. and Bowley, N. (1987) Using patient instructors to teach behavioural counselling skills. *J Med Educ*, **62**, 665–672.

28. Ogur, B., Hirsh, D., Krupat, E. *et al.* (2007) The Harvard Medical School-Cambridge integrated clerkship: an innovative model of clinical education. *Acad Med*, **82** (4), 397–404.

29. Wagner, P.J., Jester, D.M. and Moseley, G.C. (2002) Medical students as health coaches. *Acad Med*, **77**, 1164–1165.

30. Gask, L., Coskun, B. and Baron, D. (2006) Using multimedia in mental health education: the many uses of video. *Turkish Journal of Psychiatry*, **17** (2) (Supplement 1), 166. (Section of Education in Psychiatry Workshop at the WPA International Congress, 12–16 July 2006, Istanbul, Turkey.)

31. Coskun, B., Kocaaslan, C., Uzun, A. *et al.* (2004) 'Toplumsal Duyarlilik Programi' (Social sensitivity program – in Turkish) *14. Ulusal Cocuk ve Ergen Ruh Sagligi ve Hastaliklari Kongresi 21–24 Nisan, Bursa*.

32. Coskun, B. (2009) Thoughts, feelings and drawings of first year medical students before they meet their first patient – the cadaver. http://iamse.org/conf/conf13/professional_development.htm#a2 (accessed January 2010).

6

Problem-Based Learning and Psychiatric Education

Raja Vellingiri Badrakalimuthu[1], Rob van Diest[2], Maarten Bak[2] and Hugo de Waal[3]

[1]Cambridge and Peterborough NHS Foundation Trust, Fulbourn, Cambridge, UK
[2]Department of Psychiatry and Neuropsychology, Maastricht University, Maastricht, The Netherlands
[3]East of England Deanery, Fulbourn Hospital, Fulbourn, Cambridge, UK

6.1   Introduction

Problem-Based Learning (PBL) is a learning method based on a particular educational philosophy. The method involves an instructional strategy by which students, working in small groups, confront contextualized, ill-structured problems, striving to find meaningful solutions. The presented cases trigger students to detect deficiencies in their knowledge and define learning objectives. During this explorative process they are usually guided by a facilitator or PBL-tutor. PBL was first pioneered and developed in 1969 at the McMaster Faculty of Health Sciences, Hamilton, Canada, and shortly thereafter three other medical schools – Maastricht University (The Netherlands), the University of Newcastle (Australia) and the University of New Mexico (United States) – took on the McMaster PBL model and developed it further. In medicine this educational method is becoming more and more the predominant system, with around 150 medical schools across the globe using it wholly or partially as the basis of their courses.

6.2   Method and Philosophy of Problem-Based Learning

In PBL, students use triggers from case scenarios to define their own learning objectives, usually relating and mapping those objectives to a defined curriculum. The group then

Teaching Psychiatry: Putting Theory into Practice   Edited by Linda Gask, Bulent Coskun and David Baron
© 2011 John Wiley & Sons, Ltd

allocates pertinent topics and areas of study to the individual members, who subsequently carry out independent, self-directed study, before returning to the group to discuss their findings and, thereby, sharing and refining their acquired knowledge. Thus, PBL is an Enquiry-Based Learning (IBL) method, with students generating their own analyses of appropriate problems to increase their knowledge and understanding of whatever topic is being covered. PBL, whilst a practical methodology, embraces the dialectical approach associated with Socrates, as well as the Hegelian thesis-antithesis dialectic [1]. The acquisition and structuring of knowledge in PBL is thought to work through the cognitive mechanisms (Box 6.1) and is facilitated by, and dependent on, the interest and motivation on the part of the learner.

Box 6.1   Cognitive Mechanisms of PBL [2]

Initial analysis of the problem and activation of prior knowledge through small-group discussion.

Elaboration of prior knowledge and active processing of new information.

Restructuring of knowledge, construction of a semantic network.

Social knowledge construction.

Learning in context.

Stimulation of curiosity related to the presentation of a relevant real-life problem.

Though we focus on PBL as a problem solving model of teaching, it needs to be noted that the core principle of PBL includes using specific problems to gain *further* knowledge and understanding.

6.3   Problem-Based Learning: The Evidence Base in Undergraduate Training

6.3.1   Undergraduate Medicine

PBL in undergraduate medical education has received favourable systematic reviews, reporting better outcomes on clinical performance, student satisfaction and retention of knowledge in the longer term. Newble and Clarke [3] report that PBL improves retention and recall of important units of information, that it fosters life-long self-directed learning skills and encourages and strengthens hypothetico-deductive reasoning.

Student attitudes, class attendance and mood were better amongst students belonging to a PBL group than amongst those in traditional teaching institutions. PBL students deploy more productive and constructivist approaches to learning and – most importantly – their diagnostic skills are significantly enhanced [4]. They performed significantly better on the psychiatric component of examinations than a conventional 'class' [5].

A systematic review by Vernon and Blake [6] also reported the superiority of PBL over traditional methods of teaching on student attitudes and clinical performance.

Koh *et al.* [7] showed that PBL was associated with:

- stronger teamwork skills,

- a better appreciation of social and emotional aspects of health care,

- a better appreciation of legal and ethical aspects of health care,

- more appropriate attitudes towards personal health and well-being in the social dimension,

- continuity of care in the technical dimension,

- coping with uncertainty,

- better use of information resources,

- better understanding of evidence-based medicine in the cognitive dimension.

Interestingly, however, the students rated themselves less high on the possession of medical knowledge (in the 'knowledge dimension') than did the graduates in a control group.

6.3.2   Undergraduate Psychiatry

Singh *et al.* [8] found PBL to be effective in changing students' attitudes to psychiatry in general. The point has been made that with a constant and rapid expansion of information, the traditional 'coverage' model threatens to become more and more inefficient and impractical and the sheer size of the 'body of knowledge' needing to be absorbed necessitates an increasing emphasis on collective work, sharing of knowledge and communicating and refining analytic thought and decision making processes. McParland *et al.* [9] compared the effectiveness of problem-based learning in undergraduate psychiatry with traditional teaching methods. They reported that, based on exam performance, PBL proved to be superior, indicating that knowledge was at a higher level compared with traditional methods. Surprisingly, the improvement was not explained by students using more effective learning styles or having more favourable attitudes towards psychiatry. Van Diest *et al.* [10] reported different patterns of knowledge growth in psychiatry and behavioural sciences. PBL students knew more about behavioural sciences than about psychiatry when they entered medical school, but this difference vanished in the final two years of training.

Controversy often surrounds PBL, as it is thought to result in a weaker factual knowledge base, especially in the basic medical sciences. Norman and Schmidt [11] found support for this presumption that PBL is inferior to the traditional method in knowledge retention, overall knowledge and competence. However, Dochy *et al.* [12] failed to find robust evidence that PBL has negative effects on knowledge possession. This often-encountered worry about 'missed material' [13] may arise from the perception that knowledge acquisition in PBL is basically an *ad hoc* learning process. This carries less intrinsic reassurance than the more organized format in which, for instance, traditional lectures deliver the learning material.

Smits *et al.* [14] reported lack of consistent evidence that PBL in continuing medical education was superior to other educational strategies in increasing doctors' knowledge and performance.

Doubts have been cast over the reliability and generalizability of the outcomes of these studies. Smits *et al.* [15] investigated PBL in postgraduate medical education and, although the study showed students being dissatisfied with the method, PBL did show a long term trend towards improving clinical performance compared to lecture-based training. There was, however, no difference between the groups on acquisition of knowledge. Having said this, the comparison group, which mainly used lecture-based teaching, also engaged in interactive sessions, thus in effect creating a mixed model as far as educational methodology is concerned. This may explain the absence of a significant difference between both groups. Additionally, the authors mention that 'compensatory measures' used by the students, involving 'learning outside' the methods under study, may have contributed to the lack of significant differences in outcomes.

With regards to the fact that various studies appear to elicit conflicting results, Schmidt [16] argued that one of the significant confounding factors in assessing the success of the PBL method might be that the investigative process ends up detecting differences in curriculum, rather than differences in methods of teaching. It is therefore important in further studies that due consideration is given to this aspect at the stage of methodological design.

6.4 Advantages and Disadvantages

In '*Tomorrow's Doctors*', the United Kingdom General Medical Council was critical of the traditional model of didactic teaching, stating that it could be detrimental to the attitude of self-directed and life-long learning, as expected from a doctor [17] (see also Chapter 4). It also raised concern about the lack of logical interpretation of information, as gathered in didactic teaching, which could have an additional negative impact on the application of knowledge in clinical practice. PBL claims to address these concerns: being based on the principles of adult learning theory, it encourages the students to take an active role in the decisions, which not only affect their own learning but – more importantly – their clinical application of the acquired knowledge.

PBL facilitates the development of flexible, cognitive strategies that help analyse ill-structured problems to provide meaningful solutions. This is particularly pertinent to psychiatry, where diagnostic protocols tend to be less well defined and structured than in other medical disciplines. Additionally, the psychiatric approach of constructing a meaningful narrative, particular to an individual patient, is likely to be more cohesive if the practitioner is well versed in such cognitive strategies. It is therefore argued that PBL is uniquely well suited to psychiatric training.

Discomfort seems regularly to arise during the transition from traditional learning to PBL: trainees tend to raise a wide variety of questions about its applicability, insecurity of what is required of them and the above mentioned doubts about the exhaustiveness of the coverage of the curriculum. Another criticism pertains to the perceived increase in cognitive load: particularly early on in the learning process novice learners may find it difficult to process a large amount of information in a short amount of time. Traditional knowledge transfer allows for 'deferment' of absorbing and processing information, whereas the collaborative activity in PBL does so to a far lesser degree.

The other potential disadvantages are the requirement of sufficient numbers of suitably trained facilitators, the availability of general resources, such as rooms and supporting educational equipment, lack of access to a particularly inspirational teacher and, as mentioned above, information overload and redundancy [18, 19] (Box 6.2).

Box 6.2   Advantages and Disadvantages of PBL

Advantages	Disadvantages
Fosters active and life-long learning	Tutors are restricted from 'passing on' their wisdom
Development of generic skills and attitudes such as collaborative practice	Requires a different cadre of tutors or facilitators who have to be trained
Encourages active participation in a group activity	Requires access to and identification of varied sources of information
Inculcates deep learning with assimilation of knowledge and application in clinical practice	Difficulty in setting boundaries whilst engaging in self-study
Builds a constructivist approach where trainees seek actively to fill the gaps in their existing knowledge	Group dynamics can influence individual outcomes

–Adapted from Diana Wood [19]

6.5   PBL in Undergraduate Psychiatry: An Example from Maastricht University (The Netherlands)

All medical schools in The Netherlands, including the Maastricht medical school, use the Dutch Blueprint of Objectives as a starting point for their educational programmes [20, 21]. Within the framework of this national document, PBL procedures were applied to cover coherent themes in fixed length blocks during the first four years of the six-year Maastricht medical curriculum. In addition to the theoretical knowledge covered in these blocks, students were trained, using 'simulation' patients, in a variety of skills in medicine (SIM), such as physical examination, communication, professional behaviour and clinical reasoning. Exposure to actual patients was confined to fixed length rotations in traditional major clinical specialities, such as psychiatry, during the last two years of that curriculum. The abrupt change from the first four pre-clinical to the final two clinical years was quite problematic for the students and urged the Maastricht medical school to start, in 2001, a PBL curriculum in which a more gradual transition from the pre-clinical to the clinical environment was provided [22]. In this 2001 curriculum, modular blocks and a variety of SIM trainings are still provided in the first two years. Exposure to actual patients, however, is no longer confined to clinical rotations in the last two years, but starts in the third year by organizing four clusters of ten weeks each. The department of Psychiatry and Neuropsychology was offered the opportunity to organize the cluster 'psychomedical problems', which is outlined in more detail in the next section. After this third year, which comprises not only the psychomedical cluster but also the clusters 'abdomen', 'circulation' and 'locomotion', students still cycle through traditional clinical rotations in years 4 and 5 and take up the role of 'semi-physician', within legal boundaries, in a clinical department of their choice for 18 consecutive weeks in the final year. An additional period of 18 weeks in this final year is devoted to participation in a scientific project.

6.5.1 The Cluster 'Psychomedical Problems'

In comparison with educational programmes that focus on specialist trainees, undergraduate medical student programmes have the task of meeting the needs of large numbers of students, the vast majority of whom do not plan careers in psychiatry [23]. In Maastricht, the needs of about 400 students each year had to be met, so it was decided to run the psychomedical cluster, like the other clusters, four times a year to solve capacity problems and accommodate about 100 students in each of the four runs. Furthermore, to provide a gradual transition from the pre-clinical to the clinical environment, the cluster was guided by a study of Walters *et al.* in which they reported that patients with common mental disorders responded well to participation in undergraduate psychiatry teaching [24]. Most of their patients valued the time they shared with undergraduate students to talk and reflect, and some even gained a stronger, more balanced doctor–patient relationship.

6.5.2 Educational Out-Patient Sessions

These findings supported the intention to implement a series of so-called 'educational out-patient sessions' as the first major element of the psychomedical cluster. Educational out-patient sessions (EOS) are also organized in the academic hospital of Maastricht for three other clusters. Capacity problems, however, urged us to organize our EOS not only in the Maastricht academic setting but also in other settings spread across the southern part of The Netherlands. These settings not only differ in institution (general hospitals, psychiatric hospitals, ambulatory health care centres), but also in length of patients stay, patients' psychopathological characteristics and preferred modes of psychiatric treatment, thus providing a rich array of patients who are potentially willing to participate. Those willing to participate are given an initial training of the 'ins and outs' of the EOS and a refresher session once a year.

The format of the EOS is the same in every centre. As an example, an EOS may start at 9:00 a.m. with one facilitator, six students and two patients. After an introduction of about 30 minutes, in which the facilitator reflects on the current learning objectives of the students, two groups of three students are formed. Each group is coupled to a patient for unsupervised interviewing, that is the facilitator is not present. In each group, one student conducts a 45 minutes interview with the patient; the remaining two students take notes for feedback.

Reflection and feedback is provided to these two 'active' students by the facilitator and the remaining students after the interview. During the interviews by the first two groups, the facilitator restarts the process with the second group of six students. Using this 'tile construction' approach, the EOS ends at about 12:00 a.m., during which two students have actively conducted an interview with the first patient and two other students have actively conducted an interview with the second patient, the remaining eight students will have their opportunity in later sessions.

For virtually all students in the curriculum the EOS is the first occasion of a face-to-face contact with a patient with a mental disorder. In order for an EOS not to be casual but effective, students are instructed to familiarize themselves with the various elements of the mental state examination (MSE) in SIM trainings prior to the EOS [25]. It is our contention that a thorough knowledge of the MSE is not only a prerequisite for those students who plan careers in psychiatry, but for all medical students, irrespective of their future career plans. To optimize SIM training in MSE, not only are simulation patients used but a recently developed interactive DVD is also used showing the interview techniques of a number of senior psychiatrists from the department with patients suffering from, for instance, a pain disorder or an obsessive-compulsive disorder [26].

6.5.3   Psychiatry and Neuroscience

In a recent study it was reported that, 'the amount of neuroscience in (psychiatry) residency curricula has increased significantly over the past five years, and further increases are expected in each specific neuroscience content area examined. While most training directors agreed neuroscience training is important for residents, even those becoming primarily psychother-apists, relevance to future (but not current) practice was consistently cited as a motivating factor' [27]. A similar type of reasoning holds for the undergraduate psychomedical cluster. It is the contention that the rapid advances in neuroscience to unravel the biological basis of mental disorders are of sufficient promise for future doctors to familiarize the medical students with basic concepts in a number of neuroscience content areas. This led to the implementation of a series of basic lectures in neuroscience, including a neuroanatomy practicum as the second major element of the psychomedical cluster. Although the third year students find it difficult to appreciate how these brain/behaviour relationships come into play when interviewing and assessing a patient in the EOS, they do acknowledge that an understanding of the complex behaviours of patients with psychiatric disorders must be based on a thorough knowledge of cerebral physiology, biochemistry and neuroanatomy, as well as any relevant contextual and psychological factors.

6.5.4   Clinical Rotations

In the Maastricht 2001 curriculum the clinical rotations are still classically organized. During year 5 of the curriculum, students participate in the psychiatric rotation for six weeks. The first week is used to refresh the MSE and organize seminars on cognitive, affective and psychotic disorders. The last week is devoted to a clinical bedside test, a short scientific debate on a given topic and a computer-based knowledge test. During weeks 2–4 of this six-week period, students are present at one of the various participating clinical wards or participate in an out-patient clinic. Implementation of PBL procedures in these clinical situations, however, remains problematic. Firstly, clinicians find it difficult to allow students to conduct initial interviews with patients; in addition, clinicians are trained to 'think' in terms of diagnoses and treatment modalities, and are too busy to indicate and discuss learning objectives (including basic knowledge) with students after having met a patient. Secondly, students at this stage of their training are eager to gather various diagnoses and therapeutic possibilities. In other words, the reflective phase, a prerequisite in PBL, is difficult to achieve in daily practice. This is a widely acknowledged problem in all clinical rotations.

In order to foster a more intense use of PBL procedures by students during this phase of their training, Maastricht University is currently reorganizing the entire clinical rotation cycle. The duration of each rotation will be extended to six continuous weeks. In addition, students will be instructed to focus on several predefined problems. For the psychiatric rotation these predefined problems include cognitive problems like memory loss, attention and concentration deficits, anxiety, euphoria/dysphoria, depression, derealisation, addictive behaviour, compulsive behaviour, obsessive thoughts, and so on. For each patient, the student has to indicate whether the patient suffered from one or more of these predefined problems and is urged to seek explanations of these problems from a biological, psychological and/or contextual framework. In the same vein, students are urged to study therapeutic rationales from the biological, psychological and contextual framework. Finally, students reflect on learning objectives by answering the question 'what did I learn?'. It is thought that this approach is of sufficient promise to force PBL procedures into the clinical rotation phase for the student and the clinician alike, and thus to allow a format to discuss patients within the context of predefined problems, a format in which basic knowledge and therapeutic solutions are not only integrated but also help to define new learning objectives. The method described mimics the approach during the first three years of the curriculum and will hopefully give rise to PBL as the learning method in an ongoing study process.

6.6   The Use of PBL in Postgraduate Psychiatric Training

PBL takes away the focus from memorization and encourages trainees to formulate narratives and solve complex and intertwined problems. Given the holistic approach in psychiatry, this constructivist character is particularly suitable: psychiatric clinical practice almost invariably derives its formulations from a biopsychosocial understanding of the patients' problems. Thus, clinical management is not restricted to just a sound grounding in biological therapeutic interventions, but extends in interpreting the social complications arising from a wide variety of psychiatric phenomena as well as from therapeutic interventions. Managing such complex issues is unlikely to be aided by applying memorized information only: factual medical knowledge will constantly require adaptation and reinterpretation within the framework of the individual patient's idiosyncrasies. PBL can be seen as a surrogate of such clinical experience and naturally mimics such complex cognitive processes.

This becomes all the more pertinent as the mature psychiatrist, in a world of ever changing service provision, is increasingly required to provide clinical leadership to the multidisciplinary team, in a role similar to that of a PBL facilitator to the PBL group. Thus, apart from gaining knowledge from the content of the learning process, PBL in itself fosters a collaborative model, which is an essential element of multidisciplinary clinical practice and is – compared to core training – a major focus of postgraduate psychiatric training.

PBL leads not only to the mere acquisition of knowledge, but further interprets and dissects that knowledge through the discussions in the PBL group. This discursive nature is particularly suited to psychiatry, as often its scientific basis is not all that 'cut and dry', but involves shades of grey, which – in order to be made explicit – need discussion and exploration. A trainee undergoing the rituals of professional development should be exposed to different and diverging views, gathered by a number of coworkers from various sources. It is not possible to achieve this through a traditional lecture format, which comes with its own potential 'red herring': the personal and possibly slanted view of the lecturer. Thus, the method of PBL reflects a very important facet of clinical practice in psychiatry, which is to facilitate an in-depth analysis and interpretation of variable data and charting a balanced, logical and agreed path toward addressing a specific clinical scenario.

6.6.1 The Role of the Facilitator

In a postgraduate setting, the role of the facilitator becomes potentially more complex than in undergraduate training. The facilitator has to be competent not only in managing group dynamics and ensuring a reasonable coverage of the curriculum: in postgraduate training, the training runs parallel to clinical work. Unlike undergraduates, who are on the whole 'new' to medicine, psychiatric trainees will have been exposed to different specialities as part of their foundation training (in the United Kingdom; elsewhere there are likely to be other forms of postgraduate but 'pre-registration' training) and in their working life are practising physicians. Thus, they will have a more extensive and pragmatic background knowledge of the practice of medicine. They are likely, therefore, to have formed more robust opinions on all sorts of matters. Therefore, the facilitator has to be aware not only of the clinical and academic strengths and weaknesses of the trainees, but also of the actual personalities and the opinions they may hold. Such factors may have a strong impact on the successful participation of individuals in a group activity. It should be noted that facilitators may themselves benefit in their own clinical practice from their tutoring: if a facilitator can run an at times difficult PBL group successfully, then such is an excellent preparation to manage mental health teams of any description.

The facilitator has to ensure that group members have an equal opportunity to contribute to the group's work. Additionally, the facilitator should keep track of the stage of training: for instance, in the United Kingdom, trainees rotate every six or twelve months (depending on their level of training) into subspeciality placements. The facilitator needs to ensure that those trainees, who lack exposure in a particular clinical setting, are not disadvantaged by other trainees, who might have had six months of training in that particular subspeciality. Although the facilitator does not have to have, and indeed cannot have, extensive knowledge across all psychiatric subspecialities, it is important to have facilitators who have a reasonable working knowledge in a subspeciality relevant to the case scenario being studied. This is not meant to extend the role of a facilitator to be a bottomless pit of 'answers', but it does help to ensure the right focus of attention is maintained in complex areas, such as mental health law. Of course, it also inspires a vital confidence amongst trainees that they are being guided by an expert.

6.6.2   Coverage of the Curriculum or Syllabus

It has appeared necessary in postgraduate usage of the PBL method to extend the format by not just using clinical scenarios: in order to ensure an adequate and appropriate coverage of the curriculum it may be useful at times to use a 'debating' format on particular issues, the formative activity then consisting of trainees being able to formulate their positions or views, to debate these (another example of the application of the 'Socratic' method) and to subject their views to competing and diverging opinions. This can be very useful, particularly in subspeciality training, where complex but important areas of the relevant curriculum may not lend themselves easily to a case-based exploration along the lines of the 'traditional' PBL model. Even in this extended format of PBL, the onus of acquiring information remains with the trainee, with the facilitator ensuring the quality of the process.

6.6.3   The Role of Internal and External Evaluation

Evaluation in general is an important and intricate part of the PBL process: it should include not only the necessary appraisal of an individual trainee's functioning and progress, but should be used to identify the strengths and weaknesses of the various components of the PBL process. Although evaluation has to be an intricate and internal activity of the group, at appropriate intervals it needs to be validated by an external authority.

Internal evaluation should focus on process and content, as well as the participation and work ethic of the group members and their professional attitudes. Evaluation of the process should include the suitability of the case scenarios or themes, how they map onto the curriculum, how they contribute to achieving clinical competencies and how they assist the trainees in progressing through any professional examinations. Further evaluation of the process should include dissecting the methods of discussion, the use of learning aides, the effective dispersion of the information gathered through 'homework' and – last but not least – the robustness of the output. Evaluation of content is, of course, very important: it should be of the highest standard and such evaluation should ensure that the information being used is of reliable quality and from reputable sources. The trainees should also be given regular opportunities to provide feedback with regards to the functioning of the facilitator. Such exercises should be based on the important philosophy of teamwork and be conducted with due professionalism: the aim is to achieve a sensitive, but formative process, which facilitates the professional growth of both trainees and tutors.

External evaluation may consist of observations of the group's functioning by a PBL-trained observer, who should provide feedback primarily on the process and the observed participation of the group members. The evaluation reports should be available to tutors, course directors, educational supervisors and clinical supervisors to enable them to assess the impact of the group on the clinical and academic aspects of the training provided and the performance of the trainees. The educational supervisors should discuss any feedback with their trainees, relate the content to the overall performance of the trainee and provide professional guidance to them.

6.6.4   PBL in Postgraduate Psychiatry: An Example from Norfolk (United Kingdom)

PBL was introduced to the psychiatric trainees of the Norfolk Psychiatric Training Scheme in September 2007, replacing the traditional lecture-based training course, which prepared the trainees particularly for the examinations of the UK Royal College of Psychiatrists. There are usually two or three PBL groups, depending on how many trainees are preparing for which component of the examination (to gain membership of the British Royal College a trainee has to pass three written papers and one final viva examination of clinical competencies). Senior trainees have been trained as PBL tutors at the medical school of the University of East Anglia (this medical school uses PBL throughout the delivery of its curriculum); they can then function as facilitators, provided they have previously gained membership of the Royal College. The groups meet for one half-day a week. The facilitator presents a case to the group (Box 6.3) and a scribe is chosen. The scribe records the 'brainstorming' discussion and the homework is allocated democratically. Members e-mail their homework to each other, the facilitator and the college tutor, before the meeting the following week. For the following three weeks, the group enters into the discussion phase, exploring and integrating a wide knowledge base through their presentations. The case scenario ends with the group taking a test of multiple-choice questions (MCQ) and extended-matching items (EMI), set by the facilitator to evaluate their learning. When appropriate the group may decide to invite an 'expert' to provide further insight into more complex topics (for instance, a psychotherapist may attend to discuss psychological defence mechanisms), which is a deviation from the 'classical' PBL method and deemed to be of particular use when highly specialist aspects of postgraduate training are being dealt with.

Box 6.3   Example of a PBL Case Scenario

Dear Colleague

I would be very grateful to you if you could assess this 29-year-old married mother of two, who has recently moved in to our area. She told me that she has been tormented by thoughts about contamination and dirt, ever since her second son was born. This has apparently progressed to the extent that she will now not touch door handles or supermarket food packaging. Her husband is at his wits end because of her behaviour. She is obviously depressed and told me that she was on the waiting list for a talking therapy. She would not want to consider medications. Interestingly, her brother, who accompanied her to the surgery, suffers from facial tics, but I am unclear whether or not this may be relevant. Apart from a bout of meningo-encephalitis in the distant past, there is no significant past medical or psychiatric history.

Please do not hesitate to contact me for further information.

With regards

GP

Although originally designed to replace a preparatory course for the professional examinations, PBL has proved in Norfolk to provide an excellent opportunity for trainees to prepare for workplace-based assessments, which now form a central part in the United Kingdom of the formative and summative appraisal processes all specialist trainees are subjected to (for a further discussion of assessment see Chapter 17). To give an example: one of the workplace-based assessments is the so-called 'Case-Based Discussion' (CBD). It is designed to assess clinical judgement, decision making and the application of medical knowledge in relation to patient care in cases for which the trainee has been directly responsible. The method is particularly designed to test higher order thinking and synthesis, as it allows assessors to explore deeper understanding of how trainees compile, prioritize and apply knowledge. CBD is not focused on the trainees' ability to make a diagnosis nor is it a viva-style assessment: the process is a structured, in-depth discussion between the trainee and clinical supervisor about how a clinical case was managed by the trainee, what occurred, which considerations the trainee took into account and what reasoning underpinned any actions taken or considered. By using clinical cases that offer a challenge to the trainee, rather than routine cases, the trainee is able to explain the complexities involved and the reasoning behind choices they made. It also enables the discussion of the ethical and legal framework of practice. It uses patient records as the basis for dialogue, for systematic assessment and structured feedback. As the actual record is the focus for the discussion, the assessor can also evaluate the quality of record keeping.

It can easily be seen that the PBL method contains very similar aspects, and thus is uniquely placed to prepare trainees for such assessments.

6.6.5 Internal and External Evaluation

In Norfolk, the evaluation process is structured using a PBL-Assessment Scale (Pilot Version, see Appendix 6.A; assessment forms for peers are semantically adapted). In this process, each trainee completes a self-assessment and assessments on three randomly selected peers, rating performance against the standards as expected for the end of their stage of training (CT1, 2 and 3 represent first, second and third year of core training). Feedback is then provided to the trainee, with particular attention to areas of development and the concordance between the trainee's perception of their own performance and how their peers felt they performed. This is passed on to the educational supervisor and clinical tutor. The cumulative scores from the individual tests provide an instant overview of the trainee's functioning, in comparison with the general performance profile of the group.

The PBL facilitators are assessed and appraised internally by the feedback provided by the group members and externally by the use of a particular workplace-based assessment the Royal College of Psychiatrists has introduced, particularly to assess meta-competencies in senior trainees (i.e. those who already have Royal College membership status). The facilitators receive supervision from the clinical tutor and the progress of the PBL group is reported regularly to the Postgraduate Medical Education meeting.

The Norfolk experience, with PBL replacing the old style didactic lectures, has certainly been favourable: trainees report a higher satisfaction with the course, pass rates of the various Royal College examinations are significantly higher than the national average and trainees welcome taking responsibility for their postgraduate education.

6.7 Problem-Based Learning in Psychiatric Education: The Future

Psychiatry continues to evolve rapidly and postgraduate education has to keep pace with it if it is to train the next generation of psychiatrists to the highest possible standards. The drive in the United Kingdom from the General Medical Council and from the Royal College of Psychiatrists towards self-directed, life-long learning and continuous professional development necessitates educational approaches be adapted: they need to incorporate the essential elements of such a professional and cultural development. PBL as a method and as a philosophy of postgraduate education is uniquely placed to facilitate the future development of psychiatric training in line with those demands.

That does, of course, imply that the application of the method in postgraduate medical education is in need of constant revision and adaptation. For instance, though it is a convention mainly to use real-life clinical problems, in future PBL groups may benefit greatly from the inclusion of more general management scenarios and public health related issues. This follows naturally from the fact that clinicians are increasingly required to develop strategic, managerial and meta-level skills, which do not necessarily form part of the core clinical competencies.

Appendix 6.1

PILOT PBL SELF ASSESSMENT FORM

NAME TRAINEE _____

PBL Theme _____

Topic Presented _____

Mode of Presentation _____

Source/s of Presentation _____

Please rate the following aspects of your performance against standards for end of ST1/2/3: (u/c + unable to comment)

Below standard		Meets standard				Above standard		
	1	2	3	4	5	6	u/c
1. Preparation for sessions	☐	☐	☐	☐	☐	☐	☐
2. Responsibility for own learning	☐	☐	☐	☐	☐	☐	☐
3. Participation in group learning	☐	☐	☐	☐	☐	☐	☐
4. Effective group skills and awareness	☐	☐	☐	☐	☐	☐	☐
5. Discussion with pears	☐	☐	☐	☐	☐	☐	☐
6. Professional behaviour	☐	☐	☐	☐	☐	☐	☐
7. Directs learning agenda and self-awareness	☐	☐	☐	☐	☐	☐	☐
8. Effective teaching skills	☐	☐	☐	☐	☐	☐	☐

How would you rate your performance at this stage of training compared to your peers?

Below expectations   satisfactory better than expected u/c

Anything Particularly Good?	Any Particular Concern?
Self-suggestions for improvement	

Trainee's Signature _____

Date

References

1. Rhem, J. (1998) Problem-Based Learning: An Introduction. *The National Teaching & Learning Forum*, **8** (1). www.ntlf.com/html/pi/9812/toc.htm (accessed 7 March 2010).
2. Schmidt, H.G. (1993) Foundations of problem-based learning: some explanatory notes. *Medical Education*, **27**, 422–432
3. Newble, D.I. and Clarke, R.M. (1986) The approaches to learning in a traditional and in an innovative problem-based medical school. *Medical Education*, **20**, 267–273.
4. Schmidt, H.G., Machiels-Baonagaerts, M., Hermans, H.H. *et al.* (1996) The development of diagnostic competence: comparison of problem-based, an integrated, and a conventional medical curriculum. *Academic Medicine*, **71**, 658–664.
5. Kaufman, D.M. and Mann, K.V. (1998) Comparing achievement of the Medical Council of Canada Qualifying Examination Part 1 of students in conventional and problem-based learning curricula. *Academic Medicine*, **73**, 1211–1213
6. Vernon, D.T.A. and Blake, R.L. (1993) Does problem-based learning work? A meta-analysis of evaluative research. *Academic Medicine*, **68**, 551–563.
7. Koh, G., Khoo, H., Wong, M. and Koh, D. (2008) The effects of problem-based learning during medical school on physician competency: a systematic review. Canadian Association Medical Journal, **178**, 34–41.
8. Singh, S.P., Baxter, H., Standen, P., *et al.* (1996) Changing the attitudes of 'tomorrow's doctors' towards mental illness and psychiatry: a comparison of two teaching methods. *Medical Education* **32**, 115-120
9. McParland, M., Noble, L.M. and Livingstone, G. (2004) The effectiveness of problem-based learning compared to traditional teaching in undergraduate psychiatry. *Medical Education*, **38**, 859-867.
10. Van Diest, R., Van Dalen, J., Bak, M., *et al.* (2004) Growth of knowledge in psychiatry and behavioural sciences in a problem-based learning curriculum. *Medical Education*, **38**, 1295–1301.
11. Norman, G.R. and Schmidt, H.G. (1992) The psychological basis of problem-based learning: a review of evidence. *Academic Medicine*, **67**, 557–565.
12. Dochy, F., Segers, M., Van Den Bossche, P., *et al.* (2003) Effects of PBL: a meta-analysis. *Learning and Instruction*, **13**, 533–568.
13. Dolmans, D.G., Gijselaers, W.H., Schmidt, H.G., *et al.* (1993) Problem effectiveness in a course using problem-based learning. *Academic Medicine*, **69**, 207–213.
14. Smits, P.B.A., Verbeek, J.H.A.M. and de Buisonje, C.D. (2002) Learning in practice. Problem based learning in continuing medical education: a review of controlled evaluation studies. *BMJ*, **324**, 153–156.
15. Smits, P.B.A., de Buisonje, C.D., Verbeek, J.H.A.M., *et al.* (2003) Problem-based learning versus lecture-based learning in postgraduate medical education. *Scandinavian Journal of Environmental Health*, **29**, 280–287.
16. Schmidt, H.G. (1998) Problem-based learning: does it prepare medical students to become better doctors? *MJA*, **168**, 429–430
17. General Medical Council (1993) Tomorrow's Doctors; Recommendations on Undergraduate Medical Education, General Medical Council, London.
18. Guthrie, E. and O'Neill, P. (1999) Self-directed, problem-based learning for undergraduate psychiatry. *Advances in Psychiatric Treatment*, **5**, 382–389.
19. Wood, D.F. (2003) ABC of learning and teaching in medicine: problem-based learning. *BMJ*, **326**, 328–330.

20. Metz, J., Verbeek-Weel, A. and Huisjes, H. (2001). Blueprint. Training of Doctors in the Netherlands: Adjusted Objectives of Undergraduate Medical Education, University Publication Office, Nijmegen.

21. Ten Cate, O. (2007) Medical education in the Netherlands. *Medical Teacher*, **29**, 752–757.

22. Ten Cate, O. and Smal, J. (2002) The transformation of medical education - from a discipline-oriented to a problem-oriented approach, in *Health and Health Care in the Netherlands* (eds E. van Rooij, L. Droyan Kodner, T. Rijsemus and G. Schrijvers), Elsevier Gezondheidszorg, Maarssen.

23. Cutler, L. (2006) Psychiatric Education for Medical Students: Challenges and Solutions. *Academic Psychiatry*, **30**, 95–97.

24. Walters, K., Buszewicz, M., Russell, J. and Humphrey, Ch. (2003) Teaching as therapy: cross sectional and qualitative evaluation of patients' experiences of undergraduate psychiatry teaching in the community. *BMJ*, **326**, 740.

25. Hengeveld, H. (2005) Het psychiatrisch onderzoek, in *Leerboek Psychiatrie* (eds H. Hengeveld and A.J.L.M. van Balkom), De Tijdstroom, Utrecht.

26. Bak, M. (2010) Het psychiatrisch onderzoek – het status mentalis onderzoek, in *Skills in Medicine* (eds M. Bak, R. van Diest and M. de Ruijter), Mediview, Maastricht.

27. Roffman, J., Simon, A., Prasad, K. *et al.* (2006) Neuroscience in psychiatry training: how much do residents need to know? *Am J Psychiatry*, **163**, 919–926.

7

Psychiatric Residency Curriculum: Development and Evaluation

Amanda B. Mackey and Allan Tasman

Department of Psychiatry and Behavioural Sciences, University of Louisville School of Medicine, Louisville, KY, USA

7.1   Introduction

The field of psychiatry is continually evolving. To assure the development of the field, educating new generations of psychiatrists is essential. How do we accomplish such a formidable task? As cited in the text *Psychiatric Education*, Yager was astute in stating that the role of a psychiatric training director, someone charged with this duty, is 'forged and reaffirmed on a daily basis through the development and monitoring of the curriculum' [1].

For the purposes of this chapter, the focus is on the residency training curriculum. Curriculum is a complex concept. Stemming from the Latin for race–course, curriculum literally refers to the course that individuals undergo during their development. Educating psychiatrists requires navigating such a developmental course. As early as 1918, in one of the first texts on curriculum as a means of education, Franklin Bobbit's preface recognized the intricacy of such a process, reading:

> Simple conditions have been growing complex. Small institutions have been growing large. Increased specialization has been multiplying human interdependencies and the consequent need of coordinating effort. As the world presses eagerly forward towards the accomplishment of new things, education also must advance no less swiftly. It must provide the intelligence and the aspirations necessary for the advance; and for stability and consistency in holding the gains. Education must take a pace set, not by itself, but its social progress [2].

Teaching Psychiatry: Putting Theory into Practice   Edited by Linda Gask, Bulent Coskun and David Baron
© 2011 John Wiley & Sons, Ltd

While Bobbit was referring in general terms to the field of education, it could be asserted that a psychiatric curriculum exemplifies such a complex course. Through this chapter, a means of approaching this mission in a logical fashion is mapped. By providing an overview of the historical context, an understanding of the foundation on which psychiatric education lies today is given. The essential elements that compose a psychiatric curriculum from a global perspective are addressed, while acknowledging the challenges that are innate to such a broad endeavour. Finally, evaluating a curriculum as a means of assuring continual growth and development is discussed.

7.2 Historical Context

Psychiatric education has been evolving since initial lectures were documented as taking place beginning in the early part of the nineteenth century [3]. Initially, psychiatric training was primarily in the form of a clinical apprenticeship with minimal oversight or clearly stated objectives. As medical education changed, organizations developed which were charged with oversight of residency training. These formal organizations have taken different forms throughout the world. In the United States, the Accreditation Council on Graduate Medical Education (ACGME) oversees psychiatric residency education while the American Board of Psychiatry and Neurology (ABPN) determines speciality board certification upon the completion of training. In the United Kingdom, the Royal College of Psychiatrist provides both functions. The Royal College of Physicians and Surgeons of Canada is the Canadian equivalent [4]. In each of these instances, a specific organization which was responsible for oversight of psychiatric education within their given nation was formed.

Changes in transport, technology and politics have altered the geographical constraints previously present. An example of this exists with the formation of the European Union of Medical Specialities (UEMS) and its European Board of Psychiatry during the twentieth century. With the establishment of the World Psychiatric Association in the 1950s, addressing psychiatric education has become a global focus, with a shift away from addressing psychiatric education and training in a country-by-country fashion.

Simultaneously, psychiatric education has become more structured over time. It is not surprising that this structure began in regions of the world with greater resources and formal organizations in place to institute such structure. This form of organization and oversight of psychiatric education, however, is spreading to regions that previously had not experienced such change. Thus, psychiatric education is evolving to a more formalised process by which clear expectations are set as to what comprises a core psychiatric curriculum. In addition, more oversight is being implemented to oversee its implementation.

7.3 Psychiatric Curriculum's Function

Constructing a psychiatric curriculum begins with clearly outlining the clinical role of the speciality. This in itself presents challenges, as psychiatrists across the globe are faced with varied responsibilities, influenced in part by cultural considerations within the field. For initial purposes, common elements are looked at. The Psychiatric Section of the European Union of Medical Specialities created a position paper outlining the clinical profile of a

Table 7.1 Core competencies.

Locale	Organizational Entity	Competencies
Canada	Royal College of Physicians and Surgeons	Medical Expert Scholar Communicator Health advocate Manager Collaborator Professional
Europe	European Union of Medical Specialities – Psychiatric Section	Psychiatric Expert / clinical decision maker Scholar Communicator Health advocate Manager Collaborator Professional
United States	American College of Graduate Medical Education	Patient care Medical knowledge Practice-based learning and improvement Interpersonal and communication skills Professionalism Systems-based practice

psychiatrist, in which they outline psychiatry as an 'integration of biological, psychological and social aspects rooted in the scientific, intellectual and humanistic traditions' [5]. In conjunction, the ACGME describes psychiatry as focusing 'on the prevention, diagnosis and treatment of mental, addictive and emotional disorders' [6].

The creation of a curriculum allows for these general principles to be conveyed to trainees in such a way that they complete the course of training in order to be a clinically competent psychiatrist. As psychiatric curricula have become more structured, this aim has been taken on by specific organizations designating what constitutes the core competencies required to be a functioning psychiatrist in their own locality (Table 7.1).

In the United States, the ACGME has outlined six core competencies, consisting of (i) Patient care, (ii) Medical knowledge, (iii) Practice-based learning and improvement, (iv) Interpersonal and communication skills, (v) Professionalism and (vi) Systems-based practice. These six core competencies are held for all medical specialities, including psychiatry. Each speciality has additional guidelines which then specify the knowledge necessary for their own specialities within this framework.

In contrast, the Royal College of Physicians and Surgeons of Canada is organised around seven specific roles of the medical professional, known as CanMEDS. These seven roles include: (i) Medical expert, (ii) Scholar, (iii) Communicator, (iv) Health advocate, (v) Manager, (vi) Collaborator and (vii) Professional [4]. Following suit, the European Board of Psychiatry (a part of the UEMS Section of Psychiatry) in conjunction with the European Federation of Psychiatric Trainees (EFPT) has prepared a proposal for adopting a framework of competencies that is similar to the Canadian system. The UEMS version outlines the following roles of the psychiatrist: (i) Psychiatric expert / clinical decision maker, (ii) Communicator, (iii) Collaborator, (iv) Manager, (v) Health advocate, (vi) Scholar and (vii) Professional [7].

The adoption of required competencies by these organizations provides a theoretical framework in which one can approach formulating and monitoring a curriculum. There is not, however, a specified course which the curriculum must follow. Ideally, upon the completion of training, a psychiatrist is capable of serving as a medical expert with the clinical ability to diagnose and treat mental illnesses within given systems in a professional manner that further improves the quality of practice.

7.4   Curriculum Content (The Terrain)

Creating the curriculum involves creating a map by which trainees obtain the necessary skills (Table 7.2). An adequate curriculum not only conveys specific pieces of knowledge but is also carried out through various educational modalities. To begin, the content, or the terrain, that must be covered will be looked at.

The knowledge contained within the psychiatric curriculum continues to be extensively studied and debated as the profession evolves. Within the United States, the Residency Review Committee's Essentials for Psychiatry, under the auspices of the ACGME, outlines specific requirements in regard to knowledge. In conjunction, the American Board of Psychiatry and Neurology (ABPN), the United States credentialing body outlines specific parallel expectations. The Royal College of Psychiatrists in the United Kingdom outlines a specified curriculum using the same competency headings as CanMEDS (medical expert, scholar, communicator, health advocate, manager, collaborator and professional). Organized in a modular fashion, very specific expectations are outlined as a trainee advances [8]. While these are examples of specific national mandates, it must be recognized that they approach their expectations with their given national needs in mind.

In the late 1990s the World Psychiatric Association created a work group charged with outlining core training elements for use around the world. Published in 2002, the World Psychiatric Association Institutional Program on the Core Training Curriculum for Psychiatry provides a description of recommended topics in outline form [9]. Comprising various nations and cultures, the European Union of Medical Specialities Psychiatric Section initially

Table 7.2   Key elements when charting psychiatric curriculum development.

The terrain	Content
Transport modalities	Means by which knowledge is conveyed (clinical settings, didactics, conferences, supervision)
Map	Developmental considerations
Pace	Timing

refrained from creating such a specific listing aside from their initial competency framework, citing that 'elements are determined by national conditions' [7].

Consistent with the European Union perspective, it is recognized that the training terrain will clearly vary based on where psychiatric training is taking place. Thus, the initial phase of curriculum development or design requires that a programme must begin by looking at what, if any, governing body provides oversight to psychiatric training in their nation, or region. Then careful study of the requirements in regards to knowledge content assists in laying a foundation of what topics must be covered, as well as in designing appropriate clinical placements.

Knowledge is the terrain that comprises a curriculum. While the fundamentals within psychiatry are constant, that terrain may vary based on organizational requirements and needs within a given region. The particular knowledge and skill set needed has been debated in numerous venues. It has been wisely concluded that trainees must be exposed not only to an adequate breadth of information to enable work in a variety of practice settings at the completion of training, but also the appropriate level of depth necessary to be a clinical specialist [1]. Designating topics becomes more challenging as the field of psychiatry expands with advances in neurosciences and development of new modalities of all form of treatment. While competencies provide a theoretical framework within which to approach content, they do not concretely structure and encompass all the necessary clinical skills, or professional attitudes.

A commonality across the globe is the recognition that trainees must be able to obtain a history and conduct a physical examination, recognizing and appropriately diagnosing mental illness. In addition, trainees must have an understanding of disease process in regards to mental illness, with comprehension of what is known about aetiology, cultural factors, clinical course and appropriate treatment interventions. Treatment interventions must be understood from a biological, psychological and social framework. Specific expectations in regard to this content are often outlined by the governing body for a given region (Table 7.1).

However, the actual amount of time spent on a given topic and how this is conveyed to a trainee is rarely mandated or specifically addressed. This omission lends itself to further discussion of how much time should be spent on each topic or subspeciality area. The issue of timing, or the speed at which one covers the course of the curriculum will be addressed further later in the chapter. A plethora of model curricula have been developed outlining how to cover and approach specific topics from psychopharmacology to cultural issues, a few of which are listed in Table 7.3. Of course, if one were to ask a psychiatrist specializing in Bipolar Disorder how much time should be spent on mood disorders, they would have a strong argument that a significant amount of time should be spent on such a prevalent condition. Approaching a psychiatrist specializing in psychodynamic psychotherapy or another in cultural issues would likely produce an equally strong argument that their area of expertise requires an ample amount of curriculum time. Yet, the amount of time available in general psychiatry training is finite, generally 2–6 years. Attention must be paid, therefore, to assuring that the curriculum covers all crucial topics. Thus, we return to the importance that the appropriate national or local scope of practice is covered as well as determining national pertinence of what topics will be covered more 'deeply'. This requires recognition that the depth for a given topic will vary based on the region of world where training is taking place. For example, a locale with a high prevalence of benzodiazepine dependence may spend

Table 7.3 Examples of special topics for which model curricula have been proposed.

Topics
Chronically Mentally Ill Patients [12]
Compliance [13]
Consult–Liaison [14]
Culture [15–17]
Electroconvulsive Therapy [18]
Emergency Psychiatry [19, 20]
Medical Training [21]
Neurobiology [22]
Practice Management [23]
Sleep Disorders [24]
Substance Abuse [25]
Suicide [26]

more time focusing on this as opposed to a region of the world where benzodiazepines are not prevalent or even available.

7.5 Educational Modalities

While facts and skills lay out the terrain, the means by which such knowledge is conveyed may vary. These modalities range from less structured elements to more traditional didactic forms of teaching. Education takes place in a variety of informal and formal ways in every clinical setting. In addition, lectures, or didactics, serve as a means of conveying more concrete facts. The use of case conferences, grand rounds, journal clubs and morbidity and mortality conferences are further arenas for teaching content. As technology grows, the implementation of computer-based learning, both locally developed as well as Internet based, and alternative problem-based approaches are being implemented as well. Steeped in tradition, faculty supervision of residents' clinical work remains a fundamental means of education within the field of psychiatry, and is historically the format in which integration of knowledge, clinical skills and attitudes takes place. However, the amount and venue may vary widely based on the resources available. Relying on extensive supervision by senior faculty is a major problem in areas of the world with a paucity of psychiatrists or other mental health professionals.

Finding a balance between the various teaching modalities may be challenging. Further, while clinical settings provide 'hands on' learning in regards to patient care, without adequate on-site supervision a trainee may not gain the necessary knowledge. Unfortunately, programmes are constrained by the variety of clinical sites available locally.

Didactic teaching allows for a concrete means by which knowledge can be imparted. Without the use of such pedagogic approaches, basic information may not be transmitted. However, with advances in technology, traditional on-site lectures may be needed less as lectures are placed on-line for trainees to view at their leisure – a practice that is now taking place in some medical schools in the United States. In addition, this shift may allow for time to implement more interactive means of teaching, such as problem-based learning groups.

Group conferences offer yet another teaching modality. Morbidity and mortality conferences, where cases with undesired outcomes are reviewed, journal clubs and grand rounds all offer a means for assimilating information initially obtained through other teaching modalities. Group conferences allow the exchange of information in a more active process and call upon a higher level of integration of knowledge due to their inherent structure.

On-site faculty supervision of trainees remains a cornerstone of psychiatric education. This form of personal oversight and individual attention allows the trainee's unique talents to be acknowledged and sculpted. While assisting in clinical development, supervision remains one of the important means by which trainees are guided in the art of psychotherapy. The supervision process allows the trainee to begin to develop self-reflective skills, including awareness of the professional development process involved in becoming a psychiatrist. The importance of supervision is reflected in the fact that it is considered a strict requirement in terms of educational modalities by most governing bodies such as the ACGME.

Thus, once the content within the curriculum is established, the next logical step is to analyse by what means this information is shared. The specific requirements within a given region must again be considered. For example, in the United States, the ACGME has specific minimal requirements in regards to the amount of time spent in certain clinical settings. Other mandates may be present in terms of supervision and designated activities, including journal clubs and morbidity and mortality conferences.

Once the training requirements have been ascertained, the resources available must be considered. This may include looking at the quantity of available faculty as well as the given areas of subspeciality expertise represented. A limited number of faculty members may hinder the ability to provide numerous lectures simultaneously, while a large available faculty may offer the opportunity for smaller group teaching atmospheres. Programmes with the opportunity to use technology may choose to televise lectures via the Web, while using live teaching for more interactive endeavours. In contrast, there are regions of the world where accessing computerised literature searches may be challenging if not impossible due to the lack of available resources. Thus, an individual programme must look at the means by which the resources can be appropriately allocated to successfully impart the content, or essence, of the curriculum.

7.6   Developmental Considerations and Timing (Pacing the Map)

If trainees were polled on their first day, they would immediately want to know everything needed to be a fully trained psychiatrist [1]. Of course, obtaining this level of knowledge cannot be imparted overnight and is rather a process that occurs over time. The developmental aspects of psychiatric training present a number of unique challenges. While concrete information provides fundamental knowledge, there are abstract levels of understanding that must be taught as well. Ultimately, plotting the course by which trainees are educated typically means using various modalities of teaching simultaneously. In addition, the modalities chosen may reflect where the trainee is academically. Struggling trainees may require a more concrete and directive approach, while more intellectually attuned individuals may benefit from more self-directed means. This can be understood as a form of layering education as a means of transferring wisdom regarding the field.

When approaching the timeline by which the appropriate information is taught, one might well think of the adage, 'first things first' [1]. Spending a great deal of time discussing the psychodynamic formulation of a patient with major depression during a trainee's first day will likely not be as relevant as reviewing the criteria necessary to diagnose major depression or rule out medical causes. Obtaining an appropriate history and conducting a physical examination are more fundamental skills than learning how to perform electroconvulsive therapy. Thus, when approaching the timing by which material is covered, it makes sense to logically map basic skills first and then layering the knowledge, covering more complex and specialized information as a trainee progresses.

An example of this may be demonstrated in the Royal College of Psychiatry's Curriculum in the United Kingdom. The Royal College of Psychiatry has developed a core curriculum in which it recommends that the material be covered in 'modules' [8]. The core module covers basic essentials in clinical psychiatry, such as history taking, diagnosis and treatment. Once this module is completed, trainees then go on to complete models in speciality areas of psychiatry including: adult, forensic, learning disability, old age (geriatric), psychotherapy and child and adolescent. Finally, trainees address knowledge in modules on addiction, rehabilitation and liaison psychiatry. The premise of this approach is that trainees learn basic, necessary information needed for clinical practice that is then expanded upon as they move forward. Within the UK medical system, this process takes place over the course of six years. This is in contrast to other localities where training may last a minimum of 12 months or as much as six years. Thus, this modular approach may not be feasible or appropriate in every system, and certainly, if used, must be modified to suit the local situation.

Using the premise set forth by the Royal College of Psychiatry's modules, one can think of the knowledge required to be a psychiatrist as a hierarchy (Figure 7.1).

The foundation is the ability to develop rapport and conduct an appropriate physical and mental examination of the patient. Next, the understanding of the diagnoses within psychiatry should be covered. Building upon this, treatment modalities are addressed. Again, more concrete interventions, including pharmacology and types of brief supportive psychotherapy, are reviewed before learning how to perform other specific modalities of psychotherapy. It should be clear that as a trainee progresses through the hierarchy, their movement on to higher levels of understanding builds on the fundamental foundation they have learned.

While addressing timing in regards to how curriculum content is covered, attention must also be paid to which modality of education is employed. As mentioned previously, it is likely that multiple modalities are in place at a single time. For example, trainees may be clinically progressing through rotations while also receiving didactics on specific subjects, participating in designated case conferences and receiving individual clinical supervision.

The timing of clinical rotations, or settings, also must be addressed. Developmentally, trainees initially and ideally should be placed in more structured settings that provide more oversight and supervision early in training. As a trainee becomes more knowledgeable, it is important that the trainee progresses to less structured settings where less oversight is present. This increasing autonomy assists in professional growth as the skill set improves.

As noted earlier, regions with governing bodies such as the ACGME in the United States may have specific minimum requirements for given clinical experiences. For example, the

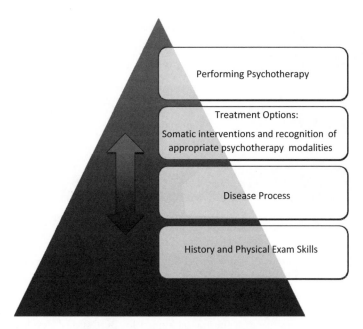

Figure 7.1 Curriculum content hierarchy.

ACGME requirements include a minimum of eight months of in-patient psychiatry and a minimum of twelve months of out-patient work. It is typical that training programmes in the United States have residents complete the majority of their in-patient training in the first year. While these are the most structured and supervised assignments, this approach often means that the most unskilled trainees are faced with the most severely ill patients. In contrast, as trainees gain experience they may be placed in clinical environments, with less oversight and more freedom regarding clinical decision making. Such rotations requiring integration of more clinical information, such as hospital consultation, take place usually later in the clinical sequence. In addition, subspeciality interests also can be pursued later in the rotation schedule once trainees have met basic clinical requirements.

As discussed, knowledge can be imparted in varying modalities simultaneously. Thus, trainees will be practising and learning in various clinical settings and with various teaching modalities throughout their training (Figure 7.2).

The timing of developmental aspects of learning must be, as discussed earlier, considered when addressing how these other means are used. For example, asking a new trainee to review a complex journal article outlining treatment outcomes in schizophrenia may be inappropriate when the trainee may lack the basic understanding of what schizophrenia is and how the disease is diagnosed and treated.

Using structured didactics early in training is usually important. Continuing with only a didactic-based curriculum later in training, however, could serve to impair learning more complex assessment and treatment processes and appropriate clinical inferences (a higher form of information processing). As acquiring the skills to make a trainee's level of knowledge grow, more advanced teaching modalities can be used. For example, advanced trainees may benefit more from analysing studies or cases and presenting within the framework of a

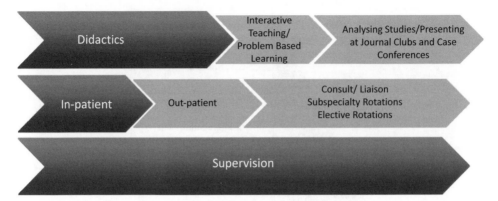

Figure 7.2   Developmental timing of educational modalities.

journal club or case conference, since the ability to intellectually process the information and present it requires a higher level of understanding.

Supervision is a key element of psychiatric training. While 'supervision' occurs throughout training, what transpires within supervision may vary. Supervision offers a unique opportunity to tailor what takes place to the trainee's need for professional development. Being cognisant of where the trainee lies along the developmental spectrum is crucial. For example, an individual at the start of training may not benefit from presenting detailed psychotherapy process notes in supervision as much as discussing the fundamentals of developing a therapeutic alliance. In fact, at the beginning some trainees may also need to discuss what it means to be a psychiatrist and require assistance in developing their identity as a medical professional. It is essential to respect the importance of such fundamental processes in the development of a psychiatrist, so trainees will be well prepared to move onto more advanced levels of supervision in which their talents in psychotherapy can be developed.

The fact that some trainees will not be able to advance as far as others in sophisticated clinical skills must also be noted. In some cases, problems in developing appropriate skills may require remediation. This is where appropriate evaluation of the trainee and of the curriculum comes in to play, a topic that will be addressed later. The development of the 'core competencies' discussed earlier has fostered development of specific benchmarks that trainees must meet to be a competent psychiatrist. While some trainees will exceed the thresholds of competency, others may barely reach them if at all. In contrast to group didactic learning, supervision more easily allows education to be tailored to the individual's needs. For example, the trainee may be an adequate clinician, yet their personality characteristics may be more suited to engage in cognitive behavioural focused treatment rather than a psychodynamic approach. While the trainee may meet the threshold regarding competency in psychodynamic psychotherapy, spending excessive time and resources working with the trainee beyond this in the situation may not be an appropriate allocation of resources. In fact, focusing supervision on likely areas of clinical work, once basic competencies are gained, allows for more personalised growth and development.

To summarize, timing issues in the psychiatric curriculum require attention to various developmental processes. This holds true not only for the order and complexity of the content which is covered (Figure 7.1), but also the means by which that knowledge is shared

(Figure 7.2). Timing should be addressed as a continuum, including recognition that the pace at which topics are covered may also vary.

Pacing may be a direct reflection of the amount of time designated to specific aspects of training. Regions where psychiatric training takes place over forty-eight months will spend more time on designated topics and will make assignments to certain clinical settings more so than programmes where only twelve or twenty-four months are required. Ideally, the pace should be altered based on the individual, but this is most often possible when there are multiple trainees in a programme. Thus, it is not only the terrain that must be mapped, the means used (Table 7.2) and the speed at which a trainee transverses the map must also be decided.

7.7 Implementing the Curriculum

Once a curriculum course has been mapped, it must be implemented and carried out. Available faculty resources and national requirements often dictate the leadership requirements for training programme oversight. A number of national standards require a specific individual be charged with programme oversight and this is highly desirable when possible. The programme director is charged with the duty of developing and monitoring the curriculum. In addition, having ample faculty to provide on-site teaching as well as assisting in other educational modalities is important. Without trained faculty who are engaged in the teaching process, trainees lack mentors, supervision or guidance. While in many countries adequate faculty resources are not available, this discussion will assume reasonably adequate resources to exist. While the programme director is responsible for developing and monitoring the curriculum, it is the faculty that is charged with carrying it out.

7.8 Assuring Continued Quality and Improvement

Providing a strong curriculum requires frequent review. There are continual advances within the field of psychiatry and the content, or terrain, of the curricular map needs to reflect this evolution with regular updates. In addition, the resources available for education, including clinical sites and available faculty members, may change. Governing bodies may alter requirements by which training programmes must adhere. Each of these changes requires the curriculum to be modified accordingly. Sustained quality also relies on monitoring deficiencies and responding to them appropriately.

In order to approach such review, there must be a clear understanding of who is involved in such a process. Training directors often will be called upon to lead this endeavour within a given programme. This process should also ideally include other faculty as well as trainees. Governing bodies, such as the ACGME, have certain requirements regarding the evaluation of all training programmes. These governing bodies must be taken into consideration when formulating a means of evaluating the curriculum.

The involvement of both trainees and faculty is important as their perceptions and experiences may vary considerably [10]. The most effective approach is often the creation of a committee whose goal is to evaluate and monitor the curriculum. Committees often include representatives from each year of training and faculty from various clinical sites, with the training director chairing the committee. Concerns and proposed changes to the curriculum are brought before the committee, allowing trainees and faculty to discuss and debate the issues. Ultimately, proposals regarding changes within the curriculum grow from this process and then are implemented and carried out under the direction of the training office.

Assuring quality education requires ongoing feedback. Within training programmes this may take the form of several outcome measures. The most obvious assessment is the trainees' completion of evaluations of clinical rotations and didactics. This affords the opportunity for trainees to give feedback about their experiences. In addition, faculties are continually evaluating trainees' performance. Yet, these subjective measures may not be the most useful attestation of a curriculum's quality.

If the goal is to test a training programme's efficacy, more objective measures may be necessary. If the ultimate goal of training is to develop competent psychiatrists, then an understanding of clinical competency must be clear. This often requires looking at expectations of governing bodies. In the United States, the American Board of Psychiatry and Neurology oversees board certification. Looking at the percentage of graduates who pass their national qualifying examination may serve as an example of such an objective measure. This measure, though, is available only after a trainee has completed a programme and only where such examinations exist. This is well past the point that interventions in the curriculum that will more quickly improve quality can be implemented. The use of written examinations throughout training, such as the US Psychiatry Residency In-Training Exam (PRITE), may provide a timelier assessment of the curriculum. Oral examinations may also provide a more objective form of feedback regarding a trainee's clinical skills. A number of clinical skill assessment tools are available (e.g. The American Association of Directors of Psychiatric Residency Training (AADPRT) Web site, http://www.aadprt.net/).

Objective measures paired with faculty evaluations of trainees' performance may be used to accurately assess the efficacy of the curriculum. If trends in trainees' shortcomings and lack of skills become evident across the training programme, this is an indication that an element of the curriculum may need strengthening. The curriculum content may require adjustment, or the make up of clinical rotations might be re-evaluated, all as part of regular curricular reviewing and updating. Quality training involves a cyclic approach to curricular changes (Figure 7.3).

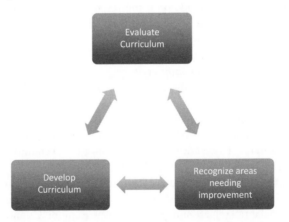

Figure 7.3 Cyclic nature of the curriculum.

Some national requirements include specific guidelines regarding the cycles in which programmes must undergo such reviews. At a minimum an overall analysis of the curriculum should occur every five years [1]. Regular, less formal assessment should occur at a minimum on an annual basis, paying close attention to objective markers as they become available throughout the academic year.

7.9   Challenges

As discussed in the introduction, the psychiatry curriculum is complex, incorporating developmental needs and constraints of available clinical systems. After reviewing how to approach developing and evaluating curriculum, it is not surprising that a number of challenges present themselves, clearly varying with available resources and national standards.

Given the nature of psychiatry, different areas of the world may have diverse needs in terms of the content that should be covered. An understanding of cultural issues is important in developing and maintaining a therapeutic alliance and will clearly vary by location. Attention to such culturally diverse needs may not only reflect wide geographical distances. The European Union of Medical Specialities' Board of Psychiatry acknowledged this in its proposed curriculum recommendations for Europe [7]. A broad mandate, it felt, was not warranted due to the diversity of nations even within a relatively small geographic area. Even within the United States, it may be recognized that a programme on the west coast may not spend as much time studying the rural eastern Appalachian mountain culture. While respect for cultural differences is paramount, the depth of study of individual cultures would vary considerably. This requires acknowledging the context in which training is taking place and the anticipated practice locations of trainees.

The availability of training resources warrants ample consideration and discussion. The availability of resources not only effects access to care for patients, but also what opportunities are available to promote the education of trainees, including the types of clinical sites and the accessibility of expert faculty. As technology advances around the globe, sharing resources may become more commonplace. The advent of telepsychiatry affords the opportunity for increased clinical exposure. Advances in technology may also increase experts' ability to share knowledge from sites at a distance to the training programme. Acknowledging that stigma may continue to play a role in the availability of psychiatric training is also relevant. Though varying in degree, stigma plays a role in lack of resources for psychiatric training in nearly every country.

Limited resources can impede educational efforts on many levels. Without adequate faculty, the most dynamic curriculum would fail. A shortage of faculty will limit how much supervision trainees receive. In addition, if faculty members have too many responsibilities, they may not have the time or ability to fully engage in the teaching process. Insufficient resources may limit exposure to varied clinical settings. Some medications are not available in various parts of the world. While a medication may be 'available', its cost may make it completely cost prohibitive. Striving to incorporate the 'latest advances' in the neurosciences is important [11]. However, if one is in a location where access to high speed Internet is not readily available, the ability to carry out a literature review to inform educational content would be quite difficult.

The means by which health care is financed may also play a role in training. In countries such as the United Kingdom, Canada and Germany, where health care is provided for all, psychotherapy continues to be reimbursed when provided by psychiatrists. Thus, psychiatrists in these regions continue to train in and perform psychotherapy as part of their routine practice [4]. In most parts of the world, however, both lack of payment and/or inadequate numbers of psychiatrists make psychotherapy an uncommon part of regular clinical practice. Thus, it would make little sense to devote a large amount of curricular time to ensuring a high level of psychotherapy skills in these regions.

While content and educational modalities present challenges, the variability in length of training across countries presents inherent difficulties. The length of medical education varies around the world and psychiatric residency training varies considerably in duration as well. Psychiatric training programmes may range from one to six years [4]. As noted earlier, some general training may be followed by fellowship training with further subspeciality emphasis, but such training does not exist everywhere. If a training programme is shorter in duration, it may be impossible to cover the entire field adequately. Decisions must be made regarding the breadth and depth with which material is covered, even with topics deemed essential. It is not reasonable to expect that a trainee will obtain higher hierarchical levels of understanding in a single year or two, but this may be all that is available. While the resources available may limit the amount of time available for training, it also must be acknowledged that this hinders the ability to easily train skilled psychiatrists. There may be distinct differences in competency levels of psychiatrists trained in various parts of the world based simply on the availability of resources and time available for training. There is no ready solution for this problem.

7.10   Model Curricula Illustrations

There are many illustrations of model curricula covering a myriad of topics within psychiatry, a few of which are listed in Table 7.3. After outlining a means of approaching the complex map that psychiatric training encompasses, the challenges appear great. However, there are examples of curricula that exemplify the model that has been described. For the purpose of illustration, two such models will be referred to: one addressing psychopharmacology training and the other psychodynamic psychotherapy.

Psychopharmacology, like most bodies of knowledge and skills, requires a basic understanding which then is expanded upon through study and clinical training. The American Society of Clinical Psychopharmacology has developed a Model Psychopharmacology Curriculum aimed at providing an accurate and clinically relevant educational resource [27]. Now in its fifth edition, the curriculum is presented in three volumes and two CDs. The first volume outlines an overview of the curriculum along with explanations, rationales and learning objectives. The second and third volumes contain lecture materials, comprising detailed PowerPoint slides on specific topics.

The curriculum is very clear in acknowledging that the materials are to be used over the course of four years in a progressive manner. There is a 'crash course' comprising seven sessions: Antipsychotics; Medicine for bipolar disorder; Antidepressants; Anti-anxiety agents; Drug–drug interactions; Therapeutic alliance; and Art of psychopharmacology, These provide an overview of key topics. Then, topics are placed under 'basic' and advanced headings.

The 'Basic Course' comprises: Psychopharmacology in the Emergency Room; Pharma-cokinetics of psychotropic drugs; Schizophrenia and antipsychotic medications; Bipolar Disorders; Bipolar depression; Antidepressant Pharmacotherapy; Treatment resistant depression; Electroconvulsive therapy; Substance abuse; Sleep disorders; Psychopharmacology of violence; and Traumatic brain injury. The 'Advanced Course' includes: Combining pharmacotherapy and psychotherapy; Mood disorders in women of child bearing age; Atypical depression; Panic Disorder; Generalized Anxiety Disorder; Social Anxiety Disorder/Social Phobia; Post-Traumatic Stress Disorder; Obsessive Compulsive Disorder; Personality disorders; Eating disorders; Body Dysmorphic Disorder; Psychopharmacology and the HIV-positive patient; Psychopharmacology of sexual dysfunction; and Sexual dysfunction associated with psychiatric disorders and psychiatric drugs (Table 7.4).

More fundamental topics such as pharmacokinetics and drug class-based lectures are covered first. Building on this foundation, more detailed presentations for specific disorders are then covered. There are further specialized series in geropsychiatry, child and adolescent psychopharmacology and substance abuse.

The reason for selecting this as an example, however, is its format and structure. This model curriculum addresses the key elements outlined earlier in this chapter. By providing clear content, the course provides a strong foundation, or terrain. The map is consciously taken into consideration in recognizing that, developmentally, trainees must learn basics before more advance topics are approached. This illustrates clearly the fundamentals of layering

Table 7.4 Psychopharmacology curricula.[a]

Crash Course	Basic Course	Advanced Course
Antipsychotics	Psychopharmacology in the Emergency Room	Combining pharmacotherapy and psychotherapy
Medicine for bipolar disorder	Pharmacokinetics of Psychotropic drugs	Mood disorders in women of child bearing age
Antidepressants	Schizophrenia and antipsychotic medications	Atypical depression
Anti-anxiety agents		Panic Disorder
Drug–drug interactions 101	Bipolar disorders	Generalized Anxiety Disorder
Therapeutic Alliance and adherence	Bipolar depression	Social Anxiety Disorder/Social phobia
Art of psychopharmacology	Antidepressant pharmacotherapy	Post-Traumatic Stress Disorder
	Treatment resistant depression	Obsessive Compulsive Disorder
	Electroconvulsive therapy	Personality disorders
	Substance abuse	Eating disorders
	Sleep disorders	Body Dysmorphic Disorder
	Pychopharmacology of violence	Psychopharmacology and the HIV-positive patient
	Traumatic brain injury	Psychopharmacology of sexual dysfunction
		Sexual dysfunction associated with psychiatric disorders and psychiatric drugs

[a] [27].

knowledge over time, with increasing complexity of content. The educational modality is outlined in didactic format, which in turn provides attention to detail and assures that necessary details are not negated. Recruiting strong faculty to use the resource is a key requirement, and will present a significant dilemma for those training programmes located in low resource areas.

Developing a curricular map may appear on the surface to be more challenging with some topics compared to others. One such area is psychotherapy, specifically psychodynamic psychotherapy, which requires developmental considerations and calls upon multiple educational modalities, including didactics, supervision and clinical experiences. Dr David Goldberg from the United States published a model for training in psychodynamic psychotherapy that maps a very articulate and clear course to follow. The model (Table 7.5) is comprised of two coordinates, deemed the 'phases of learning' (horizontal axis) and 'developmental categories' (vertical axis).

The phases of learning progress from the more concrete to more abstract: (I) observation and description; (II) conceptualization; and (III) synthesis. Simultaneously, the developmental categories progress in a similar fashion: (1) goals, roles and boundaries; (2) participants; (3) verbal flow; (4) technique; and (5) theory [28]. This model succeeds in recognizing tangible elements within a complex framework. By breaking down an intricate series of educational endeavours into finite steps that can be addressed in specific educational components, this approach enables trainees to gain further knowledge and insight while also providing feedback within the process [28].

While some may argue that model curricula may provide a too rigid, structured approach, these examples of curricula are presented here to illustrate approaches to developing a curriculum for a specific content area. Such approaches are particularly useful when approaching training from the perspective of acquiring a range of clinical competencies of ever increasing complexity. Dr Goldberg astutely states while presenting his model, 'it is not intended to impose a static structure on psychotherapy education. Rather, it adds a counterpoint to the richness and diversity contained in individualized, process-orientated, student/patient-focused teaching' [28]. Model curricula are not meant to be rigid, static, lifeless entities. Their modelling offers a structure in which to give life to the educational process. Another approach to designing a curriculum for psychotherapy can be found in Chapter 9.

7.11 Conclusion

As has been reviewed, designing, implementing and evaluating a psychiatry residency curriculum is a complex process. Mapping a psychiatric curriculum requires an understanding of key elements. The use of these various elements, the sequencing of training experiences and making decisions about the time devoted to each element all warrant careful consideration. Once a programme has been created, it must be continually evaluated and reassessed. While there have been trends regarding psychiatric training that have fostered improved quality of training, there are still a wide variety of challenges facing those charged with providing quality education to the future generation of psychiatrists. Through careful consideration, though, a well-constructed course of psychiatric training is possible, even when resources and length of training are limited. Engaging in such a process offers the most promising future for educational progress in the field.

Table 7.5 A model psychotherapy curriculum.[a]

	I. Observation and Description	II. Conceptualization	III. Synthesis
1. Boundaries, roles and goals	Boundaries: 1. Time, space and money 2. Outside relationships 3. Professional relationship 4. Privacy and confidentiality Therapist's roles: 1. Analytic attitude 2. Interventions 3. Education of patient (overt and covert) Patient's roles: 1. Active participant 2. Free association 3. Curiosity	Recognition of breaches in boundaries and roles as they occur within the context of treatment. Goals: 1. Interplay of symptoms and behaviours with process in treatment and intrapsychic life 2. Ability to assess patients and establish specific and realistic goals 3. Time (brief and long term goals)	Ability to consider breaches in the context of dynamic understanding and the overall process of the therapy. Ability to interpret and correct during hour. Goals: 1. Ability to match patient to levels of intervention and focused treatment goals 2. Integration with other forms of intervention (somatic and psychotherapeutic)
2. Participants	Therapist: 1. Attention to one's own overt thoughts, feelings and fantasies Patient: 1. Description of patient (affects, character, non-verbal behaviour) 2. Life history: development, themes, repetitions, meaning (narration) 3. Handling patient's level of anxiety and avoidance Dyad: 1. Rapport 2. Effects on each other	Therapist: 1. Development of introspection and self-reflection 2. Recognition of prominent counter-transference reactions Patient: 1. Ability to recognize and describe transference 2. Dynamic formulation 3. Ability to recognize and describe resistance Dyad: 1. Working alliance 2. Repetitive interactions (overt and covert)	Therapist: 1. Application of knowledge gained from introspection for interpretation 2. Use of counter-transference for interpretation Patient: 1. Management and interpretation of transference 2. Ability to interpret resistance 3. Use of dynamics to make interventions Dyad: 1. Ability to repair working alliance 2. Integration of repetitive interactions, transference/countertransference, and use in interpretations

[a] Reprinted with permission from the Journal of Psychotherapy Practice and Research © 1998, American Psychiatric Association.

(Continued)

Table 7.5   (*Continued*)

	I. Observation and Description	II. Conceptualization	III. Synthesis
3. Verbal Flow	1. Listening with openness and concentration 2. Ability to summarize manifest themes 3. Maintaining verbal flow 4. Tolerance to ambiguity	1. Active listening/ empathic listening 2. Identifying major latent theme(s) 3. Appropriate focusing and unfocusing	1. Matching latent theme to dynamics 2. Integrating latent theme with transference, resistance, treatment focus and stage of treatment
4. Technique	Theory: 1. Repetition of outside behaviours and relationship in the treatment 2. Overview of phases of treatment Skills: 1. Open-ended and focused questions 2. Listening/ responding/ listening 3. Supportive/ expressive technique 4. Confrontation and clarification	Theory: 1. Transference/ countertransference 2. Resistance 3. Functions of interpretation Skills: 1. Interpretation 2. Use of self with patient 3. Pacing of interventions	Theory: 1. Integration of theory, resistance, transference and interpretations 2. Working through 3. Termination 4. Therapeutic action and its comparison with other modalities Skills: 1. Subtleness of interpretation (i.e. depth, timing, content, style) 2. Different approach to patients 3. Integration with other approaches (e.g. cognitive, interpersonal, systems)
5. Theory	1. The unconscious 2. Importance of early development 3. Repetition of past in present 4. Historical and narrative truths	1. Conflicts and defence 2. Symptom formation 3. Developmental theory 4. Object relations perspective 5. Fantasy and dreams	1. Specific models: structural, ego psychology, object relations, self psychology 2. Comparison with other frameworks: interpersonal, behavioural, family, cognitive, systems, other

References

1. Andrews, L. and Lomax, J.W. (1999) Developing and monitoring the curriculum, in *Handbook of Psychiatric Education and Faculty Development* (eds J. Kay, E.K. Silberman and L. Pressar), American Psychiatric Association, Arlington, pp. 363–380.
2. Bobbitt, F. (1918) *The Curriculum*, The Riverside Press, Cambridge, pp. iii–v.
3. James (1991) Sketches from psychiatric history. *Psychiatric Bulletin*, **15**, 631–634.
4. Zisook, S. *et al.* (2007) Psychiatry residency training around the world. *Academic Psychiatry*, **31**, 309–325.
5. European Union of Medical Specialities, Section for Psychiatry (7 October 2005), http://www.uemspsychiatry.org/section/reports/2005Oct-PsychiatristProfile.pdf (accessed 12 November 2009).
6. Accreditation Council for Graduate Medical Education (1 July 2007). ACGME Program Requirements for Graduate Medical Education in Psychiatry, http://www.acgme.org/acwebsite/rrc_400/400_prindex.asp (accessed 12 November 2009).
7. European Union of Medical Specialities European Board of Psychiatry (October 2009). European Framework for Competencies in Psychiatry, http://www.uemspsychiatry.org/board/reports/2009-Oct-EFCP.pdf (accessed 12 November 2009).
8. Royal College of Psychiatrists (January 2009). Competency Based Curriculum for Specialist Training in Psychiatry, http://www.rcpsych.ac.uk/training/curriculum2009.aspx (accessed 12 November 2009).
9. World Psychiatric Association (August 2002). World Psychiatric Association Institutional Program on the Core Training Curriculum for Psychiatry, http://www.wpanet.org/v1/education/core-curric-psych-stu.shtml (accessed 12 November 2009).
10. Yudkowsky, R., Elliott, R. and Schwartz, A. (2002) Two perspectives on the indicators of quality in psychiatry residencies: program directors' and residents'. *Academic Medicine*, **77**, 57–64.
11. Rubin, E.H. and Zorumski, C.F. (2003) Psychiatric education in an era of rapidly occurring scientific advances. *Academic Medicine*, **78**, 351–354.
12. Faulkner, L.R. *et al.* (1989) A basic residency curriculum concerning the chronically mentally ill. *Am J Psychiatry*, **146**, 1323–1327.
13. Weiden, P.J. and Rao, N. (2005) Teaching medication compliance to psychiatric residents: placing an orphan topic into a training curriculum. *Academic Psychiatry*, **29**, 203–210.
14. Maislinger, S., Rumpold, G., Kantner-Rumplmair, W. *et al.* (2007) Curriculum for a course in c-l psychiatry, psychology and psychosomatics in Austria. *Journal of Psychosomatic Research*, **62**, 599–600.
15. Boehnlein, J.K., Leung, P.K. and Kinzie, J.D. (2008) Cross-cultural psychiatry residency training: the Oregon experience. *Academic Psychiatry*, **32**, 299–305.
16. Harris, H.W., Felder, D. and Clark, M.O. (2004) A psychiatry residency curriculum on the care of African-American patients. *Academic Psychiatry*, **28**, 226–239.
17. Seirles, F.S. (2005) Using film as the basis of an American culture course for first-year psychiatry residents. *Academic Psychiatry*, **29**, 100–104.
18. Dolent, T.J. and Philbrick, K.L. (2007) Achieving competency in electroconvulsive therapy: a model curriculum. *Academic Psychiatry*, **31**, 65–67.
19. Brasch, J., Glick, R.L., Cobb, T.G. and Richmond J. (2004) Residency training in emergency psychiatry: a model curriculum developed by the education committee of the American Association of Emergency Psychiatry. *Academic Psychiatry*, **28**, 95–103.
20. Bhuvaneswar, C., Stern, T. and Beresin, E. (2009) Using the technique of journal writing to learn emergency psychiatry. *Academic Psychiatry*, **33**, 43–46.

21. Kick, S.D., Morrison, M. and Kathol, R.G. (1997) Medical training in psychiatry residency. A proposed curriculum. *General Hospital Psychiatry*, **19**, 259–266.

22. Lacy, T. and Hughes, J.D. (2006) A neural systems-based neurobiology and neuropsychiatry course: integrating biology, psychodynamics, and psychology in the psychiatric curriculum. *Academic Psychiatry*, **30**, 410–415.

23. Wichman, C.L., Netzel, P.J. and Menaker, R. (2009) Preparing psychiatric residents for the 'real world': a practice management curriculum. *Academic Psychiatry*, **33**, 131–134.

24. Winkelman, J.W. (2005) Education designing a sleep disorders curriculum for psychiatry residents. *Harvard Review of Psychiatry*, **13**, 54–56.

25. Iannucci, R., Sanders, K. and Greenfield, S.F. (2009) A 4-year curriculum on substance use disorders for psychiatry residents. *Academic Psychiatry*, **33**, 60–66.

26. Schwartz, A.C., Kaslow, N.J. and McDonald, W.M. (2007) Encountering patient Suicide: a requirement of the residency program curriculum. *Academic Psychiatry*, **31**, 338–339.

27. A Committee of the American Society of Clinical Psychopharmacology (2008) *Model Psychopharmacology Curriculum for Training Directors and Teachers of Psychopharmacology in Psychiatric Residency Programs*, 5th edn, American Society of Clinical Psychopharmacology, New York.

28. Goldberg, D.A. (1998) Structuring training goals for psychodynamic psychotherapy. *The Journal of Psychotherapy Practice and Research*, **7**, 10–22.

8

Acquisition of Psychiatric Interviewing Skills

Linda Gask

School of Community Based Medicine, University of Manchester, Manchester, UK

8.1   The Salience of the Consultation

The psychiatric expert is presumed, from the cultural definition of an expert, and from the general rumours and beliefs about psychiatry, to be quite able to handle a psychiatric interview.

—Sullivan [1]

The consultation or medical interview remains the indispensable unit of medical practice. In psychiatry perhaps more than any other speciality, the interview is the key to both assessment and successful management of the patient's presenting problem. Good interview skills are essential in order to arrive at the right diagnosis, yet it has been noted that *'one often observes a greater comfort and intellectual curiosity in the discussion of the psychopathology of the patient rather than exploration of the interview process'* [2]. Furthermore, in recent years, the previous pre-eminence of psychiatry in the teaching of communication skills in the undergraduate curriculum has been overtaken by the rise of specific expertise in this domain in primary care and family medicine, and the professional development of multidisciplinary 'communication skills' teachers. However, teachers of psychiatry retain a key role in the undergraduate curriculum in teaching communication skills relating to psychiatry history taking, exploration of emotional problems and teaching of the skills of mental state examination. They also, of course, have a key role in the training of both mental health and primary care professionals (Chapter 13) in key interviewing skills for the assessment and management of people with mental health problems. In speciality training even those who desire to develop their knowledge and expertise in the field of biological psychiatry still essentially require the necessary skills to conduct a psychiatric interview.

Teaching Psychiatry: Putting Theory into Practice   Edited by Linda Gask, Bulent Coskun and David Baron
© 2011 John Wiley & Sons, Ltd

In the past, medical students received little or no training in interviewing patients other than being given lists of questions to ask in order to clarify patients' initial complaints and to ensure that no other important symptoms had been missed. This is still the case in some countries of the world, but in the curricula of many medical schools the picture is now changing rapidly. Communication skills training is a continuous process carried out alongside and within other teaching during all specialities, in hospital and in the community and not something simply carried out during general practice or psychiatry attachments.

A number of models for the learning and teaching of consultation skills (for example the Cambridge–Calgary Model [3] used in many British medical schools) have been influential in the development of *medical* interview skills training over the last three decades. These are now having a major impact at the undergraduate level and on training in general medical and primary care settings, and also have relevance to the basic tasks which a psychiatrist in training also need to master. This is not the place to review these, but *The Three Function Model* developed by Julian Bird and Steven Cohen-Cole [4], which has been very influential in the United States of America, makes the most immediate sense. The model highlights three core functions of the interaction between doctor and patient: (1) gathering data to understand the patient; (2) development of rapport and responding to the patient's emotions; and (3) patient education and behavioural management. Another important and highly influential concept in medical teaching has been *'Patient Centredness'*, a much debated concept which has been defined as 'providing care that is respectful of and responsive to individual patient preferences needs, and values and ensuring that patient values guide all clinical decisions' [5].

This chapter briefly discusses the key interviewing skills that are necessary for psychiatric history taking and mental state examination and key management skills that need to be acquired early in speciality training, together with an overview of methods for teaching these skills which hare applicable to a range of different settings (for example, in primary care, see Chapter 14). All of this must be approached with the awareness that the illnesses which we, as mental health professionals, treat still carry an enormous amount of stigma for our patients within society and that many patients are vociferously dissatisfied (often with some justification) with our performance in the consultation.

8.2   Teaching Psychiatric Interviewing

In psychiatry, the initial interview serves several quite different purposes:

(a) it is a means of asking questions to obtain factual information on historical events, happenings and activities;

(b) it serves as a stimulus to elicit emotions, feelings and attitudes; and

(c) it begins to establish a relationship which will constitute the basis for further therapeutic contact. [6].

The form of the interview is determined by the range of skills employed by the clinician in response to what the patient has to say. The content of the interview is not only determined by the patient, but also by the specific topics addressed by the clinician. Students have to learn that the skill of interviewing lies in getting the balance right between an 'open-ended' and 'checking out' style of interviewing, which can encourage a patient to talk more and may be essential in engaging a person who is finding it difficult to talk to express feelings, and a more 'probing' and systematic style of interviewing, which seems to be important in getting good quality factual information. A skilled interviewer is thus able to demonstrate flexibility and to switch between styles during the interview in order to be able to carry out the three different tasks of the assessment interview listed above, as well as to respond to cues provided by in the patient.

8.2.1 The Basic Skills

Most undergraduate textbooks of psychiatry summarize very clearly the key tasks of the psychiatric history. However, medical students, and those postgraduate students who have never received specific training in interview skills (although they may have had sometimes quite extensive clinical experience in psychiatry), still need specific guidance in:

- how to begin the interview;

- the key tasks in getting the 'history of the presenting problem';

- specific communication skills that are essential in psychiatric consultations.

These are summarized in Boxes 8.1, 8.2 and 8.3.

Box 8.1   Beginning the Interview

- Arrange seating so that doctor and patient are conveniently close – not separated by a desk. Chairs placed at right angles allow the patient to make eye contact if he or she wishes.

- Introduce yourself and say what your role is.

- Indicate the purpose of the interview.

- Explain how much time it is likely to take.

- If you are taking notes, stress confidentiality. If recording, say what will happen to the recording of the interview and obtain written consent.

- Check that patient is happy about all this.

- Do not write immediately. Learn how to both make notes and ensure eye contact, particularly at the end of a question or statement.

Box 8.2   History of the Presenting Problem(s)

For each presenting problem establish as clearly as possible:

- Nature of the problem.

- Time of onset.

- Development of the problems or symptoms over time.

- Precipitating factors or possible links with life events.

- Key events since the onset.

- Alleviating or exacerbating factors

- What help has been given or offered?

- What is the **patient's view** of what is wrong, what help they have been offered so far and what help they would like?

Box 8.3   Information Gathering Skills

Asking Open-Ended Questions

These are questions which cannot be answered in one word. It is essential to begin the interview in an open-ended manner such as *'what are the problems that have brought you here?'* A common error in interviewing is to ask too many questions which can only be answered by *'yes'* or *'no'* too early in the interview, therefore not giving the patient space and opportunity to develop a description of how he or she is feeling. **Directive questions** such as *' Tell me about how you have been sleeping'* help to direct the patient to a particular topic without closing down the conversation. Closed questions have their place nearer the end of particular sections of the interview to fill in gaps in information. This pattern of open changing to closed questions is known as **open to closed cone**.

Listening

It is essential to allow the patient time to talk without interruption both at the beginning of the interview and at crucial points where silence may be important. An effective interview, however, has periods of silence interspersed with times when the psychiatrist uses other skills to help the patient to focus on key topics or to dwell on specific experiences or feelings. These skills include:

Facilitation

Encouraging the patient to continue talking by either verbal means, for example saying *'go-on . . .'*, or by non-verbal means such as nodding.

Noticing and Responding to Verbal Cues

These are key words and phrases offered by the patient which indicate what he is worried about. These can be explored by:

- **Clarification** for example: *'What do you mean when you say you have been having panic attacks?'*. Staying with the patient's own words is often much more efficient than embarking on a check list of questions about panic attacks immediately.

- **Asking for examples** such as *'take me through the last time you had one of these attacks . . . . . .tell me exactly what happened'*.

- You may also **delay** your comment until the patient has finished a particular story before saying something like *' A moment ago you said you had been depressed before you had this attack . . . can you tell me more about that?'*

Noticing and Responding to Non-verbal and Vocal Cues

There may be changes in posture or eye contact when talking about particular problems or **vocal cues** which are significant changes in tone of voice. Comment on such cues can be very effective in helping to discover what is worrying the patient but must be offered with sensitivity, for example, *'you seemed quite tense when we talked about your father . . .'*.

Eliciting and Dealing with Emotion

- **Reflection** means 'stating or labelling the observed emotion'. Sometimes this is called **making an empathic comment** Offer this as a suggestion based on your observation rather than a firm statement about what the patient is feeling: *'you seem quite upset when you are talking about this'* rather than *'you are upset by this'* allows the patient to either confirm or refute the suggestion and enter into a discussion about it, which will further aid clarification.

- The combination of picking up a non-verbal cue, followed by an empathic comment can be a very powerful way of giving a person 'permission' to talk about his/her feelings. For example, *'You look quite sad . . . . . .I can see that things must have been very tough for you recently'*.

- **Understanding hypotheses** are used to make an educated guess about what has been happening, given as a statement, to help in clarifying how events are linked. Foe example, *'it seems like the depression got worse after you broke up with your boyfriend'*. As this is given in the form of a statement it again allows the patient to either agree with it or refute it.

- **Directly responding to emotion** by drawing attention to feelings you observe, for example, *'you look quite angry when you talk about that'*.

Checking

Allows you to review the information you have elicited and correct misunderstandings. Checking comments also indicates that you have been listening, so helps to develop rapport; they can also provide useful 'thinking space' during which you can make a decision about where to go next.

Encouraging Precision
You may need to explain that you need to be as precise as possible about information. Be prepared to say something like *'I'm still not sure that I've got this quite right, can we try and sort this out before we go any further.'*

Summarizing
Summarizing statements can be used as the patient finishes talking about each problem to check out what the patient has reported and provide a link to the next part of the interview. For example, ' *Before we talk about the panic attacks can I just summarize what you've told me about the depression, correct me as a go along'*, ending with *'have I got that right?'* Summarizing can also be useful to help control the flow of the interview if a patient presents too much information at once.

Methods for teaching these skills are discussed later in this chapter. Certain issues come up on a regular basis during teaching sessions. In my experience, both undergraduate and postgraduate students may have difficulty with the concept of 'conveying empathy'. Sometimes they may be aware of experiencing empathic feelings for the patient but fail to convey these either verbally or non-verbally in a way that the patient or their peers can recognize. Unfortunately, rather than conveying the empathic comment in the form of a suggestion they may sometimes assert that they know exactly how someone is feeling, which can be interpreted as rather patronising behaviour. Asserting appropriate control of the interview may also be difficult. Beginning interviewers may be good listeners, but fail to follow-up on patient cues or attempt to *shape* the interview, such that they do not obtain the information required for diagnosis and further management. They may not even feel that it is possible to shape an interview – they experience it almost as something which *happens to them*, sometimes because of a high level of anxiety. They need to learn the skills required to politely interrupt the patient and briefly summarize the progress of the interview so far before moving on to ask a more directive question. A good listener will still face problems if the patient finds talking difficult, and students need to learn how to *comment on the process of the interview* by picking up on non-verbal cues about how the patient is feeling and making empathic comments about how it might feel to be talking to a psychiatrist in order to gently encourage the patient to begin to talk. Other problematic situations that students may need specific help and guidance with are where a patient has a hearing difficulty, or the interview has to be conducted through an interpreter.

8.2.2   Interviewing and Mental State Examination

Students also have to learn the utility of effective interviewing skills in carrying out an effective mental state examination. In addition to the key skill of accurate observation, the set of skills in Box 8.4 is central to being able to clarify the nature of the patient's experience and get the patient to describe exactly what they are preoccupied with or concerned about in order to arrive at a psychopathological description. This means employing both sensitivity and precision when, for example, asking about the exact nature of psychotic phenomena, and when assessing the quality and severity of mood disturbance by examining the nature and intensity of depressive thoughts.

Box 8.4   Some Basic Therapeutic Skills

- How to engage the patient in a working treatment alliance of any nature.

- How to provide information.

- How to negotiate: this may involve helping a patient to stop or start any form of treatment, stop having or start to have medical investigations, and either leave or alternatively be admitted to hospital.

- How to help someone to talk freely about their thoughts, feelings, ideas, worries, concerns and expectations.

- How to manage someone who is in crisis.

- How to help a patient to change, for example stop drinking or engage in some form of rehabilitation for any type of disorder.

- How to deal with a range of potentially difficult situations where there is, for example, risk of violence, risk of self-harm or harm to others, an encounter with angry relatives and so on.

- How to be able to talk to families and couples without necessarily training formally in family therapy.

Students may not understand the value of empathic comments when exploring the nature of potentially very frightening experiences. Instead they may focus on trying to get the right information in order to be able to label the psychopathology, or perhaps make the mistake of questioning the reality of the patients experience too soon, thus appearing to be making a premature value judgement rather than 'joining with' the patient in trying to understand exactly what he or she has been experiencing and how it affects them.

8.3   Acquisition of Basic Therapeutic Skills

A range of basic skills is required by any mental health clinician whatever their orientation (Box 8.4) and young psychiatrists in speciality training need to develop many of these skills during the first year of their postgraduate or residency training.

Some trainees will want to focus on the knowledge base of psychiatry and will not necessarily see the point of taking the time to address the skills required to put this knowledge into practice taking this as 'self-evident'. Demonstration of the value of skilled interviewing by watching peers, colleagues and senior staff talking to patients (see next page) goes a long way to challenging this view. Nevertheless, most interview skills training focuses only on the psychiatric assessment interview. Formal psychotherapy training, a requirement in most speciality education, may help to develop a trainee's pragmatic understanding of what happens in the human psyche and its relationships, but may only seem to be relevant to working with a 'long' psychotherapy case. The skills learned may not appear to be generalizable to the routine of the psychiatric out-patient clinic where the reality, at least in some countries, may be less contact time than the patient is already having with their own family doctor. To acquire the skills that can be used in 'brief' therapeutic encounters with patients, trainees need to be provided with simple models that make immediate clinical sense, and provide them with a clear framework of the tasks that have to be carried out in the meeting with the patient and the skills needed to do this.

8.4   Specific Methods for Teaching Skills

8.4.1   Modelling

The use of video feedback in changing professional behaviour goes back 30 years, and the first systematic studies of teaching the skills described above came from several sources. Although watching interviews carried out by 'experts' can be informative and helpful, there is sometimes a tendency for this to add to a sense that the learner 'couldn't possibly do that, because I can never be so skilled'. So it can be really useful for the required skills to be modelled by a worker from the target group of students or professionals that are being trained (for example if the audience is medical students, having a video of a student carrying out an interview demonstrating the key skills). This isn't always possible, and it may not be easy to set up, but particularly when teaching primary care doctors who work in a very different context from that of the psychiatric unit it can be very powerful. The demonstration can be carried out *in vivo* in a role-play or using a pre-prepared teaching tape.

When using a tape previously prepared there are usually 'Discussion Points' during the tape, and most tapes also have notes for the teacher reminding them of things to elicit from the group at such points. The teacher plays the role of a 'facilitator' during such discussions, encouraging those who have not spoken to contribute, and agreeing with suggestions that seem helpful. If someone suggests something that the teacher considers unhelpful, the teacher asks how others in the group handle such moments, rather than openly disagreeing with the speaker. The teacher is generally supportive to the group, and only suggests his or her own solutions if they do not emerge in the general discussion.

8.4.2   The Use of Role Playing to Practice Skills

Role play is particularly useful for acquisition of the range of basic therapeutic skills shown in Box 8.4, where it may not be easy to observe and supervise a trainee using these skills with a real patient. Indeed many health professionals are unlikely to try their new skills out with real patients until they have practised them in safer circumstances – and this is where role playing comes in. For each role play, it is necessary to prepare three documents, one for the person who will play the professional, one for the 'patient' and one for the observer. This threesome constitutes the 'trio'.

The 'health professional' is told what the health care organization or setting they are working in knows about the patient who is about to be seen: not the actual medical notes, but the relevant information about the patient that would normally have been available.

The 'patient' is told to play someone of their own age and gender, but typically given another occupation. They are told their presenting symptoms, and any life events that may have occurred recently, which they may or may not wish to tell the health professional about. If asked questions that have not been covered, they are advised to answer them from their personal experience.

The 'observer' is given the most information: that on the other two forms, as well as the list of key behaviours they are looking out for. After the enactment the group is asked to do three things:

- to *ask the professional* how s/he felt the interview went. What pleased her/him about it? Was there anything that could have been improved?

- to *ask the 'patient'* how s/he felt about the interview, and how the problem was handled. What did they like? Could anything have been improved?

- finally, to give the health professional their *own feedback* last of all, based upon their own observations.

These tasks are derived from Pendleton's rules of feedback [7] (Box 8.5), which provide an important structure for the task and ensure that it is perceived as helpful and not unduly critical.

Box 8.5   Pendleton's Rules for Giving Feedback in a One-to-One Teaching Session [7]

1. Briefly clarify matters of fact.

2. The learner goes first and discusses what went well.

3. The Trainer discusses what went well.

4. The Learner describes what could be done differently and makes suggestions for change.

5. The Trainer identifies what could be done differently and gives options for change.

6. The learner and trainer agree on the priorities for change and a method and timescale for meeting them.

The teachers (as indicated above there should, ideally, be a ratio of one teacher to six health professionals) move from one set of health professionals to another, offering advice and help as they find it appropriate. The enactments should be quite short – not more than about four minutes, with the feedback and discussion typically taking another 10 minutes to quarter of an hour. The trio then proceeds to the next role play, changing roles so that each doctor gets a chance to play the 'professional' role. It is important that such role plays are adapted to the conditions of the culture in which teaching is occurring, and that sufficient copies are made for several trios of health professionals to use the same role-play.

8.4.3   Group Teaching Using Standardized Patients

This approach is described in considerably more detail in Chapter 14. One member of a small teaching group (ideally no more than eight students) interviews a 'patient' (played by a trained standardized patient with a pre-prepared outline history) but is able to pause the interview (as is the group facilitator – I usually introduce the idea of a virtual remote control with 'pause' and 'play' buttons) in order to ask for assistance from other members of the group. The facilitator has to ensure that the group actively participates and that the person who is interviewing the patient feels supported and not unduly criticised by the group. At the end of the session feedback should again be provided in a structured way, starting with the person playing the health professional, the 'patient' and the group members. Standardized patients are trained to give feedback and are able to provide this both in and out of their role; however, it is important not to take them out of role until the end of the session, as it is difficult for them to switch between being themselves and playing the patient and also potentially confusing for the group.

8.4.4   Using Videotape of the Trainees Own Consultations

Video and audiotape feedback have been used in the acquisition of skills for many years. When showing videotape the teacher should always ask the person who made the tape for permission to show it, and to invite him or her to comment before inviting comments from others. It will usually be found that the person playing the doctor makes the most critical remarks about his or her own performance, and that others are more supportive. If someone makes a critical comment, ask them what they would have done in such a situation, before asking others. In general, the teacher elicits responses *from the group*, rather than allowing themselves to be identified as an all-knowing 'guru'. Some suggested guidelines for group video feedback teaching, developed after many years of research and practice, are shown in Box 8.6.

Box 8.6   Guidelines for Group Video Feeback

1. **Set ground rules**

- *Check out if the person has seen him/herself on video before. Ensure that the group realizes this may be difficult and elicit support.*

- *Ensure the group knows that anyone can stop the tape but if they do they must say what they would have done/said differently at that point.*

- *Stress confidentiality: for the group and also for patient if this is a real consultation.*

2. **Set an agenda**

- *Clarify the purpose of session.*

- *Ask the person presenting the interview to tell the group about the background of the patient and what has happened before this interview.*

- *Engage group in asking questions.*

- *What does the person showing the tape want from the group?*

3. **Provide opportunities for rehearsing new skills**

- *Stop the tape regularly at key points and invite rest of group to do so if they wish with the proviso noted above.*

- *Ask the group for comments on what has happened and whether anyone would do things differently.*

- *Give the person showing the tape first opportunity to comment.*

- *Label key skills and strategies that are being used on the tape or suggested by the group.*

4. **Be constructive**

- *Comment on things done well as frequently as you can without seeming false and even if this seems very difficult!*

- *Positive comments first followed by things that might have been done differently*

5. **Make the group do the work**

- *Facilitate the group, don't demonstrate to them what you know!*

- *Summarize suggestions and keep the session flowing.*

- *Ensure that the group keeps to the agenda.*

6. **Conclude positively**

- *Summarize and ask for feedback from the person showing the tape and the group.*

- *Facilitate the development of an action plan for future consultation if this is a real patient.*

- *Assist in the formulation of new learning goals for the members of the group.*

—Adapted From Gask, Goldberg and Lewis [8]

Where videotapes of real patient material are being used, members of the group should respect normal medical confidentiality outside the group. They should also agree not to talk about other people's performance outside the group, otherwise this will detract from the group being able to relax and achieve some work. This may be particularly important if the group meets on several occasions and group members, be they medical students or experienced doctors, deal with issues they personally find particularly difficult in their consultations and take the risk to bring consultations to show which demonstrate these difficulties.

References

1. Sullivan, H.S. (1954) *The Psychiatric Interview*, Norton, New York.
2. McCready, J.R. and Waring, E.M. (1986) Interviewing skills in relation to psychiatric residency. *Canadian Journal of Psychiatry*, **31**, 317–332.
3. Kurtz, S.M., Silverman, J.D. and Draper, J. (1998) *Teaching and Learning Communication Skills in Medicine*, Radcliffe Medical Press, Oxford.
4. Bird, J. and Cohen-Cole, S.A. (1990) The three function model of the medical interview: an educational device. *Adv Psychosom Med*, **20**, 65–88.
5. Committee on Quality of Health Care in America (2001) Crossing the Quality Chasm: A New Health System for the 21st Century, Institute of Medicine, Washington, DC.
6. Rutter, D. and Cox, A. (1981) Interviewing techniques: I. methods and measures. *British Journal of Psychiatry*, **138**, 273–282.
7. Pendleton, D., Scofield, T. and Tate, P. (1984) *The Consultation: An Approach to Learning and Teaching*, Oxford University Press, Oxford.
8. Gask, L., Goldberg, D. and Lewis, B. (2009) Teaching and learning about mental health, in *Primary Care Mental Health* (eds L. Gask, H. Lester, T. Kendrick and R. Peveler), Royal College of Psychiatrists, London.

9

Teaching Psychotherapy in the Classroom and in Supervision

Glen O. Gabbard

Department of Psychiatry and Behavioural Sciences, Baylor College of Medicine, Houston, TX, USA

9.1   Introduction

Psychiatry faculty today face new challenges in teaching psychotherapy to psychiatric residents. Recent developments in mental health care delivery have shifted the field significantly. While psychotherapy was once central to the identity of a psychiatrist, it is now fighting for its life as other mental health disciplines are taking over psychotherapeutic treatments [1]. Moreover, with the remarkable advances in neurobiological and genetic research, many psychiatrists see psychotherapy as peripheral to their career interests. Psychiatric residents who observe their role models' limited investment in psychotherapy as part of their professional role may be much less motivated to learn psychotherapy than they once were. They may assume that other mental health professionals, such as psychologists, social workers and nurse practitioners, will conduct psychotherapy while psychiatrists concern themselves with biological treatments. Finally, while psychoanalytic/psychodynamic psychotherapy used to be the only game in town, there are now a number of competing psychotherapies in the market place that need to be taught as well. This development has been greatly accelerated by the recent emphasis on 'evidence-based' therapies, which has led to a flurry of activity around which treatments are indicated for which disorders [2].

In this chapter this new setting in which psychotherapy is being taught to psychiatric residents is addressed and practical strategies are suggested to deal with the many challenges that must be addressed. The material is organized along the lines of the two principal settings of teaching: the classroom and supervision.

Teaching Psychiatry: Putting Theory into Practice   Edited by Linda Gask, Bulent Coskun and David Baron
© 2011 John Wiley & Sons, Ltd

9.2   Teaching Psychotherapy in the Classroom

9.2.1   Which Therapies and When? (Table 9.1)

The first question that must be asked is how many therapies can reasonably be taught in a four-year residency when there are so many competing topics that must also be covered. In the United States the Residency Review Committee responsible for developing guidelines for the core competencies necessary to graduate from psychiatric residencies has now reduced these competencies to three basic therapies: psychodynamic (brief and long term), cognitive behavioural and supportive. This group of therapies will serve the resident well with most patients who are encountered. These three therapies ideally should be taught in successive years of the residency, so that a basic skill set is learned and practised before new levels of theory and technique are added. Hence, in the second postgraduate year, a beginning seminar on long term psychodynamic psychotherapy, one on supportive therapy and one on cognitive behavioural therapy (CBT), might be offered. In that year residents should be required to start patients in psychotherapy in their various clinics so they can implement what they are learning.

In the third postgraduate year, they should be carrying at least four hours a week of individual psychotherapy using the different modalities that they are being taught. In this year they should also start to learn group and family/marital therapy, so they can take cases in those areas. Working with a senior colleague who can function both as supervisor and co-therapist may enhance the learning. The senior person may be either a faculty member or an advanced resident. An excellent way to teach psychotherapy is to include a case conference format led by a faculty member skilled in teaching psychotherapy who encourages each member of the case conference to present a current case. The class can then benefit from hearing numerous perspectives and can hear how the faculty member leading the conference ties theory to practice. The third year should also include more advanced seminars that take the basic theory and techniques learned in the second postgraduate year and apply them to more complex situations. For example, some of the specialized cognitive behaviour approaches, such as dialectical behaviour therapy (DBT), may be presented in one of their seminars. Similarly, transference-focused psychotherapy (TFP) or mentalization-based therapy (MBT), two more

Table 9.1   A proposal for the sequencing of psychotherapy teaching.

Postgraduate Year	Type of Therapy
PGYII	• Individual therapies: basic courses in CBT, Long Term Psychodynamic and Supportive • Beginning Family Therapy
PGYIII	• Individual therapies: advanced CBT and advanced Long Term Dynamic • Brief Dynamic • Newer Therapies: DBT, MBT, TFP, Motivational Interviewing, IPT • Couples, group
PGYIV	• Advanced Dynamic and CBT

advanced forms of psychodynamic therapy, can be taught as well. Some programmes might include interpersonal therapy (IPT) or motivational interviewing techniques for patients with addictions. In psychiatric training one needs to cover the major therapies by the end of the third postgraduate year, since a significant number of residents in some training programmes will opt for transition into a child psychiatry fellowship at the end of that year. For those who continue in the fourth year, advanced courses in different types of therapy can be offered.

9.2.2 Psychotherapeutic Principles Relevant in all Settings

In teaching these seminars, it is essential to tie in the psychotherapeutic principles to all of psychiatric practice rather than suggesting that they are confined to formal psychotherapy alone. In other words, since many of the residents will not be planning a career as a psychotherapist, it is important to point out that psychotherapy is a basic science of psychiatry that applies to all psychiatric settings, whether in-patient, medication clinic or diagnostic evaluation. The therapeutic alliance, resistance, transference, countertransference, automatic thoughts, schema and other psychotherapeutic principles are needed to form a solid doctor–patient relationship within which the patient feels heard, develops trust and collaborates with the doctor in the pursuit of treatment goals [2]. In this regard the faculty should emphasize that there is inevitably some psychotherapy provided in most medication management appointments. The psychiatric faculty should also make a point of including psychiatrists on the teaching faculty of the didactic seminars in psychotherapy, rather than relegating that teaching to psychologists and social workers exclusively. Our colleagues in other disciplines may do excellent teaching, but we must also demonstrate that psychotherapy is part of the psychiatrist's identity by having role models on the psychiatric faculty involved in the teaching.

9.2.3 Content and Process of Teaching

The content of the teaching of psychotherapy must include the evidence base for each modality so there is a sense of what treatments work for what conditions. However, it is necessary also to teach the limits of randomized controlled trials in guiding what is done with patients [3, 4]. Absence of evidence is not evidence of absence and many patients seen have complex comorbidities that make it difficult to apply the research to the clinical setting. Still other patients come with complaints that are not disorder based. Human suffering does not fit neatly into a category of illness.

Didactic teaching of psychotherapy must be varied in style and process as well as in content. Lecturing can be dry after a while, and instructors should seek to include DVD or video demonstrations. Some can be with real patients but, since breach of confidentiality is a major problem, clips from film and television are also useful. They are especially instructive about what NOT to do [5]. In addition, recent textbooks [4, 6] have included DVDs with excellent depictions of psychotherapy using actors to portray real patients in actual vignettes from the therapists' practices. These are of great value for residents, who are always asking to see senior clinicians at work. In addition, the old-fashioned one-way mirror approach is also useful in teaching. As noted above, case presentations in which one of the residents presents to the others are extremely valuable, since they provide an interactive setting where clinical dilemmas can be identified and discussed amongst the class in terms of different strategies that might be viable.

An ever-present challenge is that some students will not be interested in learning and may not show up for class. Attendance should be required, with consequences attached to falling below a specified level of attendance. To deal with the well-known fact that residents often do not do the assigned reading, it is useful to begin each class with a few questions that derive directly from the reading, so that all must be involved in answering the questions presented. Finally, teachers must look for ways to inspire interest in the students. One method is to demonstrate psychotherapeutic principles by bringing in examples from psychiatric practice settings that are not specifically psychotherapeutic. Another time-honoured approach is to study a complex case and demonstrate advanced technical skills by interviewing the patient in front of the residents.

9.3   Supervision

9.3.1   Structural Considerations

Supervision provides a one-to-one learning experience where the beginning therapist can be vulnerable in a safe setting. To make this setting safe, however, the supervisor needs to work diligently at creating a climate where those supervised can make mistakes, risk making fools of themselves, ask questions that they may think are 'stupid' and share countertransference feelings. Without this climate a set of familiar problems emerge in supervision: (i) the supervisee does not show up; (ii) the supervisee tries to impress the supervisor by sounding as though no problems are occurring in the therapy (receiving a good evaluation from the supervisor may be of greater importance than learning how to do psychotherapy); (iii) the supervisee constructs an 'as if' supervision, in which the real content of the therapy is not shared for fear of being criticised or shamed. Instead, a filtered version of 'what I wish I had said' is presented for the supervisor's approval.

To avoid these common problems, the supervisor needs to spend some time at the beginning of the supervision, perhaps in the first meeting, outlining what supervision requires from both parties to make it work. The supervisor must be patient and empathic with the supervisee's learning curve. The supervisee must attend regularly and make an effort to incorporate what the supervisor is teaching. Of great importance is for the supervisee to report accurately what is happening in the therapy. It is useful, in this regard, to say to the supervisee something like: 'Effective supervision depends on your sharing as accurately as you can, what the patient says and what you say. I can help you learn to be a good psychotherapist only if you sincerely share your struggles. A good rule of thumb is this: if there is anything you feel you must conceal from me because you are embarrassed about it, the supervisory session should begin with that information. I promise you that I will not shame you or humiliate you for taking that risk. I have made mistakes, too, and I have learned from them'.

There are a number of regulatory considerations that must be taken into account when one sets out to teach therapy through supervision. In the United States, for example, the Residency Review Committee requires two supervisory hours a week with two different supervisors. This requirement makes good sense. It allows for the resident to divide up cases between two different supervisors so that a single session or two can be dissected in considerable detail during an hour of supervision. Moreover, it allows for the assignment of one supervisor who is psychodynamic, for example, and one who is cognitive behavioural in orientation. Sometimes a third supervisor is needed for group and or family/couples therapy. These supervisors should change from year to year so that the supervisee is exposed to many different points of view and therapeutic styles.

9.3.2 Techniques in Supervision

One of the major debates amongst psychiatric educators revolves around how the data from therapy should be presented to the supervisor. A substantial number of educators advocate video recordings [7]. The advantage of this approach is that the supervisor can see the non-verbal forms of relatedness in addition to what is said. Also, the transcript is verbatim rather than filtered through the process of memory. The disadvantages are several. Firstly, what one may hear and see may be different from the way one actually practices. Konrad Lorenz [8] is said to have commented that one cannot observe an animal in its natural habitat because the presence of the observer compromises the natural habitat. In a similar vein, if patient and therapist are aware of the video camera or the tape recorder, they may alter what they say accordingly. Confidentiality is a cornerstone of psychotherapy. It allows the patient to say the most shameful fantasies and painful memories openly without fearing that they will have consequences in some setting outside of therapy. The presence of a recording device may discourage that openness. Some patients may feel that their rights are violated with taping but will not have the courage to bring it up for fear of disappointing their therapists. Many in the United States think there may be a legal risk in taping sessions as well if negative consequences result from using the clips for teaching or presentations.

Some supervisors like to have more-or-less verbatim process notes from the supervisee. The obvious problem with this request is that verbatim notes are not possible. No one can write that fast or remember that well. In addition, if one were to undertake such an effort during a session, it would be almost impossible to reflect with the patient on what is being said and to observe the patient's non-verbal affective states associated with the various topics of discussion. Many supervisors suggest that the resident simply take a few notes after the session that capture an outline of what was said with particular attention to specific interventions that the therapist tried. This approach is usually a bit more manageable. It also conveys to supervisees that they can trust their unconscious to bring up the key points that occurred in the session.

Supervisory techniques and strategies must be tailored to the supervisee (Table 9.2). Different approaches are more helpful to some than to others [4, 9]. Some do well with Socratic questioning. As the supervisee reports on the process, the supervisor periodically asks open-ended questions that encourage the resident to reflect and make formulations about what is going on. This strategy teaches autonomy so that beginning psychotherapists can think for themselves. The supervisor conveys a sense of confidence in the supervisee –

Table 9.2 Supervision techniques.

- Create climate of openness
- Emphasize candid discussion of the behaviours and comments that the resident most wishes to conceal
- Discuss countertransference in the here and now
- Socratic questioning
- Role playing
- Remembering the session from process notes
- Video taping/Audio taping
- Frank discussion of areas needing improvement

---

that is, there is an implicit message to the student that he or she is bright enough to come up with compelling formulations about the patient and the process.

Role playing can also be extremely useful. When the supervisee is willing to play the role of the patient with the supervisor in the role of the therapist, both parties have a good deal of fun and many benefits arise from the 'acting' that is going on. First of all, the resident gets to see how the supervisor would handle difficult situations that arise in the therapy. They may be surprised at how direct or how humorous the supervisor is in their effort to break an impasse with the patient. It models good therapy. Another benefit is that the supervisor is provided with a first-hand experience of what it's like to be in the room with the patient. When the resident enacts the patient, many features of the patient come out that may have not been clear in a verbal recounting of a session. Hence, the supervisor's understanding of the patient and empathy for the therapist are both enhanced. Finally, when the supervisee 'gets inside' the patient to role play how the patient behaves, they may find that there is a greater understanding of the patient as a result.

Exploration of countertransference may also be a valuable technique with those supervisees who are comfortable with it. This approach must be delicate in that it brings up the dilemma of whether one is teaching or treating [10]. It is probably best to stay at the level of the here-and-now rather than delving into the supervisee's childhood problems and their current problems in intimate relationships. For example, a supervisee might gently ask, 'What were you feeling when the patient was talking about this stuff?' If the supervisee is comfortable enough admit that they had angry, sexual, envious, bored, or admiring responses to the patient, then the resident learns first-hand how countertransferences influence one's understanding, one's interventions and one's feelings about meeting with the patient. Sometimes one can open up these issues with a few direct questions, such as, 'What does this patient look like? Is he attractive?' or 'Does this patient tend to bore you with these long, rambling stories?' This approach gives the resident permission to be open about what they are experiencing. After all, a fundamental teaching point in psychotherapy education is that the therapist is free to think anything at all without censoring it. Thinking is different from enacting and often what is in the therapist's mind is a clue to what's going on in the patient.

Finally, there must be a candid discussion of areas requiring improvement along with praise and encouragement for what is going well. Otherwise, the resident will feel ambushed by any negative comments on the evaluation at the end of the year.

9.4 Administrative Issues in Psychiatry Education

Many residents will not comply with regulations and have to be monitored. Those responsible for psychotherapy training must keep track of when supervision is started and if the resident is attending regularly. Remedial assignments may be required for those who are egregious in their non-compliance with the regulations. One must also monitor how actively the resident is pursuing a patient who has been assigned or how often the resident is making appointment with intakes to look for a suitable patient. In systems where fees are payable at the time of service, it is of great value for residents to learn how to deal with the setting and collection of fees while in training. A perennial problem in such settings is that many trainees are reluctant to enforce the payment of the fee and allow a large bill to accumulate. This too must be monitored, and teaching must be done to demonstrate that there is great therapeutic value in exploring the fee and its meaning to the patient. Often beginning therapists feel they are not skilled enough to warrant collecting a fee, and the supervisor must help them with that professional self-esteem issue.

9.5 Conclusions

Teaching of psychotherapy in psychiatric residencies today requires inspiring faculty members who can help inexperienced, disinterested and naïve trainees see the value of systematically exploring the life of the mind. Classroom and supervisory teaching must be thoughtfully presented not as isolated components of psychiatric training that are split off from the rest of the curriculum. Rather, psychotherapy training should be presented as a set of skills required for all of psychiatric practice – the essence of the doctor–patient relationship without which treatments of any kind will be compromised.

References

1. Mojtabai, R. and Olfson, M. (2008) National trends in psychotherapy by office-based psychiatrists. *Archives of General Psychiatry*, **65**, 962–970.
2. Roth, A. and Fonagy, P. (2005) *What Works for Whom? A Critical Review of Psychotherapy Research*, 2nd edn, Guilford, New York, NY.
3. Shedler, J. (2010) The efficacy of psychodynamic psychotherapy. *American Psychologist*, **65**, 98–109.
4. Gabbard, G.O. (2010) *Long-Term Psychodynamic Psychotherapy*, 2nd edn, American Psychiatric Publishing, Arlington, VA.
5. Gabbard, G.O. and Horowitz, M. (2010) Using Media to Teach How Not to Do Psychotherapy, *Academic Psychiatry*, **34**, 27–30.
6. Wright, J.H., Basco, M.R. and Thase, M.E. (2005) *Learning Cognitive Behavior Therapy: An Illustrated Guide*, American Psychiatric Publishing, Arlington, VA.
7. Alpert, M. (1996) Videotaping therapy. *Journal of Psychotherapy Practice and Research*, **5**, 93–105.
8. Lorenz, K. (1997) *The Natural Science of the Human Species: an Introduction to Comparative Behavioural Research* (Trans. by R.D. Martin). MIT Press, Cambridge.
9. Lomax, J.W., Andrews, L.B., Burruss, J.W. and Moorey, S. (2005) Psychotherapy supervision, in *Oxford Textbook of Psychotherapy* (eds G.O. Gabbard, J.S. Beck and J. Holmes), Oxford University Press, Oxford, pp. 495–506.
10. Gabbard, G.O. and Lester, E.P. (2003) *Boundaries & Boundary Violations in Psychoanalysis*, American Psychiatric Publishing, Arlington, VA.

10

Teaching Psychotherapy: Case Discussion Groups

Mark Oliver Evans

Gaskell House Psychotherapy Centre, Manchester, UK

10.1   Introduction

Michael Balint, a psychoanalyst, first introduced a form of group work with general practitioners as a way of helping them to manage patients that they were struggling to help. Since these pioneering research/training seminars began in 1949, case discussion groups (CDGs), otherwise known as Balint groups, have developed and spread to many countries, including the United Kingdom, Germany, Israel and the United States of America, and they are now widely used for training general practitioners and psychiatrists. Since Balint's death, his work has continued to flourish influenced by his wife, Enid, and various national societies that have been set up. CDGs are now a part of mandatory psychiatry training in the United Kingdom.

In his book, *The Doctor, His Patient and the Illness*, [1] Balint emphasizes the importance of listening. *'The ability to listen is a new skill, necessitating a considerable though limited change in the doctor's personality.'* He therefore considered that such groups cannot only be a powerful medium for change in a doctor's skills set but also (albeit in a limited way) in their personality itself.

10.2   What are Case Discussion Groups?

CDGs are commonly used for training and continuing professional development in primary care settings. However, for the purposes of this chapter, the focus is on their application in psychiatry training.

Teaching Psychiatry: Putting Theory into Practice   Edited by Linda Gask, Bulent Coskun and David Baron
© 2011 John Wiley & Sons, Ltd

CDGs are typically made up of between six and ten trainees with one facilitator, who might be a psychotherapist or a psychiatrist with an interest and experience in psychotherapy. Training groups usually meet weekly and each session lasts between 60 and 90 minutes. There is an expectation that trainees will attend as frequently as possible and that they will give notice of absence. The lifespan of CDGs is often between six months and one year, although some 'slow open' groups exist that run over longer periods. It is helpful for the facilitator to foster the maintenance of a boundary around the group so that external pressures, such as emergency work, do not intrude. Another function of the facilitator is to keep the CDG to its task of examining the doctor–patient relationship, rather than colluding with avoidance of this by, for example, getting into diagnostic debates or allowing the group to become a therapeutic group for the trainees' own personal issues.

Typically, one or two cases are discussed at each group without the use of medical notes. Presentations are kept to about ten minutes and the presenter is then encouraged to listen to the ensuing discussion between the non-presenting trainees. Their task is to acknowledge and find meaning for feelings aroused and to focus on what is happening within the therapeutic relationship. Ground rules of courtesy, confidentiality and listening until a person has clarified what they wish to say are necessary, as are time, commitment and a willingness to look for meaning.

There is some variation around how CDGs are run. Some focus entirely on Balint's original method as described above, whereas others include aspects of theory or skills teaching in certain weeks throughout the course. In addition, there are some training groups running which call themselves CDGs but which bear little or no resemblance to Balint groups. Sackin [2] describes three categories of such groups: those where cases are selected to illustrate a topic or theme; those that are primarily supportive and do not go into any detail about the therapeutic relationship; and those that are primarily problem solving and examining evidence and quality of care. For the purposes of this chapter, these other types of group are not focused on further and here the terms 'Case Discussion Group' and 'Balint group' are used interchangeably to mean the same thing.

10.3   What Learning Takes Place in CDGs?

Previous CDG research has focused mainly on self-report measures of professional attitudes, confidence and skills, predominantly in primary care settings. Improvements in 'comfort in dealing with emotional/clinical situations' [3], 'sense of control of work' [4] and 'professionalism' [5] have all been reported. Cataldo et al. [6] found that in a family residency programme, those trainees that completed CDG training were more satisfied with their choice of speciality. Turner and Malm [7], Rabinowitz et al. [8] and Graham et al. [9] used specifically designed outcome measures and found that subjects reported increased psychological skills at the end of the CDGs. Rabin et al. [10] found that attendance at a Balint group helped a selected group of immigrant doctors with high levels of professional distress to improve their 'psychosocial skills'.

There is also evidence that CDGs can improve a doctor's ability to tune into the emotional aspects of patients. Using restricted qualitative methods, Maoz et al. [11], Samuel [12] and Pinder et al. [13] found that mental health professionals were able to reflect more on both patients and the professional–patient relationship after a CDG. Von Klitzing [14], using a more extensive text analysis, found similar results.

Graham *et al.* [9] carried out the most in depth qualitative analysis of trainee psychiatrist's involvement in CDGs, and so these findings will be discussed in more detail. In this study they interviewed seventeen psychiatric residents and counsellors in two parallel CDGs at a UK psychotherapy service. Three questions were addressed: Does change occur in a CDG? What is changing during the process of the CDG? What is the process of the change?

A coding template was developed by reading early transcripts of interviews. This was subsequently elaborated through challenge by the research group and went through several iterations before being used to code the 17 end point transcripts. Three major themes emerged: (i) CDGs are anxiety provoking for trainees; (ii) CDGs were instrumental in learning; and (iii) some trainees struggled to use the CDGs productively.

Trainees appeared to find CDGs anxiety provoking for several reasons. Firstly, being in a group situation itself can be anxiety provoking for many people; this is not specific to CDGs. However, the experience of being in CDGs is a new one for most trainees who, despite being told about what is expected of them, find the early weeks unsettling as they start to accommodate to a new way of working which combines both thinking and feeling. Some of the anxiety is about connecting with feelings and what this might lead to. Will I expose myself too much? Will it get too personal? How will I manage negative feelings? Will it be contained within the group? How will I compare to others in this way of working? Sometimes the anxiety is defended against through lateness and poor attendance; this needs to be addressed by the facilitator.

Despite these anxieties, there was good evidence that trainees changed both in the way that they thought about their patients and about themselves as health care professionals (Table 10.1). They described being better able to understand case dynamics which were generalizable to other patients that had not been presented in the CDGs. This growing

Table 10.1 Themes suggesting that change did occur.[a]

Better understanding of the case dynamics:
It's only by going to the groups that I could have an increased understanding of the issue ... 'Why did this person do this or say that?' And I think it's the accumulation of this every week, sort of, you know it will probably come to my mind whenever somebody says something like that.

Developing awareness of own feelings from others:
I think the biggest revelation was that by telling everybody else about your patient, it allowed other people to get an idea of something I hadn't even fully got an idea of myself.

Introducing a new perspective or conceptual framework:
... before psychotherapy was like a no-go area, I didn't know anything about it, but doing the group ... it's sort of opened up this field for me, and I feel now that it's not as scary.

Talking about feelings engendered by patients:
[Previously] it felt quite difficult to ... own up ... and tell a group of people how I was feeling about this patient. But I'm really glad I did because it's made a difference to the way that I dealt with this guy, a big difference actually.

Ability to stay with feelings:
When I presented a case and I got some support from the facilitator ... it was a very tricky case and I think I needed to be held ... this person had a disability and it was about staying with the awfulness of it, because actually it wouldn't change. And I was finding it quite difficult to actually stay put with the awfulness.

[a] Reprinted with permission from *Academic Psychiatry* (Copyright 2009). American Psychiatric Publishing, Inc. [9]

Table 10.2   Change Occurred Through Several Pathways.[a]

Adherence to previous model:

I don't envisage myself ever working in a psychodynamic way . . . it doesn't really fit with my sort of
  frames of reference or philosophies about things generally.

Group as a container to help process feelings:

And that did feel better . . . you take a lot home . . . the patient stays with you . . . and I've had the
  courage to bring this to the group and we've been able to process it in a way which has made it
  more manageable, and it has worked.

Development of self-reflective practice:

I think that the biggest moment of recognition was when I realized another patient did something a
  bit similar . . . [I understood this] based on the knowledge that I'd gained in the groups . . . it was
  sort of like slowly percolating through . . .

Accommodation to a new model:

but the group turned out to be a lot more than I thought, because in one way it made me realize,
  hang on a minute, perhaps there is a big gap in my skills.

Extension to thinking about own personal life:

Her [the patient's] problem was that she told her baby to 'just go away' . . . a four month old doesn't
  understand what to do in that situation? And then I realized that my husband does this with our
  kids and it really annoys me. And I think you shouldn't say that to children. It's not right to put
  your needs before their needs."

---

[a] Reprinted with permission from *Academic Psychiatry* (Copyright 2009). American Psychiatric Publishing, Inc. [9]

familiarization with a way of thinking about patients was described by some trainees as
a useful way of introducing a new conceptual framework, psychoanalytic psychotherapy,
which had been previously experienced as a 'no-go area', foreign or alien. When trainees
did present their patients, some reported surprise and increased curiosity that there was so
much to think about. By describing a case and hearing the reactions and elicited feelings
of others in the group, it allowed the presenting trainee to acknowledge their own hidden
thoughts and feelings, which might then be expressed. Also, over the course of the CDGs,
the group became more used to and able to stay with difficult feelings in the room without
resorting to defensive strategies, such as cutting off or focusing on purely medical or cognitive
aspects.

  The change appeared to occur through several pathways (Table 10.2). As learning progressed, participants moved from the comfort of their own professional mode and slowly
adopted a dynamic perspective. Initially this involved clarification of psychodynamic language and theory. With the group acting as a 'container' to process their difficult feelings,
overtime this process was internalized in the individual trainees. Reflective practice developed and meaning was increasingly found in interactions with patients. Participants reported
being better able to examine their own emotions, were better able to work at the interface
of their own and patients feelings and were more able to pragmatically use psychoanalytic
concepts. Another striking and important finding was the degree to which this way of
working impacts on trainees own personal and professional lives. There were many examples
of participants thinking about their home life in new ways that were challenging not only
for the individuals but for their families and intimate relationships. Also, there were reports
of participants re-evaluating their work roles and how individuals with their own feelings

and personalities accommodated to these. In particular, there was a sense of trainees being increasingly able to 'be themselves' within the confines of professional roles. Sometimes, traumatic incidents from earlier in their medical training that had not previously been adequately worked through were remembered and reflected on in the light of new learning. It is important to acknowledge the containing milieu of the group as being an essential background ingredient in allowing the above processes to occur. Participants needed to feel safe enough to allow a process of change, which is at once potentially exciting but also challenging.

Some participants struggled to use CDGs productively, especially if they were new to a dynamic model. They might appear to be reading 'from a script' or would not seem to be connected to their own feelings in the discussion. There was a sense of a two dimensional quality to the presentations, which would not bring the patient to life. Others appeared to feel more at ease but remained sceptical about the lack of scientific certainty in a dynamic approach. However, there was evidence that most trainees found a second (six month) CDG a different and easier experience.

10.4 Example of a Case Discussed in a CDG

The following is a brief description of the first half of a session in a brand new CDG in order to show examples of how the groups might work. Names and some detail have been changed to protect confidentiality. The group consisted of four, year one psychiatry trainees and three general practitioner (GP) trainees. They had met on three previous weeks to do some skills training before starting the Balint style groups. Dr N, a psychiatry trainee, presented the first (of two) case in the group. None of the members had had significant experience of Balint groups previously.

Dr N described with some feeling how in the first week of her post she had been asked to see a 65 year old ex-nurse with early onset dementia, who had been admitted to an in-patient ward. Dr N had attempted to manage the behavioural problems by prescribing increasing doses of antipsychotic medication at the suggestion of her consultant. She was, however, shocked to find that the nurses were critical of this approach insisting that constipation may be the problem. Dr N described finding herself striving harder and harder to understand the mixed messages she was getting from different nursing shifts about whether the patient was 'fine' or 'in distress' and spent longer and longer on the ward with the patient. She heard from the nursing staff that the relatives were 'very happy with the care' but never got to meet the relatives herself.

The facilitator was active in this session helping the group accommodate to a new way of working by getting members in turn to describe their emotional response to the material. There was a lot of initial identification with Dr N's frustration, confusion and anxious striving. This led on to some generalizations about nurses not doing their jobs properly. Sensing that that reflective thinking was being inhibited at this point and that the group was getting stuck, the facilitator intervened expressing curiosity about the mixed messages from different nurses. Dr N was then able to give more information about how the ward had only recently merged with another ward, bringing together both dementia and affective disordered patients. The group began to understand how anxiety about the out of control behaviour may have led to splits within the nursing group that followed 'lines of cleavage' determined by whether nurses saw themselves as dementia specialists or not. The facilitator remained active in wondering with the group about whether there was also splitting between the nurses and the doctors. The group began to focus on this aspect and could identify the implicit messages from some of the nurses: 'You don't know the patient like we do'; 'you don't care about her'. With some help, the group was able to begin to understand what emotions might lie behind these attitudes. Themes of envy were discussed as was the stark fact that doctors are able to leave the ward whereas nurses are required to stay with the disturbance.

The group went on to consider Dr N's striving, which allowed her to admit to her 'dread' of going on to the ward. The group began to see that this patient was getting special care from the nurses from which Dr N felt somehow excluded. Lots of ideas were being tossed around the group at this stage but the facilitator kept the discussion focussed on why this patient might be getting special care. It took a while for the group to remember that this patient had herself been a nurse and Dr N then added that she had been known socially by some of the nurses on the ward. The group then quickly came up with the hypothesis that the nursing staff were strongly identifying with the patient. The facilitator stayed with this suggestion and encouraged the group to expand on what identifying with the patient might mean and how this might explain their powerful reactions to the patient's treatment. Themes of coming into contact with one's own mortality and potential for suffering were discussed at greater length. At this point the facilitator brought the case to a close because of time pressure and it was acknowledged that there had not been time to explore other avenues, such as why only one daughter was looking after her mother with little involvement from the other siblings. There had been some discussion about 'containment', in that the patient's behaviour had not improved significantly but the relatives had seemed happy with the admission. However, the notion of how Dr N contained herself and the anxiety was only briefly mentioned. It was expected that this theme would be revisited at a future session.

10.5 Discussion

As can be seen from the above example, CDGs offer a pragmatic setting for trainees to test out and to bring alive psychoanalytic ideas about patients they are in contact with. In this case example notions of splitting, identification and containment were used to make sense of felt experience. These terms were examined and thought about with specific reference to a detailed case example and not as some disconnected theory. In this way, CDGs offer a forum in which a meaningful introduction to a psychodynamic way of thinking can be facilitated; they also offer the potential for deeper development and change. Trainees recount their experiences of CDGs as being both powerful and memorable; this can be attributed to the subject matter discussed and also to the fact that group processes are involved. These include therapeutic factors found in group therapy as described by Yalom, such as 'instillation of hope', 'group cohesiveness', 'universality' (struggling together), 'imitative behaviour' (modelling themselves on each other and the group leaders) and 'catharsis' (space to express and resonate with each others' emotions) [15]. But this process can be anxiety provoking as trainees accommodate to a new way of thinking and earlier studies in primary care settings suggest that about one third of participants will drop out [16]. However, in psychiatric training settings the groups are often mandatory.

So how are the drop outs and the significant anxiety reported in CDGs accounted for? One way of explaining this is that participants have to accommodate to what has been referred to as 'troublesome knowledge' or 'threshold concepts' [17]. Meyer and Land suggest that threshold concepts may be found in all educational fields and offer a gateway that leads to previously inaccessible understanding linking a known knowledge space to the unknown. They describe two key characteristics for such a concept: (i) it is transformative leading to a significant shift in perception or a new world view and (ii) it is irreversible, unlikely to be forgotten and more or less impossible to unlearn. When applying these concepts to psychodynamic understandings, it is worth thinking for a moment: what makes the new knowledge transformative and irreversible?

I propose that it is the fact that feelings not only matter but add essential information for interpersonal working that can be both transformative and irreversible. Perhaps because of the shocking and provocative nature of what doctors have to manage, a significant amount of medical training encourages an intrapsychic detachment of thought from feeling and it appears that this has to be re-learned. For this reason, memories of professional situations from outside of psychiatry, in which the trainee felt in some way traumatized, are often recounted in response to the work undertaken; Balint groups offer a safe space for these to be thought about and made sense of.

For some individuals with certain defensive styles, the bringing together of thoughts and feelings appears to be too challenging, leading to drop outs or disengagement with the task. However, there is a serious question about whether trainees who repeatedly struggle with this kind of work are suited to becoming psychiatrists who on a day to day basis have to recognize and manage patients' feelings. In our experience, trainees who fail in CDGs are usually also failing in other areas because of problems with their interpersonal functioning. It is therefore likely that CDGs offer a sensitive forum in which interpersonal problems are picked up at an early stage and, usually, this leads on to appropriate and successful targeted training.

References

1. Balint, M. (1957) *The Doctor, his Patient and the Illness*, Pitman Paperbacks, London.
2. Sackin, P.A. (1986) Value of case discussion groups in vocational training. *British Medical Journal*, **293**, 1543–1544.
3. Sekeres, M., Chernoff, M., Lynch, T. *et al.* (2003) The impact of a physician awareness group and the first year of training on hematology-oncology fellows. *Journal of Clinical Oncology*, **21**, 3676–3682.
4. Kjeldmand, D., Holmstrom, I. and Rosenqvist, U. (2004) Balint training makes GPs thrive better in their job. *Patient Education and Counselling*, **55**, 230–235.
5. Adams, K.E., O'Reilly, M., Romm, J. *et al.* (2006) Effect of Balint training on resident professionalism. *American Journal of Obstetrics and Gynaecology*, **195**, 1431–1437.
6. Cataldo, K.P., Peeden, K., Geesey, M.E. *et al.* (2005) Association between Balint training and physician empathy and work satisfaction. *Family Medicine*, **37**, 328–331.
7. Turner, A. and Malm, R. (2004) A preliminary investigation of Balint and non-Balint behavioural medicine training. *Family Medicine*, **36**, 114–122.
8. Rabonitz, S, Kushnir, T. and Ribak, J. (1994) Developing psychosocial mindedness and sensitivity to mental health issues among primary care nurses using the Balint group method. *Israeli Journal of Psychiatry and Related Sciences*, **31**, 280–286.

9. Graham, S., Gask, L., Swift, G. *et al.* (2009) Balint-style case discussion groups in psychiatric training: An evaluation. *Academic Psychiatry*, **33**, 198–203.

10. Rabin, S., Herz, M., Stern, M., *et al.* (1996) Improving the professional self-efficacy cognitions of immigrant doctors with Balint Groups. *Isr J Psychiatry Relat Sci*, **33**, 253–259.

11. Maoz, B., Stern, J. and Spencer, T. (1986) Developing Psychosocial Sensitivity Among Family Doctors – a content analysis of Balint Seminar Discussions. *Israeli Journal of Psychiatry and Related Sciences*, **23**, 205–213.

12. Samuel, O. (1989) How doctors learn in a Balint group. *Family Practice*, **6**, 108–113.

13. Pinder, R., Mckee, A., Sackin, P. *et al.* (2004) Conversations-within-conversation: an ethnographic approach to working across disciplines in small group work. *Work Based Learning Primary Care*, **2**, 230–240.

14. Von Klitzing, W. (1999) Evaluation of reflective learning in a psychodynamic group of nurses caring for terminally ill patients. *Journal of Advanced Nursing*, **30**, 1213–1221.

15. Yalom, I. (1995) *The theory and Practice of Group Psychotherapy*, 4th edn, Basic Books, New York.

16. Johnson, A., Brock, C. and Hueston, W. (2003) Resident physicians who continue Balint training: a longitudinal study 1982–1999. *Family Medicine*, **35**, 428–433.

17. Meyer, J. and Land, R. (2003) Threshold concepts and troublesome knowledge: linkages to ways of thinking and practising within the disciplines. *Occasional Report 4 for Enhancing Teaching-Learning Environments in Undergraduate Courses*. Economic and Social Research Council. University of Edinburgh.

11

Teaching Research Methods: 'Doing Your Own Research'

David P. Goldberg

Institute of Psychiatry, King's College, London, UK

11.1   Introduction

In this chapter the process of a one-person research project is considered from how to get an idea, to the submission of a dissertation based upon the project. Obviously, you need to adapt the talk you give to your audience: for example, if they do not wish to work on a dissertation, you will of course omit the sections on a time budget, but the section on the research protocol is necessary if your students are to have a satisfactory relationship with their supervisor. The problem that you have is how to inform them without depressing them too much with all the difficulties.

With this in mind, many more elaborate designs have been omitted, as they exceed the abilities of one-person projects. Case-control designs have been included, because they are (just about) possible for a single researcher despite the daunting problems that they have. Designs like treatment trials of drugs or psychotherapy may often involve young researchers in the fieldwork, but the assumption here is that the Principal Investigator will have control of the procedures, so that the luckless task of the lone researcher is to do as he or she is told.

The first involvement of many young psychiatrists is by acting as a 'pair of hands' is some larger study – and this may indeed whet their appetites for having a project of their own. It is to these young psychiatrists that this chapter is addressed.

11.2   Thinking of an Idea

Maybe you already have one. If so, read around your subject, including a computer search with appropriate keywords to find what has already been done about your chosen subject.

Teaching Psychiatry: Putting Theory into Practice   Edited by Linda Gask, Bulent Coskun and David Baron
© 2011 John Wiley & Sons, Ltd

Remember the mnemonic 'RUMBA' – any research by a beginner needs to be **R**elevant – that is, appropriate to problems in your clinical work; **U**nderstandable, meaning that others should be able to understand what you are trying to show; **M**easurable – preferably using measures that already exist; **B**ehaviour should be influenced; and, finally, **A**ttainable – by one person, working by themselves, with relatively little spare time. This is every bit as difficult as it sounds and that is not all, your idea should be in the form of a hypothesis that you intend to investigate.

If you haven't yet got one, ask yourself what opportunities exist either in your hospital's records system or, better still, in your everyday clinical work. It's a good idea to ask yourself what job you will be doing in six months time, as the design stage takes a good bit of time. Perhaps the consultant for whom you will be working has a problem that needs investigating – they often have, but haven't got the time or the money to do it themselves.

This leads us to the third possibility, which many people have used over the years. Find someone in your department who has a good research record and ask them whether they need your help. Whichever method you use, the need to do a literature search and express the 'aim' of your research as an hypothesis that can either be confirmed or refuted remains the same.

The other mnemonic is KISS, which stands for **K**eep **I**t **S**imple, **S**tupid. Try to avoid planning to measure one unknown variable in terms of another, it just won't work. Indeed, it would be far better to produce a new measure if one doesn't exist and try to show that you can measure it reliably. If possible, try to correlate it with some other measure as well – to produce what is called 'external validity' for the new measure. If there is a measure already, but it hasn't ever been used in the population of patients you have in mind, a useful simple step is to translate it (if necessary) and apply it.

11.3   Reading Round the Subject

You have already used a computer for a preliminary search, but you may have found that the computer produces a list of thousands of references. Ask a librarian for advice on limiting your search. You will be advised to ask for papers only in languages that you speak, and to maybe use two or more keywords, linked by 'and' (if you use 'or', the computer will of course produce an even longer list!). It may also be sufficient to ask only for the last 10 years. Your next step is to look at the abstracts of papers whose titles look interesting to you. If an abstract also looks interesting, put a checkmark against the paper and move on doggedly through the list. Most papers are clearly irrelevant from the titles, and many more from the abstracts. Try to narrow the search down to fewer than 50 papers, and then go on to the full papers. If possible, make a copy of the full paper on your computer – but also paste the full reference in a file called, perhaps, 'Preliminary notes', stating very briefly what you think is relevant about the paper. This file will allow you to remember the full reference without having to wrack your brains about why you liked it in the first place. You can also paste short excerpts from the paper into your new file, saving even more time – but maybe producing a file which is too big.

11.4   Deciding on the Method

This where you need an hypothesis, unless your research is historical, aimed at reviewing the literature on an abstruse topic. We will not be covering historical research here, but mentioning some of the designs that are possible with one person working on their own.

11.4.1   Simple Descriptive Studies

In this design either you – or your unit – has an interesting group of patients, and you decide to make a detailed study of them. Don't just look at level of mental morbidity, because by itself it does not mean very much, it needs to be related to some other variable. For example, in a group of patients with eczema to what extent does the area of skin affected vary with their mental status? In a group of patients with Crohn's disease, does mental status relate to their account of childhood abuse, or perhaps to the frequency of their diarrhoea?

11.4.2   Studies of Risk

Imagine that you divide a large group of people into four groups, those with an exposure to a possible risk factor, and those who have not. Each of these groups is further divided into those with a disorder (in our case, a mental disorder), and those who do not meet criteria for a disorder.

A *cohort study* goes forward in time, and compares all those with an exposure, reporting the risk of mental disorders, and compares that with the rate in those who have not been exposed. This is an excellent design from a research point of view, but it is not practicable for a single researcher unless he or she has access to a data set collected at some previous time point, relating to exposure. Thus, such a study compares $a/(a + b)$ with $c/(c + d)$ in the table below, and produces a figure called a '*relative risk*'.

	With mental disorder ('sick')	Without disorder ('healthy')
Exposed to risk factor	'a'	'b'
Not exposed to risk factor	'c'	'd'

However, a variant of the design is the *case-control study*, which looks backwards in time, and records exposure in those with, and without, the mental disorder. Thus, it compares a/c with b/d in the same table, and expresses this ratio as ad/cb, which is called the 'odds ratio'. If this is near unity – or to be more precise, if unity is within the 90% confidence limits of the odds ratio – then there is no significant risk within the 'sick' group compared with the 'healthy' group.

An example of such a study is that by Dworkin and his colleagues [1], who measured depression, and counted the number of different pains, in a consecutive set of patients coming to primary care.

	No. of pains: No. of patients:	Odds ratio for depression
None	371	1
One pain	346	1.04
Two pains	205	5.74
3+ pains	94	8.55

In this example, the patients who were complaining of pain are being compared with those who have no pain, but are consulting for some other reason. So, by definition, their odds ratio is unity. It can be seen that those with only a single pain are no more likely to be depressed than those without pain, but after two different pains are present the odds of depression rises very sharply. Because numbers of patients decreases with each increase in the number of pains, those with 'three or more' have been grouped together.

Such studies are very seductive to a lone investigator, and should by all means be undertaken provided that a number of problems are dealt with:

i. *Incident or prevalent cases?*
Although all those with a disorder are much easier to come by, we need to confine ourselves to new, or incident cases, since we are interested in aetiology.

ii. *Selection bias*
Do your controls, without the disorder, give you a biased estimate of risk? It is fairly easy to find controls amongst staff in your hospital, but they may have been selected for health. Ideally, friends or neighbours of patient, or non-affected relatives are much better. As a general rule, a control should become part of the index group if he or she were to develop the condition you are looking for.

iii. *Information bias*
'Recall bias' means that those with disorder recall exposure better: the remedy is to use structured questionnaires with incident cases, and interview either close relatives, or controls with a different disorder. 'Observer bias' means that you may be tempted to probe index cases more closely than your controls, but this can be avoided if you tape record the interviews, or use a computer administered interview, or 'blind' the researcher to whether the subject has been exposed to the risk.

iv. *Confounding*
Finally, you need to ensure that some other variable does not lie behind the relationship you are investigating. Confounders cannot only lead to spurious associations, but can even eliminate an association that is really present. Possible confounders include sex, age, social class, presence of children at home. An imaginary example may make this clearer.

Suppose we suspect that there is a relationship between whether one likes chocolate, and whether one develops depression.

	Depressed	Not depressed
Likes chocolate	65	500
No special preferences	25	650

The odds ratio here is (65 × 650) divided by (25 × 500) = 3.38

So, at first glance it looks as though chocaholics are more than three times as likely to develop depression. But what is we stratify the sample for gender?

Males only

	Depressed	Not depressed	
Likes chocolate	5	200	
No preference	15	600	Odds ratio = 1

Females only

	Depressed	Not depressed	
Likes chocolate	60	300	
No preference	10	50	Odds ratio = 1

So, while there is no relationship between liking chocolate and becoming depressed, girls are more likely to be depressed than boys, and are also more likely to prefer chocolate, and this is *confounding* the result of the whole study.

Do not allow these problems to put you off doing a case-control study – but please remember that they can produce misleading results! The remedies for confounding are to match the groups for potential confounders; to use multiple controls for each case (this increases the power of your comparison); to restrict the study to a narrow range of variables; and to stratify by the presence or absence of each potential confounder.

11.4.3 Two-Stage Screening Studies

Sometimes you wish to discover the patients with probable mental disorders using a screening test, since you want to interview the patients yourself, but do not want to spend most of your time interviewing non-cases. The advice that follows applies to all screening tests, whether for a specific disorder, or for global notions like 'psychological distress'.

There are two quite different ways of thinking about scores on your chosen screen: if you are using a categorical model for mental disorders, then you have to decide on a threshold, but if you have a dimensional model then an increasing score just indicates an increasing indicator of severity of psychological distress.

If the former – and you wish to identify those with a high probability of caseness – then you have to decide on the threshold between cases and non-cases. However, this threshold itself is determined by the prevalence of disorders in your chosen population, being higher with greater prevalences. (A full discussion is given in Goldberg *et al.* [2], Furukawa *et al.* [3].) A quick way with the General Health Questionnaire is to give the screen to a set of 50 or so people, and use the mean score for the whole set to determine your best cutting threshold.

	Found to be Non-cases	Found to be Cases
High scorers	False positives 'a'	True positives 'b'
Low scorers	True negatives 'c'	False negatives 'd'
Totals	All non-cases (a + c)	All cases (b + d)

Specificity = Proportion of non-cases who are true negatives = c × 100 / (a + c) Sensitivity = Proportion of cases who are true positives = b × 100 / (b + d))

Positive predictive value (PPV) = Proportion of high scorers who are cases = b × 100 / (a + b)

You can either have one threshold, and sample as many people as possible with high scores, and an equal size random sample of low scorers, or several thresholds with decreasing probability of sampling with lower score ranges. Whichever you choose, it is necessary to reconstruct the characteristics of the original sample before calculating sensitivity and specificity. The reason for this is that any screening procedure will, by definition, under-sample those with low scores, so if you use your raw data there will be too few true negatives and false negatives, and so your estimate of specificity will be too low, and sensitivity will be too high.

Original population	Total screened	Selected for interview
High scores	178	102
Low scores	375	98
Total	543	200

Of the 102 high scorers, 13 turned out to be non-cases and 89 were true positives, while of the 98 low scorers 94 were true negatives and 4 were cases. So, the high scorers were under-sampled by $178/102 = 1.75$, while the low scorers were under-sampled by $375/98 = 3.80$. We can undo the original sampling fraction by multiplying by the under-sampling (13 and 89 by 1.75, and 94 and 4 by 3.8), producing the following – which add to the total number in the original sample of 553 people:

	Non-cases	Cases
High scores	22.7	155.3
Low scores	359.4	15.3
Total	382.1	170.6

Only now can you calculate specificity, which will be $359.4 \times 100 / 382.1 = 94.06\%$, and sensitivity, which will be $155.3 \times 100 / 170.6 = 91.03\%$. These figures are independent of prevalence.

The positive predictive value (PPV) of a screening test is the value that clinicians are most interested in, since it is the proportion of true positives amongst high scorers – but it is highly dependent upon prevalence. The higher the prevalence, the larger the PPV. It follows that all screening tests are relatively inefficient in populations with low prevalence.

11.5 The Research Protocol

When contemplating a new research project, it is helpful to write out a brief document describing what you are thinking of doing. If you are preparing a dissertation, it is essential to do this. It is a document that you will show to your supervisor and re-draft as suggestions are made to you or your thinking develops. You should have your first draft of this document before going to see your supervisor; on that preliminary visit you may have to leave some of these headings blank. The document starts with your name and the name of your potential supervisor. The whole thing can be on a single sheet of A4 paper.

You'll need a *Title*, and it is safer if you use a fairly general one to start with. The next heading is *Aim*, and that is easily the most important – it should be in the form of a hypothesis, typically that some positive relationship exists between two variables. You then investigate this by trying to 'disprove the null hypothesis' that no such relationship exists. The *Background* really need not be at all long ,but it should give your supervisor some idea of why you suspect the relationship that you are investigating. Try not to write more than three sentences – you are not writing up your research yet!

Your *method* should describe what measures you intend to use, and what patients will be approached. You may need several different measures of your main variables, unless there is one that is generally accepted. Your patients might be in two different groups – perhaps different forms of a similar disorder, like bulimia and anorexia nervosa, or you may want to compare a patient group with 'normal' controls. Whichever of these are true, you need to collect demographic data such as gender, age, social class and racial group, to ensure that your two groups may be different only because they are not, in fact, comparable at all. The final headings are *Statistical treatment of results*, in which you briefly state which statistical tests you intend to use and give a power calculation to decide upon sample size (see below), and *ethical approval*. These last headings may be left blank while you first discuss your ideas with a potential supervisor, but aim to complete the whole thing before you start any fieldwork.

A new set of problems must now be addressed: Will you be able to find enough patients of the kind that you are interested in? Has the consultant(s) responsible for these patients given their permission to approach them? Have you decided exactly what you intend to tell these patients about the purpose of your research, in order that you can obtain approval from your local ethics committee? Once the protocol is in an advanced draft, obtain an application form from your local ethics committee.

11.6 Sample Size

Power is the ability of a test to show that a relationship exists, when it *does* exist. (Also called 'false negative', or Type 2 error.) Is sample size big enough?

Significance is the probability we shall make a false claim, and say a relationship exists which did so only by chance. (Also called 'false positive', or Type 1 error.) It is usual to set power at 0.80 (giving an 80% chance of showing a relationship), with significance at 0.05 (giving a 5% chance of a false claim).

How big a difference would you be impressed by? The smaller the difference you are expecting to find, the larger the sample that you will need. For example, with power at 0.80, and significance at 0.05:

Difference (%)	Sample size
30	95
15	160
10	360

There is a nomogram giving more details in Altman [4], or fuller details can be found in Machin and Campbell [5]. Alternatively, you can use either a specialized sample size package, such as 'Nquery', or an option within a multipurpose package, such as 'sampsi' in Stata.

11.7 The Time Budget

If you intend to submit a dissertation, it is quite helpful to work out how much time you have to spare if it is to be completed by a known date. To do this start with today's date, end with time research must be handed in. Allow sufficient time for instrument preparation, and maybe a week or so to try out the procedures in a pilot study. Be fairly generous in working out time for the main fieldwork, as some patients may refuse to participate or fail to keep their appointments with you. Processing your results will certainly take longer than you think at the planning stage, and you will need to start the writing up while this is occurring. Allow time for your supervisor to read it, and then more time for you to make corrections. There should also be some time allowed for 'injury time', to allow for unexpected events. It is usual to find that you have less time than you thought!

A final checklist

✓ Are you now trained in the clinical interview you intend to use?

✓ Are the measuring instruments appropriate in your setting?

✓ Are the patients available, will the nurses cooperate?

✓ Have you obtained ethical committee approval?

✓ If so, try it all out. If you have to change anything, call it a pilot study, and do not include the findings in your results.

✓ Arrange a meeting with your supervisor to report that all is now ready.

11.8 Conclusion

It is best to assume that your audience will contain some members who already know several of the topics that you choose to cover, but this should not deter you from covering them for the others. Even if you have a dim grasp of an important principle, it does no harm to hear it again. The teaching on power and significance is a good opportunity to explain the low power of most treatment trials, and the reason that multicentre designs have to be used to achieve an acceptable power for the design.

Your lecture should be illustrated with examples, not all of them drawn from your own particular interests. For example, when discussing studies of risk, it is helpful to give an example of a cohort study, taking the opportunity of explaining why they are never possible for lone researchers. Seeing the actual numbers, combined with an explanation of how long such a study takes, makes a far more vivid example than a monotonous account of the theoretical difficulties.

To achieve this aim you will definitely need to prepare a set of slides, illustrated by examples. Make sure that you leave at least 20 minutes for people to ask you questions at the end: do not plan a lecture that goes right up to the wire. It is impossible to predict what members of your audience really want to know, nor can you be sure that an explanation that was clear to you will be clear to others.

References

1. Dworkin, S., VonKorff, M. and LeResche, L. (1990) Multiple pains, psychiatric and psychosocial disturbance and epidemiological investigation. *Archives of General Psychiatry*, **47**, 239–245.

2. Goldberg, D.P., Oldehinkel, T., and Ormel, J. (1998) Why GHQ threshold varies from one place to another. *Psychological Medicine*, **28**, 915–921.

3. Furukawa, T.A., Goldberg, D.P., Rabe-Hesketh, S. and Ustun, T.B. (2001) Stratum-specific likelihood ratios of two versions of the General Health Questionnaire. *Psychological Medicine*, **31** 519–529.

4. Altman, D.G. (1980) Statistics and ethics in medical research: III How large a sample? *BMJ*, **281**, 1336–1338.

5. Machin, D. and Campbell, M.J. (2005) *The Design of Studies for Medical Research*, John Wiley & Sons Ltd (also available online).

12

Teaching Psychiatry Students About Cultural Diversity

Nisha Dogra[1] and Niranjan Karnik[2]
[1]*Greenwood Institute of Child Health, University of Leicester, Leicester, UK*
[2]*Pritzker School of Medicine, The University of Chicago, Chicago, IL, USA*

12.1   Introduction

In this chapter some of the terminology used in this area and the issues that this raises for educators is introduced. Some issues that warrant consideration when developing diversity curricula are then discussed. An educational framework that may be useful to review in the early stages of devising a curriculum is outlined. Finally, a checklist that educators may find helpful when planning diversity programmes for either undergraduate or postgraduate trainees in psychiatry is provided. In this chapter there is no differentiation between the two groups of students; instead a more general approach is taken. However, a section is included that contrasts the specific issues that educators for each group may face. Also included is a case example that illustrates the contents of this chapter. It is not within the scope of this chapter to focus on the academic debate in the area of terminology but the reader will be referred to these areas of debate and justification provided why it is an important area for educators to be aware of. As the focus of this text is teaching, the focus on the educational and pedagogical aspects of teaching diversity.

12.2   Definitions of Key Terms

Within the health care arena, there is considerable confusion about the use of key terms such as 'race', 'ethnicity', 'culture' and 'multiculturalism', as highlighted by Mulholland and Dyson [1] amongst others. None of these terms or their usage is value free. The way terms

---

Teaching Psychiatry: Putting Theory into Practice   Edited by Linda Gask, Bulent Coskun and David Baron
© 2011 John Wiley & Sons, Ltd

are used reflects underlying values and philosophies. For example, if it is believed that there are biological differences between people on the basis of their skin colour, the biological construct around race is likely to be acceptable. However, if it is believed that that skin colour is more about social reflections than biology, the use of it as a biological fact is unlikely to be acceptable. There are also many debates around the use of these terms and the contexts they have developed from. From a health care perspective, some of the debates are rather academic and forget that, at the heart of the issue, people and their lives are being talked about. Rather than think about culture and cultural identity as being based on ethnicity alone, we would like to suggest that for the purposes of thinking about patients, it is more useful to think about culture being dependent on many different factors in relationship to the group or groups with whom he or she identifies. In this regard, Ward Goodenough's [2] classic definition of culture as 'whatever it is one has to know or believe in order to operate in manner acceptable to its members' seems at the broadest level of our understanding. Culture changes and is dynamic and, therefore, can be moderated by many factors. Culture, while not always tied to race or ethnicity, defines how we interpret and interact with others through these and many other factors. This may fit more with the concept of personal identity, which is helpful for the context in which health care is usually delivered. This working definition has been derived from the Association of American Medical Colleges (AAMC) [3] which stated that:

> Culture is defined by each person in relationship to the group or groups with whom he or she identifies. An individual's cultural identity may be based on heritage as well as individual circumstances and personal choice. Cultural identity may be affected by such factors as race, ethnicity, age, language, country of origin, acculturation, sexual orientation, gender, socio-economic status, religious/spiritual beliefs, physical abilities, occupation, among others. These factors may impact behaviours such as communication styles, diet preferences, health beliefs, family roles, lifestyle, rituals and decision-making processes. All of these beliefs and practices, in turn can influence how patients and heath care professionals perceive health and illness and how they interact with one another.

This definition centres on how individuals define themselves rather than how others define them. It also suggests that individuals draw upon a range of resources and that, through the interplay of external and internal meanings, they construct a sense of identity and a unique cultural experience. Patients will therefore define which aspects of their cultural belonging are relevant at any particular point. This may change in different clinical contexts, at different stages of an individual's life and may also depend on the clinical presentation itself. For example, the issue of gender may be more relevant to a woman when she is faced with the possibility of a mastectomy because of breast cancer, than in the case where abdominal surgery may be required (although of course this may raise other issues). Such a perspective is also useful because it recognizes that both patients and professionals bring a complex individual self to the consultation. Finally, it acknowledges that people are not neat packages who reach decisions through a necessarily similar process. This is not to underplay the complexity of the term but to use it in a way that it is suitable for the context.

In the United Kingdom, there has been little consistency in the way concepts of 'cultural diversity' are addressed. In the United States, the notion of 'cultural competence' has been developed to address such issues. A widely used definition of this provided by Cross *et al.* [4] (1989: 3) stated:

> The model called 'cultural competence' . . .involves systems, agencies and practitioners with the capacity to respond to the unique needs of populations whose cultures are different than that which might be called 'dominant' or 'mainstream' American. The word culture is used because it implies the integrated pattern of human behaviour that includes communications, actions, customs, beliefs, values and institutions of a racial, ethnic, religious or social group. The word competence is used because it implies having the capacity to function in a particular way: the capacity to function within the context of culturally integrated patterns of human behaviour as defined by the group. While this publication focuses on ethnic minorities of colour, the terminology and thinking behind this model applies to each person – everyone has or is part of a culture.

However, it is striking that this definition does not emphasize working towards services that are sensitive to a patient's individual needs but highlights the needs of groups, which may or may not be as homogenous as implied. The implication is that individuals belong to a single unitary cultural group and precludes identification through any more complex criteria. In addition, there is an emphasis on difference based on being outside mainstream America. This is generally the way that diversity has been approached elsewhere too. It probably reflects a common sense of defining difference against a perceived majority or central normative group. For the educator who considers these issues in a more critical frame, it is important to challenge assumptions about the mainstream culture being 'correct' or more justified simply because of the majority status.

In the North American medical system, many educational programmes endeavoured to teach 'cultural competence' [5]. However, although the term is widely used, it often has different meanings [6]. For reasons that will become evident as different educational approaches are discussed, the authors prefer not to use the term cultural competence.

12.3   Issues That Need Consideration

A comparison of educational programmes to teach diversity in the United Kingdom, United States and Canada, three countries in which considerable work in developing diversity has been undertaken, found several similarities in all the key areas that warrant consideration when developing curricula. There has been some work undertaken in The Netherlands and there is evidence that it is now being considered in other countries [7]. Much greater work needs to be done in medical settings outside the Euro-American context, and future research will need to examine cultural diversity in non-Western contexts. There can be an impression that the principles discussed in this chapter are only relevant when there is obvious ethnic diversity. However, it should become evident through this chapter that there is diversity in every community and educators may need to help highlight where this is impacting on health care delivery.

12.3.1   Conceptual Issues

In all three countries, there is lack of conceptual clarity about what cultural diversity means and how these concepts should be framed. While governing and licensing bodies require diversity to be addressed by medical schools and postgraduate organizations, they do not offer sufficient guidance regarding how culture and diversity should be understood and embraced in school curricula or which educational approach is more effective. There is a great difference in how culture and diversity are understood by educators as well as the philosophical stance that is taken by particular institutions. Medical schools in all three countries can determine their own pedagogical methods, formats and structure for cultural diversity education, thereby making it difficult to compare curricula and effectively measure change or progress. Very rarely is the philosophy made explicit.

12.3.2 Curricular Issues

While the governing bodies require the inclusion of cultural diversity, they give sparse guidance regarding how to implement or assess the curriculum with varying degrees of prescription regarding medical school teaching. Without such clarity, the teaching is hugely varied, which is unlike subjects such as anatomy, physiology or biochemistry. While some schools understand that cultural diversity education is about developing students' knowledge, skills and attitudes when working with patients from diverse backgrounds, others use a much broader definition of difference and diversity and prepare students to deal with health and social inequalities. Student issues are discussed below.

In all three countries there has been a tendency to emphasize teaching about different or 'other' cultures rather than developing awareness of one's own biases and prejudices which might adversely influence the quality of care provided. The dominant discourse is still about students gaining 'expertise' about other cultures and wanting certainty where it may not exist [8].

12.3.3 Faculty Support and Development

The level of expertise and experience of staff involved in cultural diversity education vary greatly in all three countries. Very few staff have formal education or training in the area when compared to staff involved in teaching core medical subjects. It is evident that a biochemist might teach biochemistry but it is less clear who is qualified or skilled to teach diversity. Despite increasing evidence of health disparities in a wide range of fields of medicine, the notion that culture can be taught by well meaning practitioners still persists. Little focus or attention has been paid to the potential value of having expertise in the social sciences and education amongst health professions' educators and leaders, and training programmes to create these professionals are scarce. Steinert [9] suggests the goals of a faculty development curriculum could include assisting teachers in their understanding of their own ethno-cultural backgrounds, values, attitudes and beliefs (self-awareness); helping teachers acquire a greater understanding and empathy for their International Medical Graduates' (IMGs) cultural backgrounds and life experiences (sensitivity); and promoting the development of skills that would enable self-awareness and cultural sensitivity in their students (skill development). It is arguable that faculty need to be sensitive to the needs of their students and the needs of IMGs are no different to the needs of other students.

12.3.4 Student Issues

Perhaps not unsurprisingly there is commonality in that some students feel that because they live in 'multicultural contexts', or are members of minority ethnic groups themselves, that they do not need to learn about cultural diversity. The implication is that through belonging to one 'minority' group somehow means there is implicit understanding of other groups. This demonstrates a lack of understanding about what diversity is and that within groups there is significant heterogeneity. Some Canadian medical graduates (6.2%) believed that instruction in cultural issues in health care was excessive [10]. Cultural competence education may still be viewed as less important than the basic science courses or just 'political correctness'. In addition, the content of cultural diversity initiatives can be seen as simply extra material which the medical exams will not test or ask about in any significant way. It is worth reflecting on students' reluctance to engage in diversity education. It is sometimes cultural arrogance and an assumption the culture that is ours is intrinsically better. It is noteworthy that cultural arrogance is not limited to dominant cultures. There may also be reluctance to be challenged about their own perspectives. It is interesting that many males are keen on equality based on ethnicity but not quite so keen on gender equality. There may also be fear of being viewed in a particular way for holding particular perspectives. Students from minority groups may also have experienced discrimination based on their minority (be it ethnicity, gender or any other factor), thereby engaging them may be difficult.

12.3.5 Assessment Issues

Formal evaluation of cultural diversity education and programme remains limited and there is ambivalence that assessments are required in cultural diversity [11].

These areas are useful to consider in turn. The focus will not be on delivery methods, as those selected will be dependent on the learning outcomes set.

12.4 Educational Philosophy and Its Influence on Programmes Developed

Campbell and Johnson [12] suggested that medical education must engender a culture that is more aware and critical of educational theories and principles. Teaching must challenge the professional and disciplinary tribalism, which results in the separation of bodies of knowledge, for which medicine's positivist culture must adapt. Medical teachers do not perhaps apply the same rigour to their teaching practice as they do to other aspects of their jobs [13]. Educators may provide teaching that reflects their personal preferred approaches and beliefs as opposed to a considered overview. Doctors and/or teachers with a sociological background may be more likely to develop educational programmes that are based in some sociological concepts, and demonstrate awareness of the debate regarding the concepts of race and ethnicity given that personal beliefs and philosophy do influence teachers [14]. Teachers without sociological perspectives may be inclined to develop programmes that use more lay public concepts: there may be little or no differentiation between race and ethnicity. Race and ethnicity according to these instructors may be seen as the sole definers of cultural belonging or a sense of identity. This stems from the simplistic notion that an individual's culture is given by their biological connection to a particular racial heritage. Traditionally, race has been seen as a biological and genetic phenomenon and used by biologists to define the ancestral heritage of individuals and their relationship to other racial groups in the past and present [15]. The collective political and social upheavals to the 1960s in the United States and Europe saw racial terms used in powerfully social ways to enable and foster discrimination. In the wake of this period, ethnicity came to be used as the marker of cultural difference because it moved away from the broad over-generalizations of racial categories to greater specificity of cultural identification and a little more fluidity in self-definition. One could start to lay some claim to be ethnically tied to one group or another based on foods, music, geography and language.

For educators entering into discussions of culture, it is important to lay some context for the use of terms and markers of race and ethnicity, and also discuss the need to broaden the understanding of culture to include some of the factors outlined above in the AAMC definition. Culture is greater and more inclusive than race or ethnicity, but nevertheless includes elements of these factors. Culture is what an individual needs to know or understanding in order to be a part of the particular social group they find themselves within. Educators can urge their students and trainees to do an exercise of trying to describe the essence of their culture and what they need to know in order to be, say, a medical student or postgraduate trainee. This type of exercise can help highlight the difficult nature of culture, and its intercalation in our everyday lives.

Some people in medicine may see medicine as more of a science than do others. Those who believe there are 'correct' or 'right' answers may tend towards developing curricula that are based on helping students learn the right way of dealing with diversity and imply there is a single and correct response. That is, they take an approach referred to as essentialism, which is the belief that it is possible to discover and articulate the truth behind natural phenomena, a truth that defines their essence [16]. Essentialism when applied to culture focuses on differences, artificially simplifying individual and group identities and interactions. Those medical educators who work in less concrete fields, such as psychiatry, may be more familiar with working with not knowing and be comfortable with uncertainty. They may be more inclined to develop or support programmes that help students manage not knowing and aim to help students learn about being willing to acknowledge when they do not know. The latter approach is less likely to produce checklists and claims that students have achieved a competence, which is then never built upon. Fuller [17] suggested the need to eradicate essentialism from programmes to teach 'cultural competence'. In the next section an educational framework is provided that will be helpful to educators planning teaching in diversity. Some examples of the various educational approaches described in the literature are then provided.

12.5 Educational Models: Ideal Types of 'Cultural Expertise' and 'Cultural Sensibility'

Using Weber's construct of ideal types [18, 19] the concepts of *'cultural expertise'* and *'cultural sensibility'* were compared by Dogra [20, 21] with regard to several characteristics. The characteristics are grouped into four major areas of course development:

- Educational philosophy and policy

- Educational process

- Educational contents

- Educational and clinical outcomes.

Educational philosophy and policy usually inform all stages of course development and also affect the educational process, educational contents and outcomes. When discussing the educational process, the way that the educational philosophy is translated into practice is an important guiding principle. The question is how the values and ideologies of those developing the course are used to develop the course. Some course designers may, of course, not recognize that their underlying beliefs about the merits or disadvantages of certain approaches influence their choices. In considering educational contents, the very nature of the material is under review. This stage involves identifying the key areas that the teaching will emphasize and whether or not the programmes will focus on the attainment of knowledge, skills and/or attitudinal outcomes. Assessment is often perceived to be the major educational outcome measure but there will also be other outcomes, albeit that some are more explicit than others.

12.5.1 'Cultural Expertise'

A dictionary definition of expertise [22] is expert skill, knowledge or judgement, with expert being defined as having special skill at a task or knowledge in a subject. There is a view that through learning knowledge about 'other' cultures, one can develop *'cultural expertise'* and that much of this knowledge can be learned through didactic teaching. *'Cultural expertise'* is about having facts about other cultures. The concept of *'cultural expertise'* encompasses the well-established model of 'cultural competence'.

12.5.2 'Cultural Sensibility'

'Cultural sensibility' is proposed so as to broaden the concept of 'cultural sensitivity', which, in general, has been a tentative alternative to the idea of *'cultural expertise'*. A dictionary definition [22] of sensibility is an openness to emotional impressions, susceptibility and sensitiveness. It relates to a person's moral, emotional or aesthetic ideas or standards. 'Cultural sensitivity' is not the same as *'cultural sensibility'*. 'Cultural sensitivity' is the quality or degree of being sensitive, which is more limited than sensibility, and does not take into account the interactional nature of sensibility. If one is open to the outside, one might reflect and change because of that experience. This is not necessarily the case with sensitivity. The approach of *'cultural sensibility'* has arisen out of Dogra's work [21] in 'cultural diversity' and medical education and an experience that the *'cultural expertise'* model potentially limits the benefits of 'cultural diversity' teaching.

Cultural sensibility builds on several traditions in psychiatry. Firstly, it recognizes and expands on a developmental model [23]. Within a developmental frame, it is clear that the individual grows and matures into a sense of culture and that it is not a one-way experience where the culture is transmitted from the family into the individual as a defined package. Rather, children and adolescents grow and dynamically change their sense of self and culture over time. The development of a sense of culture takes place as an interaction between the individual and his or her family, peers, community and self-identified cultural groups. The second element in psychiatry that the cultural sensibility model builds on is the psychotherapeutic tradition. Psychotherapy by its very nature is an interactional process which requires the clinician to learn from and listen to the patient. The dyadic nature of traditional psychotherapy is an opportune moment to allow the perspective of the cultural sensibility model to enter into the work. Through this perspective the practitioner can then elicit some of the cultural understandings of the individual more fully and incorporate these understandings into the treatment plan.

The different underlying philosophies of the *'cultural expertise'* and *'cultural sensibility'* models result in differing educational process, contents and assessments, as summarized in Table 12.1.

Using the *'cultural expertise'* model, the following outcomes in each of the learning domains might be used:

Knowledge: history and culture of country of origin; pertinent psychosocial stresses, family life and intergenerational issues; culturally acceptable behaviours versus psychopathology; role of religion; cultural beliefs about causes and treatments of disease; and differences in disease prevalence and response to medicine and other treatments.

Ability: interview and assess patients in the target language (or via translator); communicate with sensitivity to cross-cultural issues; avoid under/over diagnosing disease states; understand the patient's perspective; formulate culturally sensitive treatment plans; effectively use community resources; and act as a role model and advocate for bilingual/bicultural staff and patients.

Attitudes: as evidence of understanding, acknowledge the degree of difference between patient and physician; to demonstrate empathy, recall the patient's history of suffering; have patience in shifting away from the dominant cultural view of time and immediacy; respect the importance of culture as a determinant of health, the existence of other world views regarding health and illness, the adaptability and survival skills of patients, the influence of religious beliefs on health and the role of bilingual/bicultural staff; and demonstrate humour by having the ability to laugh with oneself and others (see Lee as cited in [24]).

Possible learning outcomes for using the *'cultural sensibility'* model might be:

Knowledge: the focus of *'cultural sensibility'* is not knowledge about groups. There is an expectation that students are aware of broad psychosocial issues that can affect the way individuals perceive health and access health services. There is a need to have knowledge of the contexts information is presented or received in.

Ability: the greater focus on this model is the acquisition of a method for acknowledging difference and working with it in a constructive and positive way. Difference between

Table 12.1 Summary of comparison between the different educational components of 'cultural expertise' and 'cultural sensibility'.

Item		
Educational content	*'Cultural expertise'*	*'Cultural sensibility'*
Epistemology (i.e. the theory of knowledge)	Knowledge exists independently	Knowledge is contextual to one's environment
Categorization of knowledge	Core competency is about categorizing groups of people and that these categories can be learned, that is knowledge can be categorized	Knowledge does not need to be categorized
Use of categorization	Categorization is helpful	Categorization may be unhelpful
Ontology (the nature of being)	Positivist	Non-positivist
Conception of reality	Objective reality to be revealed or discovered	No single objective reality to be discovered
	Structuralist	Non-structuralist
	Modern	Post-modern
	Not social constructionism	Social constructionism
Analytical perspective	Reductionist	Holistic
Historical connection	Rooted in historical context of minority disadvantage and white domination	Steps outside of the historical context of race
Politics of institutions	Improve competence of providers and/or users to improve access to care/services	Does not work on a competence level
Relation to inequalities	Attempts to change and reduce health care inequalities	Acknowledges inequalities but as such does not directly attempt to change them
Role of teacher	Teacher sets the agenda	Teacher introduces the agenda
Role of learner	Primarily as receiver	Student contributes to the dialogue as well as receiving
Conceptions of culture	*'Cultural expertise'*	*'Cultural sensibility'*
Conceptions of culture	Culture is an externally recognized characteristic	Culture is an internally constructed sense of self
Conceptions of culture	Static	Dynamic/fluid
	One-dimensional	Multidimensional
	Race/ethnicity emphasized	Race is one aspect
	Unitary	Diverse/differentiated
Perception of individual's relationship to society		
Conception of difference	Generalize the differences between individuals	Sensitive to difference
Identity formation	Individuals are shaped by their social world	Individuals construct and accomplish their own social world

(Continued)

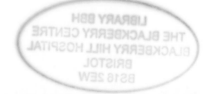

Table 12.1   (*Continued*)

Item		
Educational content	*'Cultural expertise'*	*'Cultural sensibility'*
Conception of individual identity	An individual is defined by their culture	An individual defines their culture
Individual's relationship with society (relationship of self with society)	In defining culture relationship is between groups	In defining culture relationship is between an individual and others
	Dialogue re culture takes place between groups	Dialogue re culture takes place between individuals
	Individuals remain as defined by their culture irrespective of the context	Individuals bring their own meanings and histories to different contexts that is the meanings may change dependent on the context
Educational process	*'Cultural expertise'*	*'Cultural sensibility'*
Learning process	Acquisition of knowledge	Acquisition of principles (method)
Learning outcomes	Command of body of information and facts	Command of mode of respectful questioning
Expression of learning goals	In terms of skill and competence	In terms of attitudes and self-reflection
SOLO taxonomy	Multistructural	Extended abstract
Content	Certain	Acknowledge uncertainty
	Dichotomous	Mostly grey areas
	Right or wrong	Not always right or wrong
Cultural focus	Majority view of other cultures dominant	No focus on particular groups – all individuals need to consider needs of others
	Majority whites need to consider needs of minorities	
Cybernetics theory	First order that is the teacher teaches the student	Second order that is the student and teacher learn together
Pedagogical approach	Didactic	Directed self-learning
Role of experts	There are those who are experts on understanding cultural perspectives of certain groups	No one individual has ownership of expertise of others with respect to identification of cultural belonging
Educational content	*'Cultural expertise'*	*'Cultural sensibility'*
Curriculum type (as relating to [36])	Collection type	Integrated type
Nature of content	Parochial	Global
	Specific	Non-specific
Organization of content	To meet demands of local need	To maximize student self-learning

Table 12.1 (*Continued*)

Item		
Educational content	*'Cultural expertise'*	*'Cultural sensibility'*
Curriculum	Fact acquisition to gain body of knowledge	Self-reflection and self-awareness of students
Teaching focus	Groups (treats people as groups) More service centred	Individuals (views individuals as potentially parts of different groups in different contexts More patient centred
Focus of content	Students learn about others	Students learn as much about others as themselves
Educational outcomes	*'Cultural expertise'*	*'Cultural sensibility'*
What purpose does the assessment serve?	Demonstrates knowledge of other cultures	Demonstrates some understanding of self and ability to evaluate their own learning
Which methods are used?	Paper and pencil tests ranging from multiple choice questions and short answers to long essays	Reflective journals, project work (usually experientially based)
Results of assessment	Norm referenced (i.e. students ranked against peers)	Not norm referenced
Who leads the assessment process?	Teacher assessment	Student self-assessment
Measures to check outcomes	Checklists	Self-assessment
Outcome in clinical practice	Practical in that have facts about other cultures	Practical in that have a method of enquiry to be aware that others may have different perspectives More critical and self reflective Capacity for dialogue
Applicability	Learning can only be used for *cultural issues*	Learning can apply to any context in which there are differences between the doctor and patient be they cultural, gender, education
Patient centredness	Doctor has position of expert	Doctor and patient are active partners in care
Definition of successful course	Students learn competence in other cultures and a bonus if students learn about themselves	Course is only successful if students learn about themselves as this is necessary before ability to relate to other perspectives.

the doctor and patient is potentially present in all encounters and not just those where ethnicity differs.

Attitude: the focus is on self-reflection and awareness – the interaction between two individuals, which generates effective, shared understanding and dialogue. The dialogue has the potential to change either, both, or neither of the participants. It is built on transformative learning approach.

The comparison focused on the conceptual differences between the two models at their purest. *'Cultural expertise'* models arose from the recognition that cultural influences impact on health care provision and use. The approach of *'cultural sensibility'* is presented as an evolution of the *'cultural expertise'* approach, which potentially limits the benefits of 'cultural diversity' teaching. In an environment that demands increasing evidence-based approaches, it may be time to develop tighter teaching models that have clear conceptual frameworks and can evaluate more effectively whether or not the teaching meets its objectives. This is revisited later in the chapter when the impact of educational programmes is considered.

12.6   Does Training In Cultural Diversity Improve Clinical Outcomes?

One of the reasons that educators in psychiatry might want to teach cultural diversity to students in psychiatry is the hope that in doing so the clinical outcomes for patients might be improved. Unfortunately, many programmes in diversity are politically rather than educationally driven [25]. A brief overview of this area is presented here but readers are referred to further reading that explore the issues.

12.6.1   Training In Diversity and Implications for Practice

In the United Kingdom, David 'Rocky' Bennett died on a psychiatric ward in 1998, after being restrained, pinioned, face down by at least four nursing staff for over 25 minutes. His death eventually led to an official report which concluded that there was institutional racism within the UK mental health service. This subsequently led to policy that all mental health professionals in the United Kingdom needed to have mandatory cultural awareness training to address issues of racism. Internationally there have also been some attempts to introduce a framework for the training of staff in cultural competence with most of the literature originating from North America [26, 27]. In a survey which included the commissioners of training in UK National Health Service (NHS) mental health trusts, primary care trusts, independent sector in-patient mental health service providers, a large number of their employees and providers of race equality training, Bennett *et al.* [28] reported significant variation in the training provided. The authors comment that whilst there has been considerable investment in and commitment to race related training for many years, there is little evidence of any serious attempts to evaluate the effectiveness of such training. Whilst a majority of training providers reported that training was evaluated, it was only usually subjective data that was collected. It was difficult to evaluate how much the training, as opposed to other measures, led to change, if in fact there was change.

Concerns regarding organizations attitudes to training in 'cultural competence' have also been reported internationally [29]. Staff with the lead responsibility for training in a number of North American health care organizations commonly reported a lack of clarity in the implementation of culturally competent care. In addition to the lack of a strategic overview and low priority given to this issue, commonly cited problems included a lack of leadership, difficulties accessing the whole organization and funding problems.

There is limited evidence on the effectiveness of cultural competency training and the impact on clinical practice for any approach used. Bentley *et al.* [30] reported that most employees were positive on many aspects of the training and the majority reported a positive impact on their work. However, less than half felt the training had a positive impact on service delivery or their organization. Evaluation of training was carried out by a third of statutory organizations with internal evaluation being the most common means. A review of model evaluations found that of 109 potential papers, only nine included an evaluation of the model to improve the cultural competency practice and service delivery [31]. All the studies were North American and used different methodologies with varying definitions and outcomes. A systematic literature review and analysis of interventions designed to improve the cultural competence of health professionals included thirty-four studies, most of which took place in the United States and included medical and postgraduate students [32]. There was some evidence that cultural competence training improved the knowledge, attitudes and skills of health professionals. There was also some evidence that cultural competence training impacted on patient satisfaction, although only three studies investigated this. None of the studies investigated the costs of cultural competence training. The authors concluded that cultural competence training shows promise as a strategy for improving the knowledge, attitudes and skills of health professionals. However, evidence that it improves patient adherence to therapy, health outcomes and equity of services across racial and ethnic groups is lacking. The work reviewed by both groups predates 2005. Beach *et al.*'s review [32] is useful as it identifies those programmes which are well described and may therefore be useful to other educators.

12.7   Practical Tips for Teaching Diversity

Dogra *et al.* [33] provide twelve tips for teaching diversity and embedding it in the medical curriculum. Essentially, the tips advise curriculum planners to focus on institutional policies to ensure that there is institutional ownership of cultural diversity education and to create a safe learning environment. The learning outcomes need to be clear and achievable. The following learning outcomes are suggested as a minimum requirement:

- Define 'cultural diversity' and apply this definition with respect to clinical practice.

- Critically appraise the use of key terms, such as race, ethnicity, culture, multiculturalism and inequalities of access to health care.

- Evaluate your own attitudes and perceptions (including personal bias) of different groups within society.

- Evaluate institutional prejudices and how these relate to your own perspectives.

- Identify strategies to challenge prejudice effectively and identify local policy in this area to ensure robustness.

- Evaluate and justify the approaches used in your own clinical practice.

- Assess the impact (both positive and negative) of your attitudes on your clinical practice and demonstrate respect for patients and colleagues who encompass without prejudice, diversity of background and opportunity, language, culture and way of life.

- List the different approaches there are to developing skills in meeting the needs of diverse populations and compare and contrast these.

- Describe existing equal opportunity legislation.

- Explain how you would apply the legislation to your practice as a health care provider and as an employer.

- Evaluate the relevance of cultural diversity training in health care.

They also suggest that the content be focussed on the diversity of human and to avoid reducing cultural diversity education simply to the awareness of ethnic, racial or religious differences with respect to health outcomes, health beliefs and coping skills of specific cultural groups. They also argue that diversity education should be integrated across the entire curriculum and incorporated throughout the entire curriculum including pre-clinical and clinical years. Faculty development is also viewed as an essential component, as evidence to date suggests that staff do not feel well supported in this area.

12.7.1   Issues that May be More Relevant when Training Postgraduate Doctors

Although there will be diversity within medical student groups, their experience of training to be doctors will be somewhat more similar. However, when training postgraduate doctors, there will be even greater diversity, as they will have experienced different medical training and that may raise additional issues. Majumdar *et al.* [34] is one of a few studies that specifically looked at teaching diversity to international medical graduates. The major content areas included perceptions about foreigners, gender roles, culture shock, personal losses, and behaviour and non-verbal communication. The major training methods have included small group seminars, live observation, videotape reviews and simulated patients. This was felt to help the international medical graduates to better integrate into their new society. International medical graduates may have experienced discrimination and may need support in participating fully in diversity programmes.

Finally, a case example to illustrate the application of the cultural sensibility model described earlier is shown in Box 12.1.

Box 12.1 Case Example: Teaching Cultural Psychiatry: A Curricular Experience

The approach to teaching cultural psychiatry will be defined by a number of factors. Is the course free standing or part of other courses? How many hours are devoted to this topic? How many students are in the course? At what level of experience are the trainees in the course? Here one example of a small (6–8 students) postgraduate seminar that was one hour per week for six weeks and taught by one of the authors (Karnik) is provided.

Trainees were assigned to read Anne Fadiman's book *The Spirit Catches You and You Fall Down* [35]. It is an excellent touchstone for discussion because it details the actual events of a young girl suffering from epilepsy in the Hmong community. The book is useful as a teaching tool because Fadiman carefully weaves the story by presenting both the biomedical perspective of the physicians along with the cultural story of the Hmong family. The clash of cultures emerges over time and neither perspective ultimately gains primacy – both are given a degree of respect and a degree of criticism.

By using this book as the focal point of discussion in the first class, the class begins to discuss their cultural assumptions and beliefs, especially during the clinical encounter. In this first session, it is important to create a safe classroom space where trainees feel free to express their beliefs without fear of recrimination or retribution. It is also reasonable to set ground rules for the discussion that include a degree of group confidentiality so that trainees can express their feelings openly and honestly.

The next three weeks of the course introduce the cultural sensibility framework through a case-based approach. Trainees are encouraged to bring active cases to the class to discuss and reflect upon. Throughout this section of the course, definitions and readings drawn heavily from anthropology and sociology emphasize the core definitions of concepts while also presenting a model for the trainee to incorporate into the clinical encounter. Trainees practice phrasing open-ended questions in non-directive ways so as to elicit the cultural, spiritual and identity issues that are key to the patient. In addition, due to the child and adolescent subspeciality training in this class, the trainees are exposed to ways to think about the questions they raise in developmentally appropriate ways and to differentiate between the culture of the child or adolescent and that of the broader family.

The final two weeks of the class serve as an opportunity to bring closure to the course. Discussion focuses on transference and countertransference through the lens of culture and the ways that trainees can establish ways to continue to explore their own inherent biases as well as life-long learning patterns.

The structure of this course is just one possible way of reflecting this material but it allows trainees and faculty an opportunity for self-reflection and for building a durable framework by which to approach culture in the psychiatric context. Adaptations of this structure can be made depending on the size of the class and number of contact hours.

12.8 Summary

It is important that whatever educational programmes are developed, the education philosophy, process, contents and outcomes are systematically considered. Clarity about the philosophy and the outcomes should enable a coherent programme to be developed. All programmes should include an expectation that clinicians identify their own biases and prejudices about the patients they are likely to encounter. Personal perspectives are important to recognise because they impact on the clinical consultation.

References

1. Mulholland, J. and Dyson, S. (2001) Sociological theories of 'race' and ethnicity, in *Ethnicity and Nursing Practice* (eds L. Culley and S. Dyson), Palgrave, London, pp. 17–37.
2. Goodenough, W.H. (1957) Cultural anthropology and linguistics, in *Report of the 7th Annual Round Table Meeting on Linguisticsand Language Study* (ed. P.L. Garvin), Georgetown University Press, Washington, pp. 167–173.
3. Association of American Medical Colleges (1999) Report III. Contemporary issues in Medicine, Communication in Medicine: Spirituality, Cultural Issues and End Of Life Care. Medical School Objectives Project. Association of American Medical Colleges.
4. Cross, T., Bazron, B., Dennis, K.W. and Isaacs, M.R. (1989) *Towards A Culturally Competent System Of Care*, Volume **1**, Georgetown University Child Development Center, CASSP Technical Assistance Centre, Washington DC.
5. Deloney, L.A., Graham, C.J. and Erwin, D.O. (2000) Presenting cultural diversity and spirituality to first-year medical students. *Academic Medicine*, **75**, 513–514.
6. Henry J. Kaiser Family Foundation (2003) Compendium Of Cultural Competence Initiatives In Health Care, The Henry J. Kaiser Family Foundation, California. http://www.kff.org/uninsured/loader.cfm?url=/commonspot/security/getfile.cfm&PageID=14365 (accessed 23 July 2010).
7. Reitmanova, S. (2008) Cross cultural medical education and training. *Bratisl Lek Listy*, **109**, 82–87.
8. Dogra, N., Giordano, J. and France, N. (2007) Cultural diversity teaching and issues of uncertainty: the findings of a qualitative study. *BMC Med Educ*, **7**, 8.
9. Steinert, Y. (2003) Report commissioned by the Canadian Task Force on Licensure of International Medical Graduates. http://www.afmc.ca/img/programoverview_en.htm (accessed 2 January 2010).
10. Association of American Medical Colleges (2007) Canadian Medical School Graduate Questionnaire. Association of American Medical Colleges, Division of Medical Education.
11. Dogra, N. and Wass, V. (2006) Can we assess students' awareness of cultural diversity? A qualitative study of stakeholders' views. *Med Educ.*, **40**, 682–690.
12. Campbell, J.K. and Johnson, C. (1999) Trend spotting: fashions in medical education. *British Medical Journal*, **318**, 1272–1275.
13. Van Der Vleuten, C. (1993) Evidence-based education. *Advances in Physiology Education*, **14**, S3.
14. Toohey, S. (1999) *Designing Courses For Higher Education*, The Society for Research into Higher Education and Open University Press, Buckingham, pp. 44–49.
15. Cavalli-Sforza, L.L. and Cavalli-Sforza, F. (1995) *The Great Human Diasporas: The History Of Diversity And Evolution*, Addison-Wesley, Reading, MA.
16. Johnson, A.G. (2000) *The Blackwell Dictionary of Sociology: A User's Guide To Sociological Language*, 2nd edn, Blackwell Publishers, Oxford.
17. Fuller, K. (2002) Eradicating essentialism from cultural competency education. *Academic Medicine*, **77**, 198–201.
18. Giddens, A. (1971) *Capitalism and Modern Social Theory: An Analysis Of The Writings Of Marx, Durkheim and Max Weber*, Cambridge University Press, Cambridge.

19. Morrison, K. (1995) *Marx, Durkheim, Weber: Formation of Modern Social Thought*, Sage, Thousand Oaks, CA.
20. Dogra, N. (2003) Cultural competence or cultural sensibility? A comparison of two ideal type models to teach cultural diversity to medical students. *International Journal of Medicine*, **5**, 223–231.
21. Dogra, N. (2004) The Learning and Teaching Of Cultural Diversity In Undergraduate Medical Education In The UK. PhD, University of Leicester.
22. Thompson, D. (ed.) (1995) *The Concise Oxford Dictionary Of Current English*, Clarendon Press, Oxford.
23. Steiner, H. (2004) The Scientific Basis of Mental Health Interventions in Children and 'adolescents: an overview, in *Handbook of Mental Health Interventions in Children and Adolescents* (ed. H. Steiner), Jossey-Bass, San Francisco, CA, pp. 9–34.
24. American Medical Association (1999) Enhancing the 'cultural competence' of Physicians. Council on Medical Education Report 5-A-98, in Cultural Competence Compendium, American Medical Association.
25. Dogra, N. and Williams, R. (2006) Applying policy and evidence in developingcultural diversity teaching in undergraduate medical education in the UK. *Evidence and Policy*, **2**, 463–477.
26. Fung, K., Andermann, L., Zaretsky, A., and Lo, H. (2008) An integrative approach to cultural competence in the psychiatric curriculum. *Academic Psychiatry*, **32**, 272–282.
27. Lim, R.F., Luo, J.S., Suo, S. and Hales, R.E. (2008) Diversity initiatives in academic psychiatry: Applying cultural competence. *Academic Psychiatry*, **32**, 283–290.
28. Bennett, J., Kalathil, J. and Keating, F. (2007) Race Equality Training In Mental Health Services In England: Does One Size Fit All? The Sainsbury Centre for Mental Health, London.
29. Dogra, N., Betancourt, J., Park, E. and Martinez, L. (2009) The relationship between drivers and policy in the implementation of cultural competency training in health care. *Journal of the National Medical Association*, **101**, 127–133.
30. Bentley, P., Jovanovic, A. and Sharma, P. (2008) Cultural diversity training for UK healthcare professionals: a comprehensive nationwide cross-sectional survey. *Clin. Med.*, **8**, 493–497.
31. Bhui, K., Warfa, N., Edonya, P. *et al.* (2007) Cultural competence in mental health care: a review of model evaluations. *BMC Health Services Research*, **7**, 15.
32. Beach, M.C., Price EG, Gary, T.L. *et al.* (2005) Cultural competence: a systematic review of health care provider educational interventions. *Medical Care*, **43**, 356–373.
33. Dogra, N., Reitmanova, S. and Carter-Pokras, O. (2009) Twelve tips for teaching diversity and embedding it in the medical curriculum. *Medical Teacher*, **11**, 990–993.
34. Majumdar, B., Keystone, J.S. and Cuttress, L.A. (1999). Cultural sensitivity training among foreign medical graduates. *Medical Education*, **33**, 177–184.
35. Fadiman, A. (1989) *The Spirit Catches You and You Fall Down*, Farrar, Strauss & Giroux.
36. Bernstein, B. (1971) On the classification and framing of educational knowledge, in *Knowledge and Control: New directions for the sociology of education* (ed. M.F.D. Young), Collier MacMillan, London, pp. 47–69.

13

Teaching Psychiatry in Primary Care

Linda Gask[1], Bulent Coskun[2] and Rodolfo Fahrer[3]

[1]*School of Community Based Medicine, University of Manchester, Manchester, UK*
[2]*Department of Psychiatry, Kocaeli University Medical School, Kocaeli, Turkey*
[3]*Department of Mental Health, School of Medicine, University of Buenos Aires, Buenos Aires, Argentina*

13.1   Why Teach Psychiatry to Primary Care Workers?

Primary care has, in the last twenty five years, assumed a considerable international impor-tance for both the recognition and treatment of mental health problems. The World Health Organization has defined 'primary care mental health' as follows [1]:

- *First line interventions that are provided as an integral part of general health care and*

- *Mental health care that is provided by primary care workers who are skilled, able and supported to provide mental health care services.*

Thus, in many countries where primary care services are less well developed, primary care mental health will be provided by general medical services. There is increasing international recognition of the economic and social burden of mental illness [2]. In western countries, the majority of mental health problems seen in the primary care setting fall into the category of 'common mental disorders', such as anxiety and depression, while more severe and enduring mental health problems, such as schizophrenia and other psychoses, are treated, at least initially, by specialist mental health services. Although 'common mental disorders' are, on average, less severe than those disorders seen in secondary care settings, the public health burden that they pose in terms of disability and economic consequences is considerably greater [3]. Mental health issues are the second most common reason for consultations in

Teaching Psychiatry: Putting Theory into Practice   Edited by Linda Gask, Bulent Coskun and David Baron
© 2011 John Wiley & Sons, Ltd

primary care in the United Kingdom [4] and General Practitioners (GPs) spend, on average, approximately 30% of their time on mental health problems [5].

However, even in countries where specialist mental health services are well developed, such as the United Kingdom and United States of America (USA) [6], many people with more severe and enduring mental illness receive their ongoing mental health care primarily within primary care.

In low and middle income countries specialist mental health care may be poorly developed or even non-existent such that, by default, primary care will be the primary provider of mental health care [7]. This may also be the situation at the time of natural or man-made disasters, when mental health services may become impossible to access and psychosocial interventions must be delivered alongside other aspects of essential health care [8]. There is thus considerable international variation in the way that primary care practitioners are engaged in providing mental health care. For example, in some countries GPs cannot prescribe psychotropic medication without agreement from a psychiatrist and there may be perceived to be no role for primary care in the management of people with severe and enduring mental health problems.

Psychiatrists should bear in mind that there are important differences in the way that people with mental health problems present in primary care compared with specialist mental health care. There is often comorbidity with physical illness. A common mode of presentation of emotional problems in the primary care setting is that of medically unexplained symptoms, which may or may not be recognized by the physician as indicative of underlying emotional distress, even in the presence of expressed verbal and non-verbal cues of distress. The critical point here, however, is that primary care clinicians will often encounter undifferentiated unfiltered and unrecognized symptoms, concerns, worries and problems [9], including emotional reactions to physical health problems, that may or may not be easily identifiable as mental health syndromes. Specialist mental health clinicians in contrast are far more likely to encounter filtered symptoms that are recognized and understood as representative of a mental health problem.

A number of reasons for teaching about psychiatry (and, more broadly, 'mental health') to primary care workers are suggested in Box 13.1.

Box 13.1   Why Teach Primary Care Workers About Mental Health?

- For patients

  - To improve the quality of mental health care provided

  - To influence the care of people who are not seen in mental health services

- For professionals

  - To contribute to their own continuing professional development – learning new skills, acquiring knowledge, improving enjoyment of working with people with mental health problems

  - To also provide education about their own potential needs for example stress, burnout, healthy lifestyles.

13.1.1 What Training do Primary Care Workers Usually Receive in Mental Health?

Learning about psychiatry or mental health has, for those entering primary care practice in most countries of the world, been a rather 'hit and miss' affair. In many countries, even now, those entering primary care practice will have had no training in psychiatry beyond what they learned as undergraduates in medicine, where the emphasis will have likely been on people with a diagnosis of a psychotic illness, such as schizophrenia, rather than the common mental health problems often comorbid with physical illness which are the bread and butter of primary care.

As specific vocational training in the speciality of 'general practice' has developed across Europe in the last fifty years, there has been increasing recognition of the need for specific training in mental health, but the form that this should take has not always been clear. Experience of mental health care in large mental asylums is not appropriate preparation for the reality of mental health care in the broader community. In many low and middle income countries, specific vocational training for doctors entering primary care is now underway (which usually includes periods of training in a number of different specialities, such as paediatrics, geriatrics, obstetrics and gynaecology though not always psychiatry) and the mental health content of the curricula is under consideration and thus able to be shaped.

In the United Kingdom (UK), the informal curriculum was usually based on clinical practice in specialist hospital units, covered the 'severe' end of the mental ill-health spectrum rather than common mental disorders and was usually knowledge based rather than skills based. Research looking at the needs of GP trainees in the United Kingdom [10] highlighted the gap between traditional, knowledge based, teaching and the trainees' desire for practical skills development with feedback on these skills in relation to mental health practice in primary care.

General Practice Specialist Training in the United Kingdom, developed from the original general practice vocational training programmes and, now approved by the Postgraduate Medical Education and Training Board (PMETB), has a clear curriculum defined by the Royal College of General Practitioners (RCGP). Achievement of a Certificate of Completion of Training (CCT) for General Practice involves 'time served' in appropriate and approved posts, Workplace-Based Assessments of specific competencies, a Clinical Skills Assessment at an independent centre and an Applied Knowledge Test relevant to practice in United Kingdom primary care. As all of this is 'competency' based, the curriculum has had to define the broad competencies to be achieved in each clinical area.

This education, however, needs to build on appropriate education at the undergraduate level in the knowledge base of behavioural science (for example the importance of meanings attributed to health, illness and its treatment – for further discussion see Chapter 5) and mental illness (see Chapter 4 for more discussion of the undergraduate curriculum).

However, in many low and middle income countries there is not only no formal national health system nor any insurance system that allows the luxury of time off for training. The fee for service method of payment used widely ensures, for example, that in Pakistan a GP may work from 8 a.m. or earlier to 11 at night or later, $6^{1}/_{2}$ days a week, with a good number working out of 24-hour clinics. Training in these settings has to be based on attractive and simple modules rather than extensive and complicated texts that no GP will follow in practice after the training.

13.2 Meeting the Educational Needs of the Primary Care Team

Across the world many general practitioners still work as single handed practitioners. However, in some countries, primary care has increasingly been provided by a team of professionals working together, doctors, nurses and the extended team of health care assistants, receptionists and other workers who visit the practice. They include not only a range of specialized nurses (health visitors, community nurses, midwives) but may or may not also include mental health professionals, such as community mental health (psychiatric) nurses, psychologists and also psychiatrists who may visit the team to provide supervision or work in liaison with them.

Nurses may have very limited training in mental health care, even though they are regularly seeing patients for assessment of diabetes and cardiovascular disease who are also depressed or anxious. The role of the this extended team in providing mental health care has been acknowledged and in recent years there have been specific initiatives aimed at members of the team, such as training health visitors in the recognition and management of postnatal depression [11] or primary care nurses in management of people on depot neuroleptic treatment [12].

There is a widely held view that view that medical professionals may have a tendency to miss or disregard psychosocial aspects of patients, sometimes due to their biological orientation or sometimes due to lack of necessary knowledge and skills to detect those psychological symptoms.

However, sometimes psychologically masked illnesses may need to be recognized. Grace and Christensen [13] worked with 24 psychiatrists, 20 primary care physicians, 31 psychologists and 17 social workers on 10 different clinical vignettes where patients were seeking treatment for their psychological problems. The authors suggest that non-medical health providers have the risk of not recognizing masked medical illnesses, which brings a necessity for primary care physicians and non-medical professionals to collaborate. Through the training programmes it should therefore be kept in mind that both the behavioural health care providers and primary health care physicians bring unique skills to patient care that, when combined, greatly improve the overall quality of both medical and mental health care.

Where medical professionals may not be available and other professionals (psychologists or social workers) may have the first contact with people presenting with psychological symptoms (for example in situations such as schools or older people's homes), they must be equipped to know when to consult or when to refer to physicians.

Thus, we may conclude that the education process must have a complementary structure to cover different dimensions. The planning and implementation of the training programmes should cover all related disciplines.

A case study of a multidicisplinary approach is provided in Box 13.2.

Box 13.2   Case Summary of Physician-Lead Primary Care for Mental Health in Neuquén Province, Patagonian Region, Argentina

In the province of Neuquén, Argentina, primary care physicians lead the diagnosis, treatment and rehabilitation of patients with severe mental disorders. Patients receive out-patient treatment in their communities. Psychiatrists and other mental health specialists are available to review and advise on complex cases.

This programme has increased demand for mental health care and allowed people with mental disorders to remain in their communities and socially integrated. The effectiveness of the programme is largely the result of teamwork: the primary care physicians leading the therapeutic process, supported by psychiatrists, psychologists and nurses.

In Neuquén the model for mental health care is based on four key elements:

1. Primary care physicians. Diagnosis, treatment and rehabilitation services for severe mental disorders are provided by a team of health service providers, under the leadership of a primary care physician who is trained for that responsibility. Moreover, primary care physicians frequently address life stressors and family conflicts, which they manage with brief, problem-orientated psychotherapy.

2. Out-patients. People with mental disorders receive out-patient treatment in their communities, where they enjoy the support of family, friends, familiar surroundings and community services.

3. Holistic care. Patients receive biopsychosocial care, which is responsive to both mental and physical ailments.

4. Specialist support. Psychiatrists are available to review and advise on complex cases. They also train primary care physicians and nurses:

   - Where there are few mental health specialists, they can be leveraged most effectively by refocusing their work from clinical care to training, supervision and management of complex cases.

   - With training and ongoing support, general medical practitioners can provide integrated mental health care.

   - High-level political commitment and the establishment of a national mental health commission contributed to the success of this integration effort.

   - Primary care physicians identified the importance of primary care for mental health and, therefore, were highly active and enthusiastic in the overall reform.

   - Extending and reinforcing mental health training for residents and practising primary care physicians were essential for the success of the programme.

   - Integrated primary care is important, but most effective when complemented by community-based rehabilitation. In this case, primary care physicians led the creation of an important community-based programme – the Austral – which resulted in fewer relapses and improved the quality of life for patients.

- Collaboration between the public health sector (primary care clinics) and a partially state-funded non-governmental organization (the Austral) can be effective for providing comprehensive mental health care.

- Community-based rehabilitation paid dividends, socially and economically. Patients relapsed less often and hence needed less hospital care; in addition, they remained integrated with families and friends and were able to start income-generating projects.

- Experts from outside Argentina were useful in sharing experiences and providing training. However, it was important that they did not try to impose their views or prescribe solutions to the local health team.

13.2.1 The Importance of a Collaborative Approach to Teaching

In our experience, it is essential to develop psychiatric education for primary care workers *in close collaboration* with primary care professionals in order to ensure that they are fully engaged in the process, their needs are being met and the teaching is being delivered as effectively and efficiently as possible. Unless psychiatrists have worked in or closely with primary care, they may not understand the specific requirements of and problems faced by primary care workers in delivering mental health care.

The aim should be to develop teachers within primary care who can themselves disseminate mental health training (a 'train-the-trainers' approach), so that mental health training becomes 'owned' by primary care itself. Ideally there should be some opportunities for contact between sectors (primary care, specialist services, social services and voluntary or non-governmental organizations), which often do not communicate as well as they might do. Indeed, there is a great deal of mutual learning required: many psychiatrists have very little idea of the multitude of different pressures faced in a busy primary care clinic. Teaching and learning is not a one-way process and psychiatric trainees have a great deal to learn from participating in sessions with primary care workers to learn about the key role of primary care in providing mental health care in the community. In some countries. such as the United Kingdom, much undergraduate teaching, including teaching about mental health problems, is now being carried out in primary care settings, by primary care teachers.

13.3 Developing a Curriculum: What do Primary Care Workers Want and Need to Know?

As noted earlier, the content of any training programme will be highly dependent on what has been previously learned in basic medical or nursing education by those attending any course, and the reader is directed to Chapter 4 for a further discussion of the essential contents of the undergraduate curriculum.

In the United Kingdom, the mental health curriculum of the Royal College of General Practitioners (Boxes 13.3 and 13.4) begins with the assumption that all trainees will have had a thorough undergraduate training experience in psychiatry and a basic understanding of the nature of key mental health problems such as psychosis and depression.

Box 13.3   Royal College of General Practitioners (UK) Competency Areas for GP Training: Mental Health and Illness

Bereavement

Dementia

Delirium

Alcohol and drug misuse

Chronic psychotic disorders

Acute psychotic disorders

Bipolar disorder

Depression

Phobic disorders

Panic disorders

General anxiety

Chronic mixed anxiety and depression

Adjustment disorders

PTSD

Unexplained somatic complaints

Eating disorder

Sexual disorders

Learning disability

Chronic fatigue syndrome.

Box 13.4 Royal College of General Practitioners Competency Areas for Training: Key Aspects of Care

Primary Care Management	
Knowledge	Aetiology, diagnostic criteria, management options, local and national guidelines
Coordination of care	Within practice, in local team, referral, team working and multiagency coordination
Practice 'issues' in delivering care	Team structures, skills and competencies. Protocols and pathways for care. Governance and risk management.
Problem Solving	
Ability to identify and diagnose in primary care	Apply knowledge and skills in clinical setting to produce a differential diagnosis and recognize serious diagnoses
Ability to manage in primary care	Ability to formulate a safe and appropriate management plan
Person-centred care	Effective doctor–patient communication, respecting autonomy, continuity of care, contextualizing illness in family and societal settings, awareness of values and beliefs
Comprehensive approach	Managing multiple health problems and comorbidity, prioritization of problems, health promotion, medico-legal issues
Community Orientation	Reconciling individual and community health needs, resource management, meeting local needs.
Holistic care	Assessing psychological and social aspects of illness in parallel with physical. Caring for the whole person in the context of their family, culture and beliefs
Attitudinal aspects of care	Awareness of the effects of attitudes on care delivery. Duties of a doctor.

In some parts of the world undergraduate medical education in psychiatry may have been lacking and there is a knowledge gap to close. Knowledge deficits may be concerned with the features that need to be considered in order to justify a diagnosis and a suggested intervention, the psychosocial interventions that have been shown to be effective in particular disorders, or the efficacy of pharmacological interventions for such disorders. The WHOs *Classification of Mental Disorders for Primary Health Care (ICD10-PHC)* (www.mentalneurologicalprimarycare.org), gives detailed advice on the management of the 24 mental disorders that are most commonly encountered in primary care settings. In their original form these consisted of a set of 24 cards, which was subjected to a field trial in 15 countries – the British field trial [14] showed that use of the depression card caused doctors to require more depressive symptoms before prescribing anti-depressants and added to their management strategies when dealing with a depressive episode. However, it should not automatically be assumed that a knowledge deficit is the main problem: it is far more common for doctors to have attitudinal problems and skill deficits of which they are unaware.

In their review of the literature, Hodges *et al.* [15, p. 1580] noted the mismatch between what psychiatrists wanted to teach and primary care workers wanted to learn:

> Primary care physicians most often wanted to increase their knowledge regarding somatization, psychosexual problems, difficult patients and stress management, whereas psychiatrists emphasized the diagnostic criteria of disorders such as schizophrenia, bipolar disorder, and depression ... education that is focused on diagnosis and medication may neglect the very cornerstone of psychiatric primary care, which is learning to develop and maintain effective relationships with patients who have complex problems.

The impact of this mismatch may be one of the reasons why education programmes have sometimes been less than successful [16].

Teaching can also be provided about specific psychosocial interventions – what they are and who/what they work for. For example, problem solving for depression [17], simple behavioural interventions such as motivational interviewing for alcohol problems [18], graded exercise combined with cognitive behavioural strategies for fatigue and reattribution for medically unexplained symptoms [19].

It is also important to explore how primary care workers can find out about local resources in their area and link in with the specialist services and Non-Governmental Organizations (NGOs) which can provide them with necessary expertise and support. These agencies may be invited to participate in the training, but it is essential to ensure that they fully understand the purpose of the training and do not see this as an opportunity to simply ensure referrals to their own organization. However large such agencies or institutions are, they cannot perform the essential role of front-line workers; however, they may feel unnecessarily threatened (as seems to be the case in some countries) by attempts to develop the role of primary care workers.

It is therefore essential, before delivering any type of course or curriculum of training, *to have a clear idea of exactly what the needs are of the primary care workers in that setting,* by meeting with them some time in advance. What particular knowledge and skills do they need to develop? What problems do they find most difficult on a day-to-day basis in their work? Are there any particular attitudinal issues that might need to be addressed with respect to mental health issues?

It is also crucial to work with the primary care workers to try to learn the needs of the target population of the primary health care services during the planning phase. Some existing epidemiological data may be available, but if some research can be planned and implemented together with the primary care workers, it may enhance their awareness regarding the needs of the target population they are serving and also enhance the research capacity of the professionals involved, including psychiatric residents who may be encouraged to become involved in collaborative research initiatives [20] (see also Chapter 11). Methods employed to collect data must, however, be simple and easy to implement in order not to consume too much of the limited time of the primary care workers. Sometimes asking one or two well designed questions during the routine interaction with the patient or giving out a questionnaire before or after the consultation (self-rated or filled in, for example, by a nurse or a midwife before or after their interaction with the patient or, if present, their relatives) may be sufficient. Apart from the valuable data derived from such studies about the type and extent of problems, these approaches themselves may be useful to improve the relationships between the health workers and the patients and their relatives.

Strengthening the communication channels amongst the primary care workers and also between the primary care workers and the target population may improve the quality of the health services (including the mental health services) [21].

13.3.1   Methods of Teaching

The most commonly used teaching method still seems to be continuing education meetings and workshops. In some cases organizing educational meetings is expected to solve many problems. However, as Forsetlund and colleagues [22] have commented 'educational meetings alone are not likely to be effective for changing complex behaviours'. They suggest that 'strategies to increase attendance at educational meetings, using mixed interactive and didactic formats and focusing on outcomes that are likely to be perceived as serious may increase the effectiveness of educational meetings'. Thus, the most effective educational interventions are multifaceted, offering a range of possible options for those attending to learn from and providing the possibility for a range of different needs to be met.

Medical knowledge doubles every five years and this has mandated student or learner-centred approaches to ensure life-long learning practice. These kind of learning strategies include problem-based learning, case-based learning, project-based learning, peer teaching/peer assisted learning and group work [23]. Learner-centred learning is a form of active and reflective learning that initiates and is maintained by the learners' intrinsic motivation to learn. Group activities are another helpful strategy but require more teacher-facilitators because the students are divided into several small groups. Lecturing in the classroom remains a critical component for low-resource institutions but must be interactive, well organized and coherent [24].

Advances in technology allow learning through Web-based learning or distance learning. Computer-based instruction is growing in developed countries (see Chapter 16 for a further discussion of the use of new technologies).

Clinical teaching and experience in a primary care training or residency attachment to psychiatry must include ward work, out-patient work and, particularly, community work. Every student must be involved in clerking patients in out-patient and in-patient settings. Students should observe teachers and peers interviewing patients, as well as observing psychologist, social workers and occupational therapists at work. The needs of the primary care or family practice resident in training differ from those of a psychiatrist and should be specifically addressed in their learning programme. Residents who are training in family practice and spending time in psychiatry should not be used to provide physical health care to psychiatric in-patients at the expense of their training in the speciality.

13.3.2 Practical Considerations – Where and How?

Training for working primary care professionals in the community seems to be best attended when it is provided at or near the place of work of those attending, at a time that is convenient to them and in a pattern that enables them to practice and try out what they have learned between sessions. Although sometimes it is difficult to avoid having to provide training in blocks of several days so that people can attend from some distance away, this is not ideal because of the lack of opportunity to use what has been learned and report back on progress. It is also good if invitations can be sent out from a well known and respected person, ideally working in primary care and who has helped to plan the meetings and may co-chair sessions. Experience suggests that busy workers appreciate refreshments, particularly if attending at lunchtime or in the evening.

Sponsorship from pharmaceutical companies helps to reduce costs, but can be problematic in terms of governance over the content of what is taught, as the companies may wish to have a particular lecturer on the course, or have rules about their own product not being promoted in any way in the content – which can be equally problematic if it is a useful drug that you wish to recommend! It's preferable, but not always possible, to look for alternative sources of funding from governmental or other agencies or have a range of funders, so that no single company is being promoted. Keeping costs down enables non-medical staff to attend too, as they will find it very difficult to pay for any training.

13.3.3 Knowledge, Attitudes and Skills

Lectures designed to convey essential knowledge should:

- be brief,

- be tailored to the needs of the audience (too often psychiatrists present what only psychiatrists need or want to know and do not address the needs of primary care),

- have plenty of opportunity for questions and discussion,

- provide good handouts with key references and Web links.

Many primary care workers will have attitudes that do not differ greatly from lay people with respect to mental illness. This can be perceived as less stigmatizing by some of their patients, who do not want to receive a 'psychiatric' label or treatment or to 'normalize' their problems, but for others, particularly those with severe and enduring mental illness, lay assumptions about mental health problems may be stigmatizing.

Group discussion may be useful in *challenging unhelpful attitudes*. This can be triggered by case presentations, videotaped interviews or, *most powerfully*, participation of real people telling their own stories about their experiences of mental illness and of mental health care.

However, the key component of educational interventions should be that of *developing the skills* of primary care workers to communicate with, assess and manage mental health problems in primary care more effectively. There is now considerable evidence that the skills of primary care workers can be improved by using a range of active educational methods, including role play and video feedback [25]. These are described in detail in Chapter 8.

13.4   Engaging Psychiatry in the Task

In general medical and primary care settings, consultation-liaison psychiatry, in particular, has an important role to play in education within the general hospital and in primary care and represents the application of the biopsychosocial model to medical practice [26]. However, psychiatrists in all specialities, including residents, should be engaged in liaising with primary care and a key function of this role is that of (mutual) education. This may be a local, national or even an international activity (Box 13.5) in which psychiatrists in training should be encouraged to participate.

Box 13.5   Case Study: Primary Care Mental Health Training in Sverdlovsk, Russian Federation

In a study carried out in the Sverdlovsk region of Russia, a multicomponent programme was implemented to facilitate the integration of mental health into primary health care [27].

Building on local epidemiological research carried out by a new training programme in family practice, a new course was designed in collaboration with visitors from the United Kingdom, who shared expertise in active methods of training, including role play.

The content of the course was specifically tailored for the needs of local family doctors who had little previous training in psychiatry.

Training was initially delivered by the visiting experts who trained local teachers, including GPs and psychiatrists working together, to deliver further training and then provided supervision and support on further visits. There was also an opportunity for the GP teacher to visit the UK and observe teaching.

The training was extensively evaluated resulting in a joint publication [28] and presentation by the GP teacher at an international mental health conference.

References

1. WHO/WONCA (2008) Integrating mental health into primary care: a global perspective, WHO, Geneva. Downloadable from: http://www.who.int/mental_health/policy/services/mentalhealthintoprimarycare/en/index.html (accessed 30 July 2010).

2. Murray, C.J. and Lopez, A.D. (1997) Alternative projections of mortality and disability by cause 1990–2020: Global Burden of Disease Study. *Lancet*, **349**, 1498–1504.

3. Andrews, G. and Henderson, S. (2000) *Unmet Need in Psychiatry*, Cambridge University Press, Cambridge.

4. McCormick, A., Fleming, D. and Charlton, J. (1995) *Morbidity statistics from general practice: fourth national morbidity study 1991–1992*, HMSO, London.

5. Mental Health Aftercare Association (1999) *First national GP survey of mental health in primary care*, HMSO, London.

6. US Department of Health and Human Services (1999) Mental Health: A Report of the Surgeon General – Executive Summary. US Department of Health and Human Services, Substance Abuse and Mental Health Services Administration, Center for Mental Health Services, National Institutes of Health, National Institute of Mental Health, Rockville, MD.

7. Patel, V. (2003) *Where There is no Psychiatrist: A Mental Health Care Manual*, Gaskell, London.

8. Blignault, I., Bunde-Birouste, A., Ritchie, J. *et al.* (2009) Community perceptions of mental health needs: a qualitative study in the Solomon Islands. *International Journal of Mental Health Systems*, **3**, 6 http://www.ijmhs.com/content/3/1/6.

9. Balint, M. (1964) *The Doctor, his Patient and the Illness*, Pitman, London.

10. Williams, K. (1998) Self-assessment of clinical competence by general practitioner trainees before and after a six-month psychiatric placement. *British Journal of General Practice*, **48**, 1387–1390.

11. Holden, J.M., Sagovsky, R. and Cox, J.L. (1989) Counselling in a general practice setting; controlled study of health visitor intervention in treatment of postnatal depression. *BMJ*, **298**, 223–226.

12. Gray, R., Parr, A.M., Plummer, S. *et al* (1999) A national survey of practice nurse involvement in mental health interventions. *Journal of Advanced Nursing*, **30**, 901–906.

13. Grace, G.D. and Christensen, R.C., (2007) Recognizing psychologically masked illnesses: the need for collaborative relationship in mental health care. *Prim Care Companion J Clin Psychiatry*, **9**, 433–436.

14. Goldberg, D., Sharp, D. and Nanayakkara, K. (1995) The field trial of the mental disorders section of ICD-10 designed for primary care (ICD10-PHC) in England. *Family Practice*, **12**, 466–473.

15. Hodges, B., Inch, C. and Silver, I. (2001) Improving the psychiatric knowledge, skills, and attitudes of primary care physicians, 1950-2000: a review. *Am J Psychiatry*, **158**, 1579–1586.

16. Gask, L., Dixon, C., May, C. *et al.* (2005) Qualitative study of an educational intervention for general practitioners in the assessment and management of depression. *British Journal of General Practice*, **55**, 854–859.

17. Mynors-Wallis, L. (2005) *Problem Solving Treatment for Anxiety and Depression: A Practical Guide*, Oxford University Press, Oxford.

18. Miller, W.R. and Rollnick, S. (2009) *Motivational Interviewing: Preparing People to Change Addictive Behaviour*, 2nd edn, Guildford Press.

19. Goldberg, D. Gask, L. and Sartorius, N. (2002) Training Package for Mental Health Skills in Primary Care Settings, World Psychiatric Association.

20. Ried, K., Farmer, E.A. and Weston, K.M. (2006) Setting directions for capacity building in primary health care: a survey of a research network. *BMC Family Practice*, **7**, 8.

21. Coskun B. (2006) *Development of a Program for and with Primary Health Care Workers.* Unpublished study presented as a poster at the 4th World Conference on the Promotion of Mental Health and Prevention of Mental and Behavioural Disorders, 11–13 October 2006, Oslo.

22. Forsetlund, L., Bjorndal, A., Rashidian, A. *et al.* (2009) Continuing education meetings and workshops: effects on professional practice and health care outcomes. *Cochrane Database of Systematic Reviews*, 2 (Art. No.: CD003030). doi: 10.1002/14651858.CD003030.pub2

23. Fardouly, N. (2001) Principle of Instructional Design and Adult Learning. Learner-centered teaching strategy, University of New South Wales, Australia.

24. Amin, Z. and Eng, K.H. (2003) *Basics in Medical Education*, World Scientific, New Jersey.

25. Gask, L., Goldberg, D. and Lewis, B. (2009) Teaching and learning about mental health, in *Primary Care Mental Health* (eds L. Gask, H. Lester, T. Kendrick and R. Peveler), Royal College of Psychiatrists, London.

26. Engel, G.L. (1977) The need for a new medical model: a challenge for biomedicine. *Science*, **196**, 129–136.

27. Jenkins, R., Bobyleva, Z., Goldberg, D. *et al.* (2009) Integrating mental health into primary care in Sverdlovsk. *Mental Health in Family Medicine*, **6**, 29–36.

28. Zakroyeva, A., Goldberg, D., Gask, L. and Leese, M. (2008) Training Russian family physicians in mental health skills. *Eur J Gen Pract.*, **14**, 19–22.

14
The Standardized Patient

Michael Curtis[1] and David Baron[2]

[1]William Maul Measey Institute for Clinical Simulation and Patient Safety, Temple University School of Medicine, Philadelphia, PA, USA
[2]Keck School of Medicine, University of Southern California, Los Angeles, CA, USA

14.1 Introduction

The education of medical students consists of didactic (classroom) and clinical (bedside) components. Future physicians worldwide traditionally spend the beginning of their training learning the basic science of medicine, with the latter part of their medical education focusing on the acquiring of clinical skills and the application of didactic knowledge. Becoming a competent physician requires the integration of complex cognitive, affective and motor skills. Knowing *how* to take adequate history and perform a clinically relevant physical exam on a patient is as knowing what to ask and where to palpate. The development of clinical competency requires much practice and extensive 'real time' feedback on the students' performance. This is particularly true for the cognitive specialities, such as psychiatry. The ability of the student to get immediate feedback from the 'patient' on the impact of a clinical encounter is a powerful learning experience. Developed nearly 50 years ago as a clinical teaching tool for medical students, Standardized Patients (SPs) are now an integral component of assessment as well as teaching technique. The ability to target specific learning objectives in a controlled environment and provide students with immediate feedback and the opportunity to practice new skills in a less stressful environment are the strength of this teaching strategy. It is one of the only techniques which addresses cultural competence, regardless of the culture. The use of SPs should be an integral component of all undergraduate medical education. Advances in educational technology can be beneficial, as discussed in the chapter, but are not required. An effective SP programme can be developed and maintained with limited financial resources and does not require expensive equipment to be functional.

Teaching Psychiatry: Putting Theory into Practice   Edited by Linda Gask, Bulent Coskun and David Baron
© 2011 John Wiley & Sons, Ltd

14.2 The Standardized Patient

The Standardized Patient is a person, usually a lay person, who has been trained to portray, in a realistic, disciplined and standardized manner, a patient, for the purpose of training or assessing medical professionals. While they are often referred to as 'actors', and many SPs are in fact actors by profession, they need not necessarily be actors, and the use of the term can lead some to infer that the SP methodology is more related to performance and dramatics than to professional education.

There is a paradox connected with standardized patients: it would seem at first that what makes an SP useful is that they are 'just like a real patient', but in fact the real value of an SP is that he or she is not a real patient. With an SP an educator can create a specific learning situation for a particular level of student; one can present a situation that would be potentially harmful to the real patient, especially in the hands of an inexperienced trainee clinician, without any risk to the SP, and thus create as safe situation for the student, allowing them to make mistakes and to learn from them. In particular teaching situations the educator can halt the simulation to discuss the student's work, or re-direct them to more productive ends; and one can do all of these at a convenient time, place and situation. None of these would be feasible with real patients. In particular, psychiatric patients may be less willing or less able to function in a teaching situation with students, making the SP all the more valuable.

It must be emphasized that the SP must never be considered a replacement for the necessary experience students must have with real patients. Rather, they should be considered both preparation and enhancement to that experience. The preparation will allow them to be at a better, more advanced skill level when gaining clinical experience, and thus to be able to benefit more from that experience. As an enhancement, SP methodology allows the student's training to be directed and controlled more closely, ensuring that they are exposed to particular types of clinical situations, patient problems and patient affects that will be needed to gain a fully-rounded training. As a practical matter, there are greater opportunities for faculty observation and involvement in the training than would be possible if training is restricted to work with real patients.

The history of the use of SPs in teaching is, in fact, closely related to deficiencies in medical education. Two of the pioneers in the field in North America, Dr Howard Barrows and Dr Robert Kretzschmar, saw opportunities to use SPs for the direct and controlled observation of student skills that was not happening as much as it should have for complete training. In the 1950s and 1960s, with hospital in-patients being more ill than in the past, and with lengths of stay dropping, clinical material for student practice was becoming harder to come by, so educators turned to simulating the necessary range and extent of patient experience. Lately, Ziv *et al.* have written of the use of simulation in medical education as an ethical imperative, that simulation enables learning that must happen and that can happen in no other way [1].

While SPs can be, and increasingly are, used in the assessment of clinical skills the emphasis here must be on the use of the methodology in teaching, and any new SP programme should start with use in teaching before moving to assessment. The potential benefits from the use in teaching are very high, more so than those of assessment. As well, faced with SPs for the first time in an examination, learners will find the concept distracting and artificial, and that will compromise the value of the demonstration of their behaviour.

14.3   Teaching Formats

Again, it is the artificial nature of SPs that allows their use in a wide range of teaching formats:

- Group sessions: An SP works with a small group of students, five or six would be the largest workable size, under the direction of a teaching faculty member. One student at a time will interview or otherwise encounter the patient, with the others observing. The faculty member may wish to use a 'time-out', that is, pausing the encounter and taking the student out of the simulation temporarily, to discuss the student's work, impart useful information, to re-direct them, answer the student's questions, or engage the other members of the group. The SP does not engage in this teacher–student exchange, but rather behaves as though the physician had left the room to consult with a colleague. Students in turn each engage the patient, having learned from the observation of their classmates.

- Use of feedback by the SP: Following an encounter, either in group or individual sessions, the SP speaks to the student of the experience of being the patient. That is, they talk of how they believe the student's actions would have made the patient feel. It is usually framed as 'When you did/said that, as the patient, I felt...'. It is not evaluative and does not speak of the content of the encounter, but rather simply shares information with the student, with the SP saying directly what the real patient rarely, if ever, would.

- Direct teaching by the SP: A well trained SP can follow up simulation by coming out of their role as the patient and speaking with the student to provide constructive criticism about the tasks of taking a history, doing physical examination and developing a therapeutic doctor–patient relationship.

- Individual sessions, in which the student is alone with the SP: Students often find this very involving, as of course it more closely resembles actual clinical situations than do group sessions.

- Faculty observation and discussion: Following such individual sessions, a faculty member who has observed, either in real time or afterwards via recording, meets with the student for critical discussion of their work.

- SP discussion/teaching: Following the session the student meets with the SP, who steps out of their patient role to discuss the student's work, in more of a direct teaching role. If this is done without faculty present it frees up the faculty time, but must be done with great care to ensure the lay person SP adheres to appropriate teaching protocols and the necessary curriculum. Significant effort must be put into training for this purpose.

- Self-assessment and critique by the student: These can be in written or verbal form. It can be useful for the student to reflect on their work, and assess their progress from a baseline.

- Audiovisual recordings can be incorporated into these formats, with review separately by the student, or in conjunction with the SP and/or teaching faculty (see Chapter 8 for more discussion of how to do this).

- Longitudinal series of encounters, covering an extended period in the patient's life, rather than a single moment. The patient can be seen repeatedly at selected intervals in the development of illness or in the progress of recovery, with the patient presentation varying according to the actions taken in the previous encounter. This can be highly appropriate for psychiatric training, given the long term nature of some psychiatric care, and the ability of the SP to portray variations in patient manner.

14.4   The Case

As one great strength of SP methodology is that the educator can present a specific learning opportunity, it follows that the patient case must be developed carefully to achieve that goal. High quality case development is, therefore, a critical element in the use of SPs. Criteria for a good case include:

- It must be based on clinical reality. What the educator is presenting is intended to be accepted by the learner as being a representation of reality. The SP can be so convincing in a realistic portrayal of the patient that whatever the student sees they will take as being an accurate representation of clinical reality. There is, therefore, the ethical requirement that it in fact adheres to what would be seen clinically.

- The case must be descriptive of the patient, not prescriptive of any student behaviour. That is, it cannot be expected to result in the student doing anything specific. One hears faculty saying 'and then the student will do thus-and-such'. But in fact one wants to simply create a situation where the student can do whatever they might do. That may involve mistakes, but they will be ones from which the student will learn.

- It should have a clear teaching goal. Whatever the content and form of the case might be, a lesson will be taken from it, therefore that lesson must be controlled, and in that way it will better serve the curriculum. It can be very useful to provide specific learning points within the case, for the use of the teaching faculty. The very process of noting these will help to focus the case writers on the teaching goals.

- The teaching goal must be appropriate for the level of student involved.

- The case should allow the student to succeed at what is expected of them. There is no value in having a student make an honest attempt, use the appropriate techniques with great skill and still be unable to achieve the necessary goal. The lesson would then be that such effort is futile, leading only to cynicism on the part of the student.

- It must be complete, in the sense that no matter what the student does the SP will be able to respond with material that is consistent with the patient history and the teaching goals.

- It should describe fully the patient affect and use of language. Specific examples of language can be provided as illustrative guides for the SP.

- If there is a physical simulation required it must be described precisely.

- If other clinical materials are to be incorporated, such as imaging, or props, such as medicine bottles, they must be described exactly.

- It should be written in lay language for use by the SPs.

- It should be written in the third person, to enhance the separation between the patient and the SP.

- The case must be feasible, in the sense that it can in fact be portrayed convincingly. Here the psychiatric context enables a very broad range of what could be feasible. The patient affect and history are so much a part of the psychiatric clinical experience that the skills of a well-trained SP can be put to good use in simulating them, even when the affect can be quite extreme. The accompanying physical findings, which are most often neurological in nature can often be simulated by SPs to a high degree of verisimilitude [2].

- It should not require the student to do anything other than what they would do clinically. For example, the student should not be required to 'role play' by imagining any previous encounter or relationship with the patient which they have not had. To expect this is to invite problems, for many students will not be able to create such a 'back story' that is consistent with the case. What should be expected of them is clinical behaviour, not improvisational acting, a skill they may not have and should not be required to have. The simulation should be entirely on the part of the SP.

- The information that the clinician would have prior to seeing the patient, and that would be given to the student prior to encountering the SP, should be specified.

- It must present a situation in which it is clear what the clinician is to do. This can sometimes be problematic in very acute cases, where some immediate intervention may be the most appropriate action, but that may require something that cannot actually be done within the simulation. As non-human simulation technology (controlled robotic devices, virtual reality etc.) improves, this may become less of a restriction. Chronic cases can also be difficult, for it may not be at all evident why the patient is seeing this doctor now, for the first time (See the material above regarding the problems of requiring a previous encounter). But chronic cases can actually be unusually well suited to psychiatric use, for very often the history may be of periodic psychiatric illness, or long term recovery from an illness. Consider the use of longitudinal encounters for chronic cases.

- The case should not require the use of the SP's own history, for doing so would weaken one of the very strengths of using the SP, that one can do no harm through the simulation. There must be a strong separation between the patient and the SP. This could be particularly true in a psychiatric context, as there could be significant danger in dealing with a fragile, damaged personality.

- The case should incorporate a 'challenge'. This is simply a scripted statement made by the SP at some time during the encounter, regardless of what else may or may not have been discussed. The purposes behind it are multiple. It makes the patient portrayal more realistic, for every patient will have something on their mind that they will express spontaneously, and which they will state, rather than only responding to questions. By scripting the challenge, rather than leaving it up to the SP, there is greater standardization and adherence to the educational goals. The challenge should be at least slightly provocative, as the nature of the student's response, or lack of response, can be highly revealing of their skills and attitudes. It should not be a simple request for information, such as a diagnosis, for it is more interesting to see if such information is offered by the student without prompting.

14.5   Training SPs for Teaching

- The SP needs to understand the educational goals of the programme. In general, they must always know that the exercise is not for their benefit – whether obtaining medical care or engaging in performance – but for the student, and everything they do must be devoted to that end. This has to be made clear at the very start of recruiting SPs to a programme, with applicants who do not accept it refused positions. Specifically, they should understand what the goal is of the specific project or session. For example: Is it to allow the students to practice interviewing skills? – then they need to limit their affect, and not introduce new and extraneous material; Is it to learn how to advise the patient how to take medication? – then they must listen more than speak, and respond to specific language cues.

- The emphasis must be on actually doing the simulations. Training must never be only passive, with SPs simply observing others doing case portrayals or reading materials. These can be useful steps, but unless the SP has actually done the simulation before working with students, the quality of that work will be limited and inadequate.

- Practice must emphasize different approaches by students, so that SPs understand how to vary their responses appropriately to the variations in students' work. It can be very damaging if an SP adheres to a narrowly limited range of responses no matter what the student does. The result can be, at worst, quite inconsistent with what the real patient may say and contrary to the teaching goals of the exercise, but even if this does not happen, the responses may simply end up being generic, not specific to what the student actually did, and thus neither reinforcing correct clinical skills nor discouraging poor skills. It can be useful for the trainer to prepare a listing of possible different types of student behaviours or approaches to the patient problem. Thus, the SP is prepared for whatever might happen.

- The SP must know the material thoroughly. In fact, this is one of the easier parts of the job, though it may not appear so to new SPs.

- The patient affect must be completely realistic. Frankly, this is a matter of the skill that the SP must bring to the work. The trainer should not be expected to be an acting coach. If the SP cannot produce the necessary affect without basic direction, they cannot be allowed to continue. With the broader range of behaviours that might be seen in a psychiatric context, even into extremes of behaviour, the skills of trained and experienced actors may be needed more often than in programmes in, for example, family practice.

- The SP must be able to elaborate on the case material in a neutral manner as needed. Inevitably there will be a question from a student that cannot be answered with material in the written case.

- If direct teaching is expected of the SP, then specific protocols must be developed. For example, the SP should not speak to the student in an evaluative manner, but rather simply explain what happened, what worked, what did not. Nor should they be giving advice, which can only come from a clinician.

14.6 Assessment with Standardized Patients

As noted previously, it is probably wiser to start the use of SPs in psychiatric teaching, rather than in assessment, but there is great value in assessment.

What is the educator attempting to achieve with assessment? Is it a merely pass/fail summative exercise? If so, one should question whether it makes sense to put the necessary significant resources into assessment for only that. Or is there a formative goal and, if so, what? Are the learners who have not achieved a minimum standard of work to receive remediation? Or do all learners receive further assistance, targeted to specific deficiencies, to maximize improvement? All of these will affect the structuring of the assessment and, therefore, should be determined in advance.

The most common form of assessment using standardized patients is the OSCE, the Objective Structured Clinical Examination, in which the learner encounters a series of patients, as portrayed by SPs, presenting with a range of patient problems. The reader is advised to consult Turner and Dankoski for an excellent review of the current state of the art [3]; there is also more discussion of OSCEs in Chapter 17.

The advantage of simulation-based assessment in an OSCE format is that it can test actual clinical skills, not knowledge, though of course the two are not readily separated. The premise is that one creates situations in which learners need only do what they have been trained to do, what they would actually do when seeing a patient. That is, a situation in which clinical skills can be assessed because it is those skills that are being exercised, rather than artificial exam-taking skills. Within a psychiatric context there can be a very wide range of skills that can be assessed. These may include:

- history taking, both in the sense of obtaining the correct information from the patient, and the process by which that information is obtained;

- physical examination, which in psychiatry would include close observation of patient affect;

- therapeutic counselling;

- medication use and substance abuse counselling;

- skills in interacting with a wide range of patients and patients affects;

- working with family members;

- recognition of life-threatening situations, including suicide risk;

- recognition of threat to safety of others;

- ethical problems;

- recognition of varying patient acuities;

- communication with other health care professionals (either verbally or in writing through post-patient encounter exercises).

The design of an effective OSCE would involve a sufficient variety of cases, so as to give the opportunity to assess a wide range of skills in a balanced examination form.

The OSCE has come to stand in for direct observation and, perhaps, highly subjective assessment by expert observers – senior clinicians and faculty – of work done in actual clinical settings, which, due to time constraints, usually is limited to small samplings, replacing it with high sampling of behaviour assessed by non-expert observers and objective data gathering. In fact, an OSCE creates enormous amounts of data. The psychometric work of Paula Stillman and David Swanson effectively established the potential validity and reliability of OSCE data [4]. Remember, too, the assessment is not only of the learners, but of the teaching institution.

14.7   Technology and the Standardized Patient

Not so long ago one could say that the use of SPs was very much a 'low-tech' approach to medical education, in the sense there was nothing more needed than the SP, the learners and the teachers. In recent years, however, there has been an explosion of technology surrounding SPs, in three areas: (i) physical facilities, (ii) audio/video recordings and (iii) data gathering, analysis and reporting. The developers of a start-up SP programme should not feel intimidated by these developments.

14.7.1   Physical Facilities

Many institutions have built very elaborate facilities dedicated to simulation-based teaching and assessment, but it remains true that any space can be a classroom if the most important activity in it is the simple meeting of doctor and (simulated) patient and the meeting of instructor and learner.

More complex modified or purpose-built facilities can allow the incorporating of viewing facilities, such as one-way windows or unobtrusive installation of audio/video recording equipment, and may permit more efficient work flow for assessment activities, but these advantages must be carefully weighed against expense and extent of use. Smaller programmes may do best by using clinical space or non-specific spaces when available.

14.7.2   Audio/Video Recordings

There can be definite value in having recordings by which learners can view their work, and the use of simulated clinical encounters through standardized patients means that issues of patient confidentiality are minimized. Certainly the subtle aspects of patient affect, and language use and professional manner and language use on the part of the clinician that are so critical to psychiatric practice, would be well observed by means of recordings.

However, it is important to retain a sense of scale. How much time can be devoted to the viewing of the recordings? Can learners benefit from viewing their own work if that work is not also viewed by, and in conjunction with, teaching faculty who can provide critical insight from clinical experience?

Programmes should consider carefully the technical format for making recordings. The field has advance with great rapidity in recent years. There are now available software packages that allow digital recordings be compiled on servers for online viewing at any time and from any place. They also permit instructors to bookmark critical incidents and enter written commentary on notable aspects of the encounters. But they are expensive and cannot always be justified if use is limited by other resources. They also require significant and expensive support in the way of operation, technical maintenance, upgrading and hardware infrastructure. It may be much more cost effective, and not significantly less educationally effective, to use the simplest and cheapest materials at hand, even those that may be considerably short of the most modern standards. For small scale projects, an inexpensive or even obsolete system may be every bit as useful.

One should also consider if there would be better educational results from real time observation by teaching faculty and immediate discussion, which the availability of recordings may simply discourage.

Finally, understand that much of the cost of such recording will come from the video aspect, while the greatest value may be from the audio recordings. Again, one must be cautious about the expenditure of resources not matched by benefit.

14.7.3   Data Gathering, Analysis and Reporting

In an OSCE the actual documentation of the clinician's skills is done either by an observer – sometimes a second SP, sometimes a physician – or by the SP who themselves portrayed the patient. Whichever method is chosen, there will be a need to record the data obtained, and there will be a need to analyse and report those data. While there are many technological approaches to the collecting and recording of the data, one should not assume that these are essential for the operation of an OSCE. Indeed, depending upon local conditions, human resources may be more readily available, more economical and their use more community-supported, than would be the more technically developed resources.

14.8 Conclusion

The use of simulation is one of the most important innovations in medical education. The high degree of verisimilitude possible, and the controlled techniques of standardized patient methodology, make its use in the intimate arena of psychiatry increasingly valuable.

References

1. Ziv, A., Root Wolpe, P., Small, S.D. and Glick, S. (2003) Simulation-Based Medical Education: An Ethical Imperative. *Academic Medicine*, **78**, 783–788.
2. Barrows, H.S. (1987) Simulated (Standardized) Patients and Other Human Simulations, Chapel Hill, NC, USA.
3. Turner, J. and Dankoski, M. (2008) Objective Structured Clinical Exams: A Critical Review. *Family Medicine*, **40**, 574–578.
4. Curtis, M. (1992) Not the Real Thing: The Standardized Patient, (unpublished) Hannah Institute for the History of Medicine.

15

Patients as Teachers: Involving Service Users

Rex Haigh[1] and Kath Lovell[2]

[1]*Berkshire Healthcare NHS Foundation Trust, Bracknell, UK*
[2]*Emergence Community Interest Company, London, UK*

15.1   Distant Origins

The Winterbourne Programme in West Berkshire in the United Kingdom (UK) has been evolving since its origins in the heyday of social psychiatry [1]. Originally it was part of the 'unlocking the wards' movement and it functioned as a mixed diagnosis therapeutic community admission ward, under the consultant Dr David Duncan. By the 1990s it had closed its beds and become a non-residential group therapy programme, based on Gestalt and Group Analytic Psychotherapy [2]. An informal arrangement with the acute wards allowed a patient to be admitted to a bed overnight, or over a weekend, if their mental state demanded it. However, this arrangement stopped in 1995 when the unit moved from Fair Mile Hospital, an old Victorian asylum on a quiet stretch of the River Thames fifteen miles upstream from Reading, to a suburban home shared with the district psychotherapy service, close to the town centre. Here, various programmes evolved into what the consultant psychotherapist Jane Knowles wrote up as 'The Reading Model' [3]. This described it as an intensive treatment programme, run as a non-residential therapeutic community, alongside a dynamic psychotherapy service specializing in group analytic therapy, but also offering a range of psychodynamic and humanistic interventions – both individually and in groups. Throughout the 1990s, a number of trainees from different disciplines gravitated there to participate in different parts of the clinical programmes, and to be learners on various levels of training courses. Without being described as such, it had become a specialist personality disorder centre, based in the community.

   The relevance of this is that the training of all the different National Health Service (NHS) mental health professionals continued through the different phases of Winterbourne's

Teaching Psychiatry: Putting Theory into Practice   Edited by Linda Gask, Bulent Coskun and David Baron
© 2011 John Wiley & Sons, Ltd

evolution – and this was increasingly done as a partnership between professionals and service users. Equally relevant was the close working relationship between mainstream adult services and the Winterbourne unit: the local consultants all had a good idea who would benefit from its programmes, and referred accordingly. These were often people who had 'come to the end of the road' and had no simple therapeutic options left.

15.2   Royal College Examinations

Because of this close link, while the unit was still out in the countryside with the acute wards, the medical staff were involved in the Royal College of Psychiatrists membership examinations. The patients on the day programme would always be asked whether they wanted to be part of a young doctor's psychiatry examinations – and earn a small honorarium by doing so. Every six months, two or three subjects were supplied for the clinical part of the exams. It was while preparing the case summaries for these that I (Haigh) first realized that we were, predominantly, a borderline personality disorder unit: I remember, about 1994, that borderline personality disorder was at the top of the differential diagnoses for all five summaries I had prepared for that exam. Is it really that common, I wondered? The patients thoroughly enjoyed this experience, and usually came back to us with tales of how they had told extreme stories of their bad behaviour to mental health staff in the past, and exaggerated their symptoms. They also explained how they helped the candidates if they were 'nice' (presumably meaning that they behaved respectfully, or perhaps were quivering with nerves), and had been really awkward to the ones who were being 'uppity'.

The next educational activity evolved from our regular invitation to take our turn presenting the hospital's clinical case conference. Before, this had been a case of our Senior House Officer (SHO) presenting a case in standard psychiatric format, and discussing the psychotherapeutic as well psychiatric as aspects of the case. A particularly brave SHO thought we could take several patients to the meeting, and the idea evolved over a week or two into taking all 18 members of the group, and running the whole event as a role played community meeting. We never did another 'straight' case presentation; each time our turn came round it became an opportunity to do a teaching session – with an assembly of junior and senior colleagues to do it for. Although it was slightly nerve wracking for us, I think it was much more so for our colleagues! Again, much benefit was felt by members, many of whom never believed that they could have conducted themselves in such a confident way in front of strangers. For some this discomfort followed by triumph was even more acute, as the SHOs or consultants who had previously looked after them were present at the meeting. Occasionally, it was 'too much' for the group members, and others supported and sat with them away from the teaching session. But however difficult or playful it was for the participants, it always produced good material to explore in future therapy sessions.

Various specific activities were developed from these sessions, such as teaching new junior doctors how to talk to difficult and angry patients, how to prevent difficult situations arising and how to start to gain the trust of a very hesitant and silent patient. These are very easy to arrange with members of a well-functioning group who are in an intensive treatment programme: people are usually keen to use their own understanding of 'what goes wrong' to help prevent it for others who follow them.

15.3   Hitting the Road

Recognizing the use of these role plays of large group therapy, we soon developed them into a suitable format for taking elsewhere. One of the things I (Haigh) rarely had time to do was much preparation for occasional invited lectures, such as the Monday evening lectures at the Institute of Group Analysis where I myself trained. With some trepidation, I asked the members of the group whether anybody was interested: we would have to go by train to Paddington, and thence by tube (Metro) to Swiss Cottage. With about ten volunteers (more than half the group), I clucked around like the proverbial mother hen about meeting times, meeting places, mobile phone numbers, train tickets, how to pay, train timetables, preparation sessions and debriefing sessions. The first we did was an 'easy' group of students – on the introductory course, not the advanced level – so we were all quite confident that we knew enough about group therapy not to make fools of ourselves. However, it is also a fact about the introductory course that it has more students on it – about seventy the year we were first invited. I let this fact out about a week before we went and, despite some anxiety, everybody who originally signed up was there for it.

We had a large room with three concentric circles and an hour and a quarter to fill. In all my anxiety about the practical preparations, I had completely forgotten to prepare a 'lesson plan' for what we were going to do. But I need not have worried, as the group members had discussed it amongst themselves and decided to do a role play of a half hour community meeting (using exactly the same structure and agenda as we did every day), and have several 'stooges' who would act in role about a tricky situation of threatened self-harm. We were each given roles, and we sat in the inner circle of the room, about 20 chairs, and padded it out with volunteers from the students who were willing to act as if participants in our community meeting. After we had explained it all to the students, and done the role play, we received a loud round of spontaneous applause. I doubt if most of the group members had ever experienced anything like that before – and were immensely proud of what they had done, both in the teaching session and in their daily group therapy. It was moving for the two of us there as staff – people who said little in our therapy groups in Reading explained just what they were getting out of it, others described exactly what psychodynamics the role play demonstrated and those working through painful emotions described the process of therapy with precision and deep insight. Needless to say, this was with a clarity and cohesion that few professionals ever manage when describing their work.

15.4   'Patients Teaching Doctors'

In the staff team, we soon realized what a wonderful resource this was: both for teaching trainees, referrers and colleagues about what we do, and for being used as a part of people's therapy itself. It had great benefits on self-esteem, was generally experienced as fun – often essential alongside the heaviness and intensity of depth analytic therapy – and often gave people the sense that they were doing something positive for future generations of patients and the care they might receive. Because the day programme is intensive psychotherapy, with strong sense of containment, it is possible to do this with this sort of programme – but probably not for other settings where the group relationships do not exist.

We subsequently did similar 'performances' for most lectures, talks and teaching sessions that I and others on the staff team were invited to give. The fee for such events was usually enough to cover the travel expenses and leave a little over to go into the group's own funds. Nevertheless, an opportunity arose to develop it further with a proposal to the Oxford Postgraduate Medical Education Deanery in 2002. A call was put out for projects to join up clinical work and theory; we duly submitted 'Patients Teaching Doctors' and received £8000 to advance the work. We could now establish support systems and ask ex-patients to participate. This was the early stages of the STARS programme. (STARS is a term which was invented by the ex-service users themselves, to mean 'Support, Training And Recovery System').

In this, we formalized our policies and procedures, were able to fund attendance at a few conferences and had part-time administrative support. Thankfully, this was in the person of the medical secretary who had previously dealt with and known the patients in the therapeutic programme. We started to take ex-members of the group to various national events, and run large group role plays illustrating our group's approach to the theme of the conference. Notable ones included a Royal College Psychotherapy Faculty Residential Conference in Leeds, where the group members simply described their experiences in different forms of psychiatric treatment and psychotherapy, and an international group psychotherapy conference in Athens (two weeks after the 2004 Olympiad), where we illustrated our understanding of therapeutic boundaries. In Leeds we were not well received, and left with the general impression that such events were not welcome; it may not be unrelated that I was called to reception by the hotel staff who were concerned that one of the participants' bed sheets were heavily bloodstained from self-harm. In fact, she was self-harming very much less than previously – but did so the evening of the presentation. This is the only such occasion that has happened over nearly ten years of this large group teaching, and the person concerned has since made great progress. In Athens we did a very large group dramatisation where I (Haigh) played a rather inebriated patient coming late into a therapy group, and being asked to leave. The gentle Europeans were quite distressed that I was dealt with so harshly!

15.5   Thames Valley STARS

The 'Thames Valley Initiative' was the largest of the eleven community pilot project services for personality disorder which were funded by the National Institute for Mental Health in 2004, covering Berkshire, Buckinghamshire and Oxfordshire. As well as providing new services around the Thames Valley, loosely based on the 'Reading Model', the bid included funding to support the 'recovery' function. Although it has since been questioned whether 'recovery' is a valid concept in personality disorder (because people are trying to attain a level of functioning and well-being that they have never had before), the team has done a great deal of work to involve service users, ex-service users and 'long-time ex-service users' in training, and much besides, as the basis for work thereafter. The range of training activities in which our 'experts by experience' have been involved is shown in Table 15.1.

'STARS' (Support, Training And Recovery System) is the semi-autonomous organization that has accomplished this. It started in 2005 as a group for those who were at least six months post-therapy, upstairs in a rather sleazy Reading nightclub for three hours on a

Table 15.1 Teaching activities with service users.

Case study material

- Personal history, with or without discussion
- History of mental health care and reflection about it (These two can also include family and friends)

Action and experiential methods

- Dramatisation of clinical groups
- Role play of difficult interviews
- Participation as co-trainer in work discussion groups
- Participation in students' project groups
- Co-facilitation of other training groups

Lectures and talks

- Delivering own pre-written presentations
- Delivering standard teaching materials

Development of teaching and training

- Planning teaching sessions
- Planning courses and programmes (These can be done alone or in partnership)
- Seeking new areas to offer training
- Committee work: local, regional and national training strategy

Developing others to undertake this work

- Mentoring service users who are new to teaching and training
- Training service user in presentation skills etc.
- Administration of service user-involved sessions

Friday afternoon. The venue was owned by a lottery winner who was well known to one of the founder members, and was hired to us pro-bono; sadly, it has since closed, and the group has moved. STARS is open to anybody who has been through a therapeutic programme for personality disorder and wants to get involved in teaching, research, consultancy, lobbying or co-therapy. Detailed specifications have been drawn up for what members need to do before any particular role is offered to them, and there is a system of references, Criminal Records Board checks, regular individual reviews and training. There are honorary contracts available for those working regularly in NHS settings and a few members have transferred to permanent STR (support, time and recovery) contracts in the personality disorder services. All STARS work is paid at a level which started at the Royal College level for service user involvement, but has evolved into a more complex structure as the types of work are so varied. All expenses are paid in advance or immediately afterwards, through various means such as rail vouchers and petrol money. Lack of easy access to credit for expensive train fares otherwise causes people to drop out or become unnecessarily anxious.

Each meeting is a mixture of administration, feedback and review and explicit support – but not therapy. The organization of STARS is run by a programme administrator and training lead, both NHS staff doing this work part-time. Although the training lead is a qualified psychotherapist, she does not attend STARS in that role. People arrive early for a sandwich lunch if they want, then the first hour is a review of all the training activities undertaken in the month (used as a learning opportunity to see what has worked well and what has not). After a short break, the list of forthcoming activities is populated with names, and it is decided whether mentoring or specific support is needed. The last hour is supportive – people often talk about unrelated matters, but there is an understanding that therapeutic needs are out of bounds. It is easy for those who might have therapeutic needs to talk to one of the organisers, and decide whether to have a review brought forward: they normally happen every six months, but can be arranged at short notice when needed. In very occasional extreme circumstances, an urgent referral to a clinical colleague in one of the Thames Valley services is made.

Since its inception, there have been several hundred activities for STARS to get involved in – teaching and training are the commonest, but research, committee work and direct clinical involvement are also handled through STARS. For example, there are several small-scale research projects that have needed administrative help; all the clinical services in Thames Valley have some 'social therapists' who are often STARS, and all their 'friends and family groups' have STARS in the support and psychoeducation groups; members also sit on various relevant local, regional and national committees, task forces and boards. The teaching is most commonly about various aspects of 'Personality Disorder awareness' – and it is done for all levels of all professions across relevant sectors. Examples include General Practitioner training days, voluntary service councils, third sector organizations, police officers, NHS administrative staff, housing 'floating support' workers, night shelter – as well as an Oxford professorial academic meeting in the Department of Psychiatry, and presentations at Department of Health conferences. In the forthcoming years, much of this work is likely to be subsumed under the national 'Knowledge and Understanding Framework', which is being implemented across the country with Department of Health support (Section 15.6).

Some members have gone on to become NHS employees and are now on permanent contracts and training as health professionals. Others have used it as a stepping stone to other occupations, including academic research, advocacy and accountancy. Of course, there are also significant numbers who have not wanted to join the process, for various reasons. Perhaps the healthiest of these is sometimes heard as: 'I want to get as far away from therapy and mental health services as I can'!

15.6   The National Knowledge and Understanding Framework for Personality Disorder

In 2003, the National Institute for Mental Health published 'Breaking the Cycle of Rejection: Capabilities Framework for Personality Disorder' [4]. Workforce development was seen as central to the governmental intention to improve personality disorder services, as declared a few months previously in 'Personality Disorder: No Longer A Diagnosis Of Rejection' [5]. In it, the staff needed to work in the personality disorder field were going to be predominantly defined by their capabilities and aptitude for the work, and less by their formal qualifications and professional background. Indeed, it envisaged an escalator which anybody could join at suitable points, and be carried up to senior levels of responsibility in the field; it notably included the possibility that service users and ex-service users were as likely to be good at this work as were highly trained clinicians. Since then, the concept of 'expert by experience' has been widely used by those in the field to emphasize this value of knowing the condition 'from the inside'. This is in contrast to 'experts by training' who would have different but complementary capabilities. This pairing, of service users working closely in partnership with clinicians, is central to the intentions and work of the National Personality Disorder (PD) Programme: it goes well beyond the often cited need for 'service user involvement', in requiring a particularly honest, open and balanced *relationship* between service users and clinicians. There are clearly defined different responsibilities, but shared ownership of the work. As in personality disorder clinical work, anything that accentuates an 'us and them' nature of relationship is likely to lead nowhere – or, worse, to destructive feelings, thoughts and behaviour.

The intentions of the Capabilities Framework were realized through the development of the Knowledge and Understanding Framework ('KUF'), between 2008 and 2010. The successful proposal for delivering the framework (including detailed training materials to cover all sectors and levels) was from a partnership of four organizations. The Personality Disorder Institute, based at Nottingham's Institute of Mental Health, project managed the process, in which all four partners worked closely together, met frequently and were treated as equals. The other organizations were Borderline UK, the Tavistock and Portman NHS Foundation Trust in London and the Open University. Borderline UK is the country's most prominent and longest standing personality disorder service user group. Since 2008 it has expanded its remit, including extensive and comprehensive participation in writing the KUF programmes. This has substantially involved a number of service users and ex-service users from different settings in the governance, planning and production of the KUF programmes. In 2009, it merged with 'Personality Plus', an arts-based social and anti-stigma campaigning group for personality disorder (motto: 'celebrating creative personalities'), to become 'Emergence', a social enterprise incorporated as a Community Interest Company.

The overarching philosophy of the KUF programme is 'to improve the experience for service users' and this is at the heart of its design. This is perhaps most visible in the way the awareness course is delivered: the three day-long seminars are always conducted by a team of two: and 'expert by qualification' and an 'expert by experience'. The former is usually (but not exclusively) a clinician and the latter a service user or ex-service user, or carer. This necessarily changes the teaching format from a didactic delivery of factual material to a discursive and reflective exercise in which different points of view are considered and worked with – often in very creative and imaginative ways. At its best, the crucial importance of getting beyond the 'us and them' dynamic is clearly demonstrated to the trainees by the live relationship in front of them, between the two different trainers.

15.7 Partnership in a Learning Network

Another successful and collaborative activity of the National PD Programme has been the development of the Learning Network, where staff and service users from all eleven community pilot projects meet two or three times each year to discuss and learn from each other's issues about setting up and sustaining new services. This started in 2004, and at first service user representation was minimal. However, with each Learning Network the number of service users attending increased, and by the last event at the end of the pilot phase in 2008 the balance was fairly even. A number of the service user participants 'belonged' to the participating pilot projects, but a growing number of others, who came as part of other service user organizations, also started to show an interest.

The service user section of the event has proved to be very popular and quite a powerful experience for those attending, with interest and effective partnership also growing with each event – not just the number of participants. The impact of service user involvement at these events has wide reaching effects, both spurring on the service providers and the national team to promote and extol the benefits of working in partnership with users. Service users themselves find comfort from meeting other users from different services, and inspiration from users working on a national scale to improve provision in a hitherto poorly provided field.

15.8   Building Capacity in the Regions

From the outset, the direction of movement has been towards setting up local groups of service users who can participate in training programmes and receive the necessary support, training and supervision that goes with it. This is still patchy, in 2010, with some areas and regions having active and effective service user groups, while others have none. The ideological question about the extent to which it should be integrated with mainstream mental health service user involvement has largely been resolved by the success of specialist PD service user networks, and general dissatisfaction from service users when they were expected to work in the same way as 'generic' service user groups. This differentiation was not always supported by regional and local development staff, and held up progress in some regions.

As the pilot projects have been devolved and become embedded in their local health economies, particularly in the domain of Primary Care Trust (PCT) commissioning, the idea of competition with existing services for provision of training has arisen, but also the possibility that the PD programme's service user involvement could provide stimulation or exchange of ideas to assist with the growth of more meaningful and widespread service user involvement in other ways. Many existing services find the involvement problematic, struggling with the considerable array of ways which users can be involved in their care and the tricky issue of doing so in a meaningful way.

Much can be learnt from the experiences of the National PD Programme, in showing innovative and dynamic involvement in a variety of contexts that have proved useful and beneficial to both users and service providers. Throughout the life of the programme, service user involvement has always been a prerequisite – and a lack of it has been deemed unacceptable, but in more significant ways than just as a 'tick box exercise'. The nature and quality of the partnership must also be considered: it is easy to aim criticism at services which appear to have little amounts of involvement in terms of numbers, while other services may reap praise for the number of users involved while the quality of the interaction may be dubious.

The essential qualitative component is the nature of the relationship between the staff and the service users: it must be respectful yet able to be thoughtful and critical (both ways), and creative within explicit boundaries. A competitive or adversarial relationship is not likely to work well in the PD field. There was a good example of this between a long-standing advocacy group and a provider organization with whom the advocacy group had a long history of acrimonious conflict; when the two were expected to work in partnership, it did not prove to be possible and a different partner was recruited after about a year of dissatisfaction to all involved.

To establish suitable conditions, several carefully developed policies and procedures are needed. These include capability requirements, a code of conduct, criteria for 'wellness' and shared understanding of dealing with difficulties – but these alone are not sufficient. On both sides, a commitment to the work, a passion for it and belief in the importance of working together are indispensable.

15.9   The Impact of Service User Involvement

For many years, the delivery of mainstream services to those in need of psychiatric intervention was usually seen as something done to or done for the patient, with the patient having little involvement or choice in how these services were delivered. With the advances that have been seen be in service user involvement, a new relationship has grown between those who receive the services and the clinicians and managers who deliver them. This is perhaps most easily seen and understood in the training of staff in the detailed understanding of individuals' experience of personality disorder. Simple descriptions of the different 'levels' of service user involvement are given in Table 15.2.

This 'change of the nature of relationship' has not been an easy transition, and understandably there are profound differences in the quality of this relationship in different services. Bearing in mind that many service users with a diagnosis of personality disorder have traditionally suffered expulsion or exclusion from mainstream services, the positive power of this new collaborative relationship that has ensued is all the more remarkable.

The benefits for the user are clear. Service users are involved in training with either the service they have used directly or otherwise on a local, regional or national scale, they gain much in terms of confidence and generally reap the rewards of what is, for most, a

Table 15.2   Levels of service user involvement in teaching and training.

Minimum	Describing personal narrative without discussion, as case study for example	Little interaction
Medium	Discussing insights from personal narrative in a group setting, and being willing to be questioned about personal material	Considerable interaction and involvement but no strategy involvement
High	Designing and implementing training sessions and programmes	Includes planning and strategy, can be alone or in partnership
Highest	Training other service users, bringing about systemic change through policy etc.	Whole-system view and strategic involvement

validating and worthwhile experience. This is especially important, since many users of services may have a complex history of abuse, neglect or rejection – and the opportunity to embark upon activities that shape and direct the services they receive promotes inclusion and therapeutic growth in itself. Many service users exceed expectations, not only in terms of their individual contribution, but other work with services and in their ability to sustain work and meaningful activity in the future. The social implications are phenomenal and cover numerous areas: pathways back to work or education become realistic; appropriate use of other NHS services provides substantial financial saving; problems with housing and social services can be resolved; offending behaviour can be reduced or stopped; and, most importantly, the quality of life for the user improves dramatically, with new-found social inclusion and a life felt to be worth living.

But the involvement is not without controversy and opposition, even within reputable and distinguished organizations. Many ask the question of whether service user involvement in the best interest of that individual and are concerned that it might interfere with the task of treatment or overshadow the therapy. To answer this question, it is important to assess whether the involvement is 'authentic' and whether the type of involvement is appropriate to the *wellness* of the individual user. Authenticity is crucial, since a re-enactment of invalidating experiences (for example, feeling that one is not being taken seriously) will be likely to cause distress and reduce trust in other relationships.

Tokenism is a word that has been inextricably linked with service user involvement for some time, with some statutory services and the Mental Health trusts in which they sit paying 'lip service' to service users through an illusion of listening to their views, but not following through with any meaningful action that reflects those views. It is crucial that the involvement has meaning and is followed through with appropriate action or explanation.

In terms of the appropriate level of involvement, it needs to be gauged in terms of the individual's robustness to the activity demanded. It would seem foolish to suggest that a user who perhaps is engaged in very destructive behaviour participate in high-level involvement where the demands and strain of the activity may precipitate further destructive behaviour towards themselves and towards the activity itself. As a general rule of thumb, it is possible to offer an indication of the type and intensity of the involvement, for different stages of an individual's progress through therapy and beyond:

- Individuals who are using a service directly benefit most from being involved on a local level, and there is much to be gained by including evaluation exercises and forums as part of the therapeutic programme. Any training activities need to be psychologically contained within the programme in a coherent way which uses its support and risk management functions.

- As users leave the service, they can then engage in a higher level of involvement, perhaps engaging with operational issues, with semi-independent training and in research projects.

- With increased time away from therapy and a certain level of wellness attained, users are more able to work on a regional or national level, and in matters of strategy and policy. Services which make a policy of employing ex-service users in clinical work generally specify a minimum length of time after therapy before people can be considered for these roles.

However, there will always be times where the work may become 'too much', life events intercede or resilience is diminished, and so the wellness of the user may be under threat. This can often be best preserved by taking time away from the work when this looks possible. In the development of wellness criteria, we would not see them as rules for exclusion (where somebody experiencing a dip in wellness is excluded from the activity), but as an opportunity to take time away to preserve one's personal resources, and return to the activity when feeling more robust. Much can be learnt from the idea of taking time away to preserve wellness, when, traditionally, society terms this as taking time off sick – and negative attitudes or punitive measures often ensue. The emphasis on the positive nature of taking time out makes the return to the activity easier, and does not bring the negative associations of emotional or mental ill health that generally pervade the workplace.

But what is the impact on staff? There are many benefits, some obvious and others more covert; there are also many concerns and fears. Staff from a variety of disciplines who have 'taken the plunge' have shown initial surprise at the gains from involving users, but time after time have gone on to remark upon the way in which this involvement has dramatically shaped and improved the quality of their work and subsequent interactions with users. The nature of their relationships, and particularly the way power and authority are held, are irreversibly changed. Users involved at an operational level offer an unique perspective to the work and often free up time and expense by being honest and frank about what will work in practice, and offer insight as to why things are acceptable or not.

Where service users are involved in consultation exercises, the unique perspective of-fered by the service user provides a 360° vision of the impact of the clinical work: the result is a more thoughtful delivery of therapy and psychological intervention. The staff is therefore better equipped to do the work, and this increased robustness can translate into less staff sickness and burnout, which are two areas that can affect many service users in a very painful way, as they have a tendency to feel rejected by staff who are not utterly dependable.

The main focus of this chapter is on training: here the impact on staff has two aspects. For those who are being trained, the inclusion of service users is often at first uncomfortable, particularly if the service users are taking an active and leading role in delivering, debating and discussing clinical material. Many clinicians feel challenged as to the integrity of their professional expertise. However, when this 'professional expertise' includes defensive strate-gies for dealing with uncomfortable situations, such as the use of pejorative language or dismissive opinions, the need to interact with service users in a learning situation can bring about a rapid and substantial change of attitudes.

The other aspect of training is for staff working with service users as co-trainers (and this is generally the preferred format in the National PD Programme). Here, trainers, who have generally seen their role as the efficient delivery of facts and information, are suddenly immersed in a situation where the subject of those facts and information is working as a colleague, and often a close one. As well as having some effect on the way material is generally delivered (such as being more sensitive about the use of diagnostic terms, and being prepared to be challenged about matters such as symptoms and psychopathology), this soon leads to considerable enrichment of the clinician trainer's understanding of the conditions he or she is describing. It also facilitates the easy introduction of discussion and controversy into dry teaching sessions, and sometimes brings complex issues to life with moving personal accounts.

The growth of the national programme, with the many types of involvement described for service users, has been seen to do much to dispel some of the myths and misconceptions that have long existed in the minds of many professionals – about mental health in general as well as personality disorder. Stigma is a prominent and provocative issue: the fact that many have subscribed to the view of untreatability is a strong factor determining the historical lack of service provision for users with personality disorder. The work of the National PD Programme, particularly through its extensive and innovative involvement of service users, has done much to reduce practice that excludes and stigmatizes many people – and it promises much more to come.

15.10   Recommendations

1. If you already have an intensive therapy programme, discuss with the members whether they would like to get involved in training.

2. Always ensure practical arrangements are watertight, payments are made in advance or at the time and all arrangements are written down and sent out well in advance. A personal phone call to participants often helps alleviate everybody's anxiety.

3. Develop systems for remuneration of service user teaching and training work.

4. Always plan sessions and programmes in partnership.

5. Meet shortly beforehand to brief everybody what they are doing and discuss any likely problems.

6. Always have a short debriefing session afterwards (minimum 10 minutes, or longer with more people involved).

7. As far as possible, ensure that there are some playful parts to the event.

8. Involve ex-service users in reaching new audiences.

9. Let experienced trainers develop their own ideas.

10. Whenever asked to take a teaching session, think 'would this be better if I could do it with service users?'

Web Resources

www.personalitydisorder.org.uk
www.emergenceplus.org.uk
www.personalityplus.org.uk
www.exclusionlink.co.uk
http://www.communityofcommunities.org.uk

References

1. Haigh, R. and Lees, J. (2008) Fusion TCs: divergent histories, converging challenges. *Therapeutic Communities*, **29**, 347–374.
2. Clarke, S. (1999) History of Winterbourne Therapeutic Community, unpublished Masters thesis, Open University.
3. Knowles, J. (1997) The Reading Model. *Psychiatric Bulletin*, **21**, 84–87.
4. Department of Health (2003) Breaking the Cycle of Rejection: Capabilities Framework for Personality Disorders, Department of Health (National Institute for Mental Health for England), London.
5. Department of Health (2003) Personality Disorder: No Longer a Diagnosis of Exclusion, Department of Health (National Institute for Mental Health for England), London.

16

Technology for Psychiatric Educators

Sheldon Benjamin[1] and Maria Margariti[2]
[1]*Department of Psychiatry, University of Massachusetts Medical School, Worcester, MA, USA*
[2]*Eginition Hospital, Department of Psychiatry, University of Athens, Athens, Greece*

16.1   Introduction

Prior to the internet era, technology served to record, copy, print, catalogue and access written and spoken communication. Information technology has achieved global penetration with astonishing speed. Radio existed for 38 years before its audience reached 50 million. Television achieved the same benchmark in 13 years, and the personal computer in 16 years. Only four years after becoming publicly available, the internet crossed that threshold [1]. As of 2009, 24.7% of the world population has obtained internet access, with penetration differing by country (Table 16.1). By giving every user access to massive amounts of information, the internet has, in effect, levelled the playing field and democratised information. Web 2.0, the evolution of the internet from a mode of accessing static information stored on servers around the world, to an interactive system involving information sharing, collaboration, interoperability (across platforms), and user-centred design [2], has had a dramatic impact on both education and medical practice.

Technology can add excitement, efficiency, interaction, and evidence to teaching. There is no technology that can substitute for excellent pedagogic skills, however, and care must be taken not to allow educational technology to distract us from education. As psychiatric educators we are obligated not only to teach our trainees psychiatry, but the skills necessary for a modern psychiatrist to use technology to benefit patients. In this chapter, the theory and practice of using technology to enhance learning and patient care are reviewed.

Technology well applied increases access to knowledge, enhances learner motivation, increases participation and generally makes learning easier. Resistance to becoming adept at

Teaching Psychiatry: Putting Theory into Practice   Edited by Linda Gask, Bulent Coskun and David Baron
© 2011 John Wiley & Sons, Ltd

Table 16.1   Internet penetration by country (World Internet Stats, 31 December 2009).

World Internet Use and Population Statistics		World Internet Penetration Rates by Geographic Region (% population)	
World population	6.77 billion	*North America*	76.2
Internet users (31 December 2009)	1.8 billion	*Australia*	60.8
Penetration (% population)	26.6	*Europe*	53.0
Users growth 2000–2009 (%)	399.3	*Latin America*	31.9
		Middle East	28.8
		Asia	20.1
		Africa	8.7

source: Internet Usage Statistics as of 31 December 2009. © Miniwatts Marketing Group. Available from: http://www.internetworldstats.com/stats.htm (accessed 14 May 2010).

the use of educational technology may be rooted in any number of beliefs or assumptions. The assumption that their post-millennial trainees are hopelessly more skilled than they in the application of technology to learning is one such belief held by psychiatric educators. There may also be a feeling that using technology renders training superficial or introduces too many variables that can go wrong and sabotage learning. It is the job of psychiatric educators both to help their faculty overcome these resistances and assist in 'taming' the technology to make its use by both faculty and trainees more user friendly and efficient. Hilty provided an overview of issues inherent in facilitating technology change amongst psychiatric educators [3].

16.1.1   Pedagogic Models

The ADDIE model of instructional system design can be a useful concept for thoughtful curriculum innovation, including that involving technology. The ADDIE model includes Analysis, Design, Development, Implementation and Evaluation phases [4]. The analysis phase includes establishment of instructional goals and objectives, assessment of the learners' current knowledge level and assessment of curriculum options. In the design phase, the learner's experience is created, media and technology selected, and the didactic offering mapped out. This approach reminds us that curriculum design should be intentional and that evaluating its effect must always be part of any innovation.

According to Bloom's taxonomy [5], a hierarchy of pedagogic objectives can be constructed, ranging from passive to active learning. This system organizes learning into affective, psychomotor and cognitive types. The impact of affective learning increases as the learner moves from receiving, through responding, valuing and organizing to the level of characterizing what has been learnt. Similarly, cognitive learning can be seen as moving from simply receiving knowledge, through comprehension, application, analysis and synthesis to evaluating knowledge. Technology for education may also be evaluated in this light.

The twenty first century phenomenon of 'continuous partial attention' refers to the increasing tendency of learners and, indeed most others who carry technological tools with them, to scan one information technology while doing something else out of a drive to 'stay connected' [6]. It has become commonplace for medical school lecturers to look out upon students who appear to be attending to laptop computers or smart phones during seminars. The teacher cannot ascertain whether they are communicating with friends, surfing the internet or just checking facts related to the seminar online, as has become common practice. An exciting and interactive seminar leaves little time for the above distraction, however.

Blended learning, or the combination of human interaction and e-learning or technology-assisted learning, has become commonplace. In the hands of a skilled educator, a blended learning approach can both challenge learners to discover information and engage the learners in classroom discussion.

16.2   Classroom Tools

The wide range of hardware, software and online applications for medical education has placed powerful tools in the hands of psychiatric educators. In this section, the tools for educational administration, evaluation, content creation and learning beyond the classroom are reviewed.

16.2.1   Administration and Evaluation

Educational administration has been greatly facilitated by Learning Management Systems (LMS), now widely used in undergraduate and medical schools. These systems are typically purchased by an institution for use in all its course offerings; They typically include: a course calendar; the ability to post handouts, slides, supplementary learning materials; a grading module; internet links; access to online publications; a chat room and/or discussion section; and a communication module for e-mailing learners and educators [7]. A list of some LMS vendors is provided in Table 16.2.

The advent of online evaluation systems has greatly enhanced our ability as educators to determine the efficacy of our curricula, the skill of our teachers and the progress of our trainees. More than simply a way to post old paper evaluations onto computers, these systems allow the flexibility to track various methods of competency assessment and give both trainees and faculty open access to feedback. In addition to online evaluation forms, typical evaluation systems provide: trainee and faculty tracking; a training calendar; automated reminder e-mails; an electronic learning portfolio; seminar attendance tracking; storage and downloading of handouts; and case, diagnosis or procedure tracking [8]. Different systems allow differing degrees of flexibility for users to create their own forms, assessment tools and portfolios. At least one system allows the training director to create his/her own front page with URL links or downloadable files as needed. Table 16.2 lists some online evaluation systems.

Dedicated online survey tools allow educators to create their own evaluation instruments, survey trainees and faculty on important issues, or quickly and efficiently gather survey data with a minimum of effort. A number of online providers offer survey tools, often with a

Table 16.2   Online resources for psychiatric education.

Examples of Learning Management Systems

Proprietary Systems

Blackboard Vista (includes former WebCT)[a]	http://www.blackboard.com
Desire 2 Learn	http://www.desire2learn.com
Learning Activity Management System	http://www.lamsinternational.com
Sharepoint (for MS Office Sharepoint Server)	http://www.sharepointlms.com
Pegasus (Pearson)	http://pegasus2.pearsoned.com

Open Source Systems

Claroline	http://www.claroline.net
eFront	http://www.efrontlearning.net
Dokeos (based on Claroline)	http://www.dokeos.com
ILIAS	http://www.ilias.de
Moodle	http://www.moodle.org
Sakai	http://www.sakaiproject.org

Examples of Online Evaluation Systems

E*Value[a]	http://www.advancedinformatics.com
My Residency	http://www.eresidency.net
Webesprit	http://www.webesprit.net
Meditrek	http://www.meditrek.com
Medhub	http://www.medhub.com
New Innovations	http://www.new-innov.com
VerinformRM	http://www.verinform.com

Examples of Online Survey Tools

Survey Monkey[a]	http://www.surveymonkey.com
Zoomerang	http://www.zoomerang.com
Survey Gizmo	http://www.surveygizmo.com
Poll Daddy	http://www.polldaddy.com

Examples of Online Meeting Scheduling Tools

AgreeADate	http://www.agreeadate.com
Doodle[a]	http://www.doodle.com
Meeting Wizard[a]	http://www.meetingwizard.com
Set A Meeting	http://www.setameeting.com
Time Bridge	http://www.timebridge.com

Examples of Mind Mapping Tools

Stand Alone Software

Free Mind	http://freemind.sourceforge.net
iMind Map	http://www.imindmap.com
Mind Manager	http://www.mindjet.com
Nova Mind[a]	http://www.nova-mind.com
X Mind	http://www.xmind.net

Table 16.2   (Continued)

Collaborative Web-based Mind Mapping	
Bubbl	http://bubbl.us
Mind 42	http://mind42.com
Comapping	http://comapping.com
Mapul	http://mapul.com
Mind Meister[a]	http://www.mindmeister.com
Mindomo	http://mindomo.com
Examples of Audience Response Systems	
Comtec	http://www.comtecars.com
e instruction	http://www.einstruction.com
Quizdom	http://www.quizdom.com
Turning Point[a]	http://www.turningtechnologies.com
Examples of Free Video Teleconferencing Solutions	
iChat (Mac only)[a]	http://www.apple.com
Oovoo[a]	http://www.oovoo.com
Skype[a]	http://www.skype.com
Examples of Wiki Platforms	
Metadot	http://www.metadot.net
MindTouch	http://www.mindtouch.com
PBwiki[a]	http://pbworks.com
Wetpaint	http://www.wetpaint.com
Wikispaces	http://www.wikispaces.com
Examples of Psychiatry Blogs	
Carlat Psychiatry Blog	http://carlatpsychiatry.blogspot.com/
Clinical Psychiatry and Psychology	http://clinpsyc.blogspot.com/
CorePsych Blog	http://www.corepsychblog.com/
Dr Shock: A Neurostimulating Blog	http://www.shockmd.com/
In Practice	http://www.psychologytoday.com/blog/in-practice
Shrink Rap (podcast: My Three Shrinks)	http://psychiatrist-blog.blogspot.com/
Examples of Social Network Sites of Interest to Psychiatry Educators	
Social Bookmarking	http://delicious.com http://digg.com http://www.stumbleupon.com http://www.yattle.com
Social Cataloguing	http://www.librarything.com http://www.shelfari.com http://www.goodreads.com
Social Lecture Slide Sharing	http://www.slideshare.net

[a] Indicates software used by one of the authors.

limited free version and a more full-featured paid version. It is strongly suggested that surveys be tested on a few people before sending them out to the full survey population. It is also a good idea to plan the data analysis before construction of the survey instrument itself, so that the survey can be set up to allow data to be parsed according to desired variables. Examples of online survey providers are given in Table 16.2.

A perennial headache for academic administrators is identifying meeting times that suit the various participants needed for meetings locally, by teleconference or online. A number of online tools have emerged that greatly facilitate finding common meeting times. A commonly used internal mechanism for identifying meeting times is built in to Microsoft Outlook's^{TM} calendar function. Examples of online meeting scheduling tools are given in Table 16.2. Most are free for up to a given number of participants and require subscription for higher numbers.

16.2.2 Content Creation

A myriad of tools exist to assist the psychiatric educator in creating seminar content, limited only by one's imagination. A number of vendors make electronic mind mapping tools, either in stand-alone or online collaborative versions. Mind mapping is a way of tracking ideas and rearranging them as needed in a kind of freely mutable outline. Attributed to Tony Buzan, this technique can be used many different ways – as a way of outlining for writing or teaching, in group problem solving or brainstorming, in note taking, in collaborative projects or to help in team building [9]. Argument maps, concept maps, semantic networks and cognitive maps are related tools. For background information and details on mind mapping and mind mapping software see http://www.mind-mapping.org. Table 16.2 includes examples of mind mapping tools. Figure 16.1 shows the online mind map used by the authors to facilitate international brainstorming in creating this chapter.

Audience response systems can both engage learners in classroom settings and provide a means of evaluation. These systems use hand-held devices to allow learners to respond in real time to questions posed by the presenter and immediately display the distribution of the group's answers in graphical form either through stand-alone software or via a presentation program like Microsoft PowerPoint^{TM}. In addition to keeping learners engaged and assessing participant grasp of the material being presented, audience response software can allow lecturers to build branch points or optional content into their presentations, adapting the lecture on-the-fly to the needs of the participants. Learners can either be anonymous or identified and can respond independently or in teams. Many LMS applications can incorporate audience response data, including data from quizzes or examinations. As with any pedagogic tool, it is important for the presenter to exercise restraint, so that the tool adds excitement and interaction without being over-used [10]. Table 16.2 lists several audience response systems.

The speed with which older film-based projection slides have been supplanted by computer generated slides is testament to the ease of use of the latter. With ease of use, however, has come over-use. Educators must take care that their visual aids augment and clarify their presentations while engaging learners, rather than just projecting an outline of the words being spoken, in a manner that has been described as *'death by PowerPoint'* [11]. Edward Tufte characterized the way pedagogic principles have fallen victim to computer

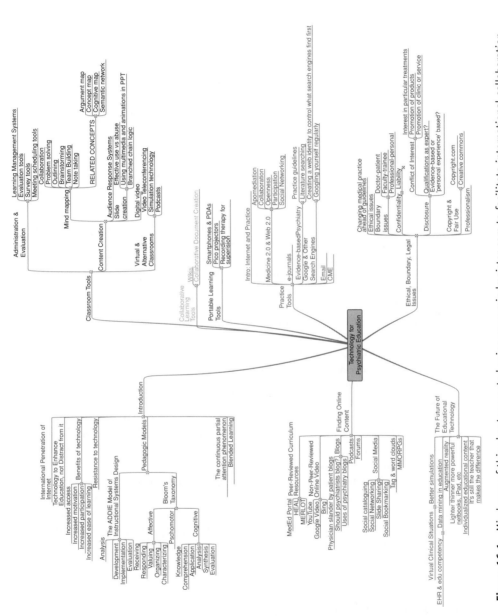

Figure 16.1 Mind map of this chapter created using www.mindmeister.com to facilitate international collaboration.

Table 16.3 Guidelines for creating effective slides.

Avoid using slides just to outline your talk	Use large font sizes (22 point or larger)
Do not put every thought you present on your slides	Avoid using more than eight lines of text
Use slides to clarify, give examples, or present data or evidence	Use bullets in only one outline sublevel
Blue backgrounds with white or yellow text are easiest to read	Use art or graphics to clarify or strengthen points; avoid distracting graphics
Avoid red or green fonts for viewing ease and to avoid disadvantaging colour-blind learners	Make sure tables can be read from back of room
Avoid textured backgrounds or graphically elaborate slide templates	Compare numbers in columns rather than rows
Avoid using all-capital text. Upper and lowercase text is easier to read.	Use the appropriate type of graph to illustrate your data [12]
Keep titles short (one line if possible)	Use animations sparingly

slide over-use, saying 'audience boredom is usually a content failure, not a decoration failure' [13]. That having been said, slide creation software can be used to create engaging presentations. Commonly used applications, such as Microsoft PowerPoint™ and Apple Keynote™, allow the user to embed audio, video, graphical elements and internet links into presentations. These applications also include colour tools, automated transitions and computer animation. Over-used, these can engender resentment in learners. Used well and timed appropriately, they can enhance learning. Table 16.3 gives several 'rules' for creating effective slides. Computer slide software can be used to create animated cartoons (e.g. illustration of neurotransmission) or scientific posters. Other tools, such as audience response systems and mind maps, can be easily incorporated into presentations.

The inclusion of video examples can be a memorable adjunct to computer slides. In almost every case, embedded video should be edited for presentation to segments of sufficient brevity and impact to hold audience attention. For computer editing and import to slide presentation programs, video material must be in digital format. Consult the manual for video file types that can be imported by specific slide software (e.g. .MOV, .WMV, .AVI, .MPEG) and make sure to convert the video to that file type before importing.

Another powerful tool found in computer slide programs is the ability to insert automated 'buttons' containing hyperlinks either to other slides in a program or to external internet links or files. This allows the presenter to use only selected groups of slides depending on the needs of the learners, to plan optional materials in case particular questions are raised, to go directly to particular internet sites to further illustrate a point made in a slide or to engage the class in seeking evidence.

16.2.3 Learning Beyond the Classroom

Video teleconferencing has become more frequent in psychiatric education, enabling online courses, interactive meetings amongst geographically distant participants, virtual attendance at core curriculum presentations by trainees at off-site rotations and the 'broadcasting' of grand rounds or other seminars to affiliated institutions. The enabling technology varies from freely available online tools using computer webcams to dedicated hardware and software platforms capable of providing high quality audio and video, and remote camera control. Examples of free online video teleconferencing systems are given in Table 16.2. Free systems typically limit the number of participants to six or fewer. The widely used Skype program currently allows only two-way video conferencing.

Simulation technology, now part of the curriculum at many medical schools, has been slow to be adopted in psychiatry. Evaluation of trainees using standardized patients has become relatively common, with many institutions using computer-assisted learner evaluation techniques. Simulations may also be presented in a team-based learning format as written clinical scenarios in which the learner group is faced with decision points critical to patient outcome. Though not yet widely available in psychiatry, simulations using computer-enhanced anatomically accurate mannequins are often used in other fields to help trainees become proficient at managing emergency situations or practising medical procedures. In psychiatry, such simulations could be adapted to rehearse medication treatment decisions, evaluation of serious side effects or emergency management of inpatient suicide attempts, amongst other things [14].

Educational podcasts have grown rapidly in popularity since Apple's iPod and iTunes store made the distribution and downloading of MP3 audio content widely accessible. Podcasts may be audio only, or include video (with slides for example). Creating a podcast requires a reasonably good quality USB microphone, sound capturing software (a commonly used free solution is Audacity) and, if video is desired, some form of digital video capture or lecture capturing software. Camtasia^{TM} (www.techsmith.com) is an example of an easy-to-use lecture-capturing product that allows users to randomly access slides and their associated audio and/or video. iTunes University (accessed via the iTunes application for Mac or Windows) allows training programs to easily post educational podcasts either for the public or for authorised users without charge (information at http://www.apple.com/support/itunes_u/). The Harvard Graduate School of Education has posted detailed public-access podcasting tutorials at http://isites.harvard.edu:80/icb/icb.do?keyword=k1967&pageid=icb.page23750.

16.3 Collaborative Learning Tools

Collaborative learning tools are amongst the most powerful educational benefits of the internet. Collaborative software can facilitate group projects, studying, writing, data analysis, problem solving and information sharing. Collaborative software is one aspect of 'cloud computing', in which the user accesses virtual resources in cyberspace (stored on internet servers), rather than resources physically stored on one's own hardware. In this section, collaborative content creation tools and wikis are discussed.

The term 'wiki', from the Hawaiian *wiki* meaning quick, entered the public consciousness in 2001 with the advent of Wikipedia.org, an enormous online encyclopaedia. A wiki allows multiple authors to collaborate in the creation of online content in a fashion that allows users to track the changes that have been made. The quality of information found on a wiki is dependent on the care taken by its authors and editors, and publicly editable sites like Wikipedia have been criticised for overly focusing on popular issues and for the variable expertise of its many authors. A limited access wiki, however, can be an excellent platform for teams of learners to work together to study for an exam, evaluate a clinical case and collect useful notes, documents, media or internet links. As of this writing there are well over 100 wiki platforms available, both free (generally supported by advertising) and by paid subscription. Table 16.2 contains examples of wiki platforms. An excellent source of information about this technology, including a wizard to help select the best platform for a given application, can be found at www.wikimatrix.org.

One of the most popular collaborative document creation systems, Google Docs, is available at no charge to anyone with a gmail (Google mail) address, though many other systems are available both free and by subscription. A lead author can assign reading or editing privileges for forms, word processing, spreadsheet or presentation documents to any number of participants. The system operates much like similar stand-alone applications, so is easy to learn. Major manufacturers of stand-alone software are also entering the collaborative document market so choices will continue to increase.

Also, see collaborative mind mapping, discussed earlier.

16.4 Portable Learning Tools

The proliferation of portable electronic devices has naturally resulted in the proliferation of portable medical education tools. eBook readers (e.g. the Amazon Kindle) make it possible for students to carry a medical library of hundreds of references in their pocket. Many physicians have some sort of electronic drug reference on their smartphone or personal digital assistant. A growing number of medical apps are being created for smartphones (the most, by far, being available for the Apple iPhone as of this writing). In addition to the nearly ubiquitous prescribing information apps, there are apps for anatomy, neuroimaging, medical calculations, electronic journals and textbooks, and many other uses. Interested educators who search online for 'medical apps' will be rewarded with many web sites specializing in reviews of these applications, so we will not attempt to list them here. Many educators/schools distribute or suggest suites of smartphone/PDA applications for students to use. The availability of so-called pico projectors has made it possible to carry an LCD projector in one's pocket. Paired with a smartphone, these can allow an educator to project data stored on the phone onto any nearby projection surface, allowing impromptu educational conferences.

An application of portable video technology unique to psychiatric training is the recording of psychotherapy sessions for later use in supervision. Reviewing actual film of trainee psychotherapeutic encounters provides a more direct measure of competency than does a trainee's recollection of the encounter. A number of different recording methods are currently used. Pocket digital video cameras have become quite inexpensive. Smartphone video capture technology has improved to the point of being an acceptable alternative for training use. Webcams (inexpensive digital add-on cameras for computers) can easily be deployed on laptop or desktop computers in outpatient clinics. Some teaching clinics have opted to build video cameras and microphones into clinic rooms, with the option of live observation or recording for later supervision. The trainee and supervisor can view the video samples together from either a server, or a storage device brought to supervision. Pocket video cameras also enable physicians to photograph or record signs and symptoms for later study or consultation. When recording patient videos, two measures are of paramount importance to preserve patient confidentiality – a method of secure storage (and scheduled deletion if appropriate) of all patient video samples; and the obtaining of informed consent that truly anticipates the intended use(s) of the material.

16.5 Finding Online Content

Most physicians are now familiar with the use of internet search engines such as http://www.google.com or http://www.bing.com to find online content apart from that in medical journals. The universe of online content relevant to psychiatric education includes many other resources, however, that educators may find useful.

16.5.1 Peer Reviewed Curriculum Resources

A few peer reviewed online resources have emerged to allow medical educators to download curricula and teaching materials. MedEd Portal (http://www.aamc.org/mededportal), a project of the Association of American Medical Colleges, publishes stand-alone resources, such as tutorials, virtual patients, simulation cases, videos, podcasts and assessment tools. HEAL, the Health Education Assets Library (http://www.healcentral.org), in association with the International Association of Medical Science Educators (IAMSE), publishes images, video clips, animations, presentations and audio files for use in medical curricula. Psychiatric educators may submit their curricula to these sites for peer review and online publication, thus allowing educators to claim 'academic credit' for their work. Though not specific to medical education, MERLOT, the Multimedia Educational Resource for Learning and Online Teaching (http://www.merlot.org) contains downloadable resources both on psychology and on pedagogic skills, and includes an online content creation tool. A number of medical schools are now posting high quality multimedia curricula on their public web sites as well.

16.5.2 Non Peer Reviewed Resources

Amongst the millions of video clips posted to the internet in ever growing numbers are many resources of potential use in education. Sites such as YouTube (http://www.youtube.com), Google Video (http://video.google.com) and Bing (http://www.bing.com/videos) offer text-based searching to help locate potentially useful clips. A large quantity of personal experience video material is posted by individuals suffering from neuropsychiatric conditions. Consent for viewing is implied but the ethics of using a given video example should be individually considered. Posted videos vary from useful to completely inappropriate or unreliable, so educators are cautioned to preview all material before recommending its use. In YouTube and Google Video, the user can employ 'deep links' to allow play to begin at any point in the video. Many videos are posted in flash format (.FLV) but can be downloaded and translated into video formats compatible with slide presentation software using free tools readily available online.

16.5.3 Blogs, Podcasts, Forums

Blogs, podcasts and forums are better used as a way of keeping up to date than specifically searching for curriculum content. A blog, short for web log, is an online journal posted by one or more people or representatives of an organization who make regular entries containing their own news, commentary, writing, links to web sites and so on. The democratisation of the Web inherent in Web 2.0 means that anyone can post information of any quality. The source is, therefore, of paramount importance in assessing the value of a blog. Table 16.2 contains examples of a few of the many current psychiatry blogs aimed at clinicians rather than patients, without any intent to rate their value. Whether psychiatrists should blog is a complex question (Section 16.7, Ethical, Legal and Boundary Issues). Many medical journals now offer podcasts either as narrated highlights of a journal issue or as audio presentations related to particular publications. iTunes University is a major source of medical education podcasts, including psychiatry grand rounds from many medical centres. A number of blogs have related podcasts. Forums, in which users post comments in running strings of conversation in response to questions or postings by others, are more popular as sources of information for patients than for psychiatrists. But forums can be good places to ask questions, such as how to troubleshoot software or hardware problems, how to assess employment prospects or how to do certain procedures. Search for forums using a web browser and the appropriate topic with the word 'forum'.

16.5.4 Social Networking

Social media refers to the online sharing of text, images, video or other user-generated content. This resource sharing, a core aspect of Web 2.0, has given rise to a number of related social networking tools. The use of social networking tools raises unique questions for physicians, and particularly psychiatrists (Section 16.7, Ethical, Legal and Boundary Issues). Though Facebook, MySpace and LinkedIn may receive more press attention than others, Wikipedia lists over 175 social networking sites (http://en.wikipedia.org/wiki/Social_networking_web sites). Many of these offer users the ability to post a profile containing information about themselves and their interests for the purpose of updating friends, relatives and colleagues or for discovering other individuals for the purpose of forming networks for social, educational or business purposes. Social network sites exploit the ability to plumb the contacts of an online 'friend' for contacts in common or with common interests. Different levels of security are offered defining who may view the information one posts. Some training programmes have created social network 'groups' as a way for alumni to keep track of one another or to post news, as a recruitment vehicle or as a service to trainees. The social networking phenomenon has spawned sites for sharing of lecture slides, library holdings, web bookmarks, media resources and other things of interest to educators. Table 16.2 lists some of these resources. Many social networking sites allow users to create keyword 'tags', which can be aggregated by the site to create 'tag clouds' in which the size of the tag font indicates the frequency of that keyword. These in turn can help the user discover alternative search terms. Word clouds are a version of tag clouds that can become an intuitive form of indexing that facilitates brainstorming. Figure 16.2 is a word cloud generated from this chapter using freely available online software.

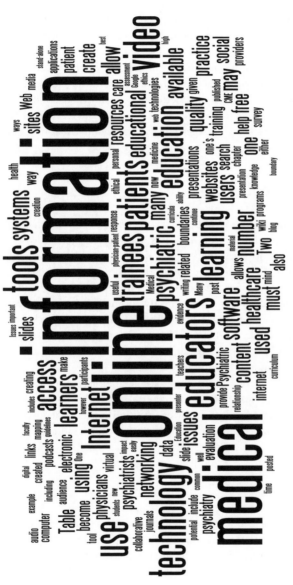

Figure 16.2 Word cloud of this chapter created using www.wordle.net. The size and boldness of the words reflect their frequency in the chapter. This is analogous to 'tag clouds' used to reflect keyword frequency in social media sites.

16.5.5 MMORPGs

Massively Multiplayer Online Roll Playing Games (MMORPGs) are best known as virtual worlds for online fantasy role playing. But this technology is also commonly used in the service of education. One of the most popular of the many MMORPGs is Second Life (http://secondlife.com), a 3D virtual world in which some 750 000 regular users create avatars that move, interact and even conduct business. Some medical school educators have created interactive exhibits, virtual clinics or educational centres in Second Life (SL). Hundreds of universities use SL as a distance learning platform or even as a place for professors to hold virtual office hours. SL is increasingly being used as a platform for virtual grand rounds, experiential sites to help patients better understand their condition or as ancillary educational venues for students. (Peter Yellowlees of UC Davis Medical School created a site in Second Life to allow users to experience auditory and visual hallucinations – search for Virtual Hallucinations in Second Life).

16.6 Practice Tools

The evolution of the internet into 'Web 2.0' has created a host of mechanisms for increased interaction, collaboration and networking, thus allowing learners to cast a broad net for information they might not have otherwise obtained. Gunther Eysenbach, of the University of Toronto, coined the term 'Medicine 2.0' to describe the impact of Web 2.0 on medicine [14]. Eysenbach defines Medicine 2.0 as including apomediation, collaboration, openness, participation and social networking. By apomediation, he is referring to the way in which internet users can be guided to health care information by intermediaries other than their health care providers, who by collective effort can discern quality information. This is the environment in which our patients obtain information, and this reality should be acknowledged in our training programmes.

Psychiatrists entering practice today enjoy accelerated access to new research findings regardless of distance from academic health centres. With this also comes rapid access to opinions and anecdotal information of lower quality. Psychiatric education must include instruction in interpretation of evidence to properly equip graduates to sift through the mountains of online data.

16.6.1 e-Journals

Almost every major psychiatric journal is published both in print and online, with several journals now appearing in electronic form only. Use of print journals is decreasing rapidly in favour of e-published journals, with a consequent decrease in the cost of information. Access is a primary determinant of which published information is used by health professionals [15].

16.6.2 Practice Guidelines

Widespread rapid access to published treatment guidelines creates a reasonable expectation that practitioners will consult them. Patients, too, can consult the latest guidelines, so psychiatrists can anticipate more patient challenges to their treatment plans. With increasingly rapid access to published evidence it is anticipated that practice guidelines will be updated more frequently in the future [16].

16.6.3   Literature Searching

The evolution of medical literature searching tools from published volumes of Index Medicus to the National Library of Medicine's (NLM) paid online Medline database in 1992, to the 1997 launch of free PubMed access to the Medline database, to the many subsequent access improvements, has been accompanied by evolution of online medical literature searching from a tool primarily for physicians to one easily accessible by patients as well. In 1998, the NLM introduced Medline Plus (www.nlm.nih.gov/medlineplus), providing full-text consumer health information from the National Institutes of Health (NIH) and other government agencies. Medline Plus was visited 31.5 million times in the third quarter of 2009 alone. By 2003, 40% of internet users were accessing health-related information online [17]. The NLM continues to release new educational and research tools. The National Centre for Biotechnology Information (NCBI), launched by NLM in 1988, for example, provides a free powerful educational tool, My NCBI, that allows users to save searches, collections and bibliographies within PubMed and have newly published citations e-mailed at any frequency desired (http://www.ncbi.nlm.nih.gov/sites/myncbi/). A large number of tools exists to facilitate searching for medical evidence, the techniques for which are beyond the scope of this chapter [18].

16.6.4   Search Engines

That patients search for information about their doctors online is a fact. Psychiatric educators in the era of Web 2.0 should help trainees to carefully consider their online persona, assuming that any personal information posted online will be available to their patients and colleagues. Trainees should learn to routinely search for themselves using the major search engines and take steps to control their presence online. Creating one's own practice web site with information specifically tailored to one's patients, learning to 'scrub' one's web profile and taking care not to post personal information to searchable social networking sites are all techniques that psychiatry trainees should learn [19, 20].

16.6.5   E-Mail

Once a novelty, now a necessity – often a headache – electronic mail at once both simplifies and complicates medical practice. Psychiatric educators must not only supervise trainees in the protection of health care information in e-mail communications, but must help trainees anticipate their patients' desire to communicate with their physicians by e-mail. Electronic communication is rife with boundary issues that are best managed by anticipation in training and by talking through the ramifications. Some psychiatrists have embraced e-psychiatry, obtaining pre-consultation history, administering questionnaires and rating scales, and communicating with patients outside the bounds of the appointment. Others attempt to steer all communication back into the appointment [21]. Either way, the subject should not be ignored in education.

16.6.6   Continuing Medical Education

By facilitating access to psychiatry Continuing Medical Education (CME) from office, home or mobile devices, the internet reduces the importance of proximity to academic medical centres in determining access to information, and increases the educational programmes available to rural physicians in a given country. Hardware availability and connection speed are determinants of access. Issues that affect psychiatrists' use of internet CME resources include: awareness of online programmes; interest and motivation to use technology; ease of use, quality and intellectually engaging nature of content; cost; registration requirements; CME credit availability; time commitment [16]; and industry sponsorship.

16.7   Ethical, Boundary and Legal Issues

The recent pace of emerging technologies has exceeded by far the speed with which medicine has been able to evolve principles, boundaries and guidelines for their ethical use. Psychiatric educators in the age of Web 2.0 must create ways of helping trainees understand the ethical and boundary issues raised by new technologies, and help them consider the challenges posed to existing values.

The internet is substantially altering the way medicine is practised, from e-mail communication to billing, consultations at a distance and routine patient care. At the same time it has created a culture in which patients no longer depend on their physicians for health information. A Google search in early 2010 revealed 108 000 000 web sites related to 'health care', 242 000 000 related to 'medicine' and 24 000 000 related to 'psychiatry'. The merger of e-commerce with health care has spawned a multitude of online business models – physician rating services, health care products, health care portals, concierge medicine and online services for health care providers, to name a few. Unlicensed or unqualified providers and disreputable sources are waiting in the wings to provide their version of health care information to patients if medical providers don't provide easily accessed, high quality information [22].

At least six categories of online medical behaviour have been identified as needing codes of ethical conduct: the doctor–patient or therapist–client relationship; the provision of medical care or therapy online; online research; the quality of information provided on health care web sites; the manner in which health care web sites operate; and privacy/security concerns [23, 24]. The American Medical Association (AMA) has begun the work by creating principles for medical web sites, online privacy and medical e-commerce that may be useful as guides for others [25].

16.7.1   Ethical Issues

Although the ethics issues raised by physician online behaviour are extensions of the core tenets of medical ethics – beneficence, respect for autonomy, non-maleficence and justice – psychiatric educators should create forums to discuss these issues specifically as they relate to the internet. On the one hand, training psychiatrists to provide high quality information to patients or to refer their patients, perhaps by linking from their own practice site, to health care web sites known to provide high quality information, would certainly support the patient's autonomy as they gather information to inform medical decision making. On the other hand, failure to respond when a patient cites information of questionable merit obtained online that could, in turn, lead to making a poor decision, could be seen as a failure of non-maleficence. One could argue that creating a web site or writing a medical blog is an example of beneficence in guiding the patient to the highest quality information available. Yet we must also caution our trainees to avoid inadvertently creating a physician–patient relationship, and its attendant liabilities, as they dispense medical information via the internet.

Dispensing medical advice via a blog or web site is a more complex and risky undertaking in the absence of a pre-existing physician–patient relationship [26]. Since internet medical information may be accessed outside the confines of a pre-existing relationship, it has the potential to replace rather than merely augment traditional medical care. This effectively changes the setting and nature of the physician–patient relationship, and thereby alters the practice of medicine [27].

16.7.2   Boundary Issues

Of tremendous importance to both psychiatrists and their patients are clear and consistent boundaries. Proper boundaries – physician–patient, professional–personal, faculty–trainee – allow the work to go forward with the focus clearly on the issues brought by the patient. Yet the very existence of the internet has changed the boundaries of practice. Careless participation by psychiatrists in social networking sites allows patients, by dint of their friendship with a mutual contact, to gain access to lists of their physician's 'friends', to obtain information they would not have otherwise obtained, and to place both parties into situations in which interactions occur outside of the usual therapeutic boundaries. A recent study of 813 students at residents at a United States medical school found that 44.5% had a Facebook account, with most accounts revealing personally identifiable information and only one third using privacy settings [28]. Privacy and boundary issues for physicians using social networking sites are complex and bear thinking through with trainees [29]. At this point, it is not yet clear whether a physician even has an ethical obligation to answer a question posed by e-mail when this service is not explicitly offered [26]. Physicians may also circumvent the boundaries of the traditional physician–patient relationship by seeking out information online about their patients, a practice that may not only violate their patient's privacy, but could negatively impact treatment.

16.7.3   Confidentiality

Studies have shown that most adult internet users believe they can visit a site anonymously and obtain information about controversial subjects such as AIDS, venereal infections or suicide without their information being exposed. Medical and health care web sites should follow strict security measures to ensure that their users' personal medical information remains private and does not involuntarily enter the hands of marketers, employers or insurers.

Physicians who blog should take care not to include information about individual patients and should assume all online information associated with their names will be available for any potential future legal interactions.

16.7.4 Disclosure

Disclosure is an important issue for physicians dispensing information online. The Accreditation Council on Continuing Medical Education requires disclosure by CME presenters of potential conflicts of interest. There are no such disclosure requirements for blogs, Web sites, podcasts, forums or other venues in which patients seek health care information. With the exception of web sites that both provide information and sell related products, it can be difficult for a health care consumer to determine the promotional advantages garnered by online information providers, or the corporate entity behind the information. By incorporating recognition of potential conflicts of interest in ethics seminars, psychiatric educators can help raise the quality of online psychiatric information provided by graduates.

16.7.5 Copyright/Fair Use

Psychiatric educators routinely create slides and multimedia presentations for presentation within their own educational programme, at medical meetings or as part of CME courses. Ironically, at a time when it appears that freely available online information is rapidly expanding, content providers and patent holders are pursuing legal remedies to protect their intellectual property with increasing frequency, effectively shrinking the pool of free information. Although some universities purchase licenses for use of electronic scientific information within their own institution (e.g. from the Copyright Clearance Centre at www.copyright.com) copyright permission must be purchased to use figures, text or other media in presentations outside one's own institution at CME meetings, lectures for which remuneration is received and so on. Freely available images and media on the internet should not be assumed to be free of copyright unless they are specifically licensed for free use by an entity such as Creative Commons (www.Creativecommons.org). It is suggested that educators who make frequent use of downloaded media familiarize themselves with fair use doctrine and copyright law. Often the medical library at one's institution can be helpful in this regard.

16.7.6 Professionalism

As psychiatric educators we are obligated to vouch for the professionalism of our graduates. How this obligation extends to the online behaviour of trainees is still being worked out. Should educators actively search for professionalism-related behaviours? How should we respond to evidence of non-professional online behaviour brought to our attention by others? What are the boundaries between protected free expression and professionalism concerns by certifying bodies? Numerous instances of trainees blogging or posting to social networking sites their uncensored criticism of institutions or individuals have emerged [30, 31].

The internet brings both a wealth of resources and some potential challenges to psychiatry. The current generation of psychiatric trainees regards the internet more as an appliance than as something new and wonderful. They are thus less likely to be concerned with the complex issues discussed herein than are their teachers. Psychiatric educators must include discussion of online ethics, boundaries and liability in seminars dealing with other aspects of these topics.

16.8   Future Trends in Education Technology

That technology will continue to play an important role in psychiatric education is certain. Predicting the dominant educational technologies of the coming decade is much less certain. Social networking, replete with the difficult issues described in this chapter, will likely continue as an important tool for learners and patients alike. Hopefully, psychiatrists will come to agree on appropriate boundaries and guidelines for its use and engage psychiatric trainees in exploration of the difficult issues raised by the technology.

The incorporation of better and more sophisticated simulation systems into medical education should result in physicians better prepared for critical decision making. While the use of simulations in pharmacologic decision making may already be within our grasp, the maturation of computer language systems could one day lead to entirely new ways of learning psychotherapy as well.

As electronic health records become more universally adopted, education will be facilitated by mining physician performance data and creating direct links between findings, diagnoses and treatments in the record and external resources.

Augmented reality, the superimposition of data from the internet onto targets observed locally using camera-equipped transportable devices (smartphones, display glasses, tablets, etc.) is a promising technology for medical education. One can envision, for example, observing a congenital craniofacial malformation through one of these devices and immediately seeing a list of possible syndromes for genetic investigation superimposed over the appropriate structures.

Lighter, thinner and more affordable internet-connected tablet computers will make it possible for trainees to carry a library of books and journals, search online databases, record clinical information and access electronic health records at any time, bringing evidence-based practice to the bedside.

The technologies explored in this chapter can all be seen as leading toward increasing individualisation of medical education. The role of the educator will gradually move from presenter of information to presenter of novel ways of interacting with information. Even as technology continues to evolve in directions our own teachers could never have predicted, skilled educators will continue to challenge learners to confront information in ways that increase their knowledge, just as the best teachers have done for millennia.

References

1. Margherio, L. (1998) The Emerging Digital Economy, http://govinfo.library.unt.edu/ecommerce/EDEreprt.pdf (accessed 25 July 2010).
2. DiNucci, D. (1999) Fragmented Future. *Print*, **52** (4), 32.

3. Hilty, D. (2006) APA summit on medical student education task force on informatics and technology: Steps to enhance the use of technology in education through faculty development, funding and change management. *Academic Psychiatry*, **30** (6), 444–450.

4. Molenda, M., Pershing, J. and Reigeluth, C. (1996) Designing instructional systems, in *The ASTD Training and Development Handbook*, 4th edn (ed. R. Craig), McGraw-Hill, New York, pp. 266–293.

5. Bloom, B. (1956) *Taxonomy of Educational Objectives: The Classification of Educational Goals*, Susan Fauer Company, Inc., pp. 201–207.

6. Stone, L. (2008) Continuous Partial Attention – Not the Same as Multi-Tasking. Business Week Online, 24 July 2008; http://www.businessweek.com/business_at_work/time_management/archives/2008/07/continuous_part.html (accessed 11 January 2010).

7. Chan, C. and Robbins, L. (2006) E-learning systems: promises and pitfalls. *Academic Psychiatry*, **30** (6), 491–497.

8. Benjamin, S. and Robbins, L. (2006) Online resources for assessment and evaluation. *Academic Psychiatry*, **30** (6), 498–504.

9. Farrand, P. *et al.* (2002) The efficacy of the 'mind map' study technique. *Medical Education*, **36** (5), 426–431.

10. Robertson, L. (2000) Twelve tips for using a computerized interactive audience response system. *Medical Teacher*, **22** (3), 237–239.

11. Garber, A. (2001) Death by Powerpoint. Small Business Computing Online [serial on the Internet]; http://www.smallbusinesscomputing.com/biztools/article.php/684871 (accessed 25 July 2010).

12. Tufte, E.R. (1997) *Visual Explanations: Images and Quantities, Evidence and Narrative*. Graphics Press, Cheshire, CT.

13. Tufte, E. (2003 September) PowerPoint is Evil. Wired Magazine, 11.09.

14. Srinivasan, M. (2006) Assessment of Clinical Skills Using Simulator Technology. *Academic Psychiatry*. **30** (6), 505–515.

15. Eysenbach, G. (2008) Medicine 2.0: Social networking, collaboration, participation, apomediation, and openness. *J Med Internet Res*, **10** (3), e22.

16. Obst, O. (2003) Patterns and costs of printed and online journal usage. *Health Information and Libraries Journal*, **20** (1), 22–32.

17. Styra, R. (2004) The internet's impact on the practice of psychiatry. *Canadian Journal of Psychiatry*, **49** (1), 5–11.

18. Baker, L., Wagner, T.H., Singer, S. and Bundorf, M.K. (2003) Use of the internet and E-mail for health care information: results from a national survey. *JAMA*, **289** (18), 2400–2406.

19. Taylor, C.B. (2010) *How to Practice Evidence-Based Psychiatry: Basic Principles and Case Studies*, American Psychiatric Press, Inc., Washington, DC.

20. Banjo, S. (2008) Washing your web face. Wall Street Journal Online. 17 February 2008.

21. Gorrindo, T. and Groves, J.E. (2008) Web searching for information about physicians. *JAMA*, **300** (2), 213–215.

22. Seeman, M.V. and Seeman, B. (1999) E-psychiatry: the patient–psychiatrist relationship in the electronic age. *Canadian Medical Association Journal*, **161** (9), 1147–1149.

23. Anderson, J.G. (2004) The role of ethics in information technology decisions: a case-based approach to biomedical informatics education. *International Journal of Medical Informatics*, **73** (2), 145–150.

24. Dyer, K.A. (2001) Ethical challenges of medicine and health on the internet: a revierw. *Journal of Medical Internet Research* [serial on the Internet], **3** (2).

25. Childress, C.A. (2002) Ethical issues in providing online psychotherapeutic interventions. *Journal of Medical Internet Research* [serial on the Internet], **2** (1).

26. Winker, M.A., Flanagin, A., Chi-Lum, B. *et al.* (2000) Guidelines for medical and health information sites on the internet: principles governing AMA web sites. *American Medical Association.* *JAMA*, **283** (12), 1600–1606.

27. Eysenbach, G. (2000) Torwards ethical guidelines for dealing with unsolicited patient emails and giving teleadvice in the absence of a pre-existing patient-physician relationship – systematic review and expert survey. *Journal of Medical Internet Research* [serial on the Internet], **2** (1).

28. Berg, J.W. (2002) Ethics and e-medicine. *Saint Louis University Law Journal*, **46**, 61–83.

29. Thompson, L.A., Dawson, K., Ferdig, R. *et al.* (2008) The intersection of online social networking with medical professionalism. *Journal of General Internal Medicine*, **23** (7), 954–957.

30. Gross, R. and Acquisti, A. (2005) Information revelation and privacy in online social networks (The Facebook Case). Workshop on Privacy in the Electronic Society (Association for Computing Machinery), Alexandria, VA, pp. 71–80.

31. Farnan, J.M., Paro, J.A., Higa, J. *et al.* (2008) The YouTube generation: implications for medical professionalism. *Perspectives in Biology and Medicine*, **51** (4), 517–524.

32. Chretien, K.C., Greysen, S.R., Chretien, J.-P. and Kind, T. (2009) Online posting of unprofessional content by medical students. *JAMA*, **302** (12), 1309–1315.

17

Assessment in Psychiatric Education

Brian Lunn[1], Maria R. Corral[2] and Adriana Mihai[3]
[1]School of Medical Sciences Education Development, The Medical School, Newcastle University, Newcastle upon Tyne, UK
[2]Department of Psychiatry, University of British Columbia, St Paul's Hospital, Vancouver, BC, Canada
[3]Psychiatric Department, University of Medicine and Pharmacy Tg Mures, Mures, Romania

17.1 Introduction

Assessment is seen as a necessary and expected aspect of structured learning activities in most educational endeavours. While some learners may view assessment as an unnecessary evil, medical schools and speciality training programmes must demonstrate that students are learning what is taught. In addition, and some would argue, more importantly, students must demonstrate that they have acquired the necessary skills and knowledge before they are granted the privilege of practising independently. The medical profession needs to demonstrate good educational outcomes in order to remain accountable to society and the general public [1, 2].

Many training programmes and accreditation councils introduced the concept of specific competencies in the hope of standardizing requisite behaviours and skills (Accreditation Council for Graduate Medical Education (ACGME), European Board of Psychiatry (2009 Draft) [3], Royal College of Psychiatrists, Royal College of Physicians and Surgeons of Canada) for competent practice (Chapter 7). One of the first organizations to do so was the Royal College of Physicians and Surgeons of Canada, which introduced the CanMEDS Competencies over a decade ago [4, 5]. Consequently, a parallel movement to develop valid and reliable measures of student achievement based on these competencies flourished. In the Canadian Fellowship oral examination, for example, the more reliable Objective Structured Clinical Examination (OSCE) replaced the traditional single patient interview a number of

Teaching Psychiatry: Putting Theory into Practice   Edited by Linda Gask, Bulent Coskun and David Baron
© 2011 John Wiley & Sons, Ltd

years ago [6]. Some organizations have suggested that the use of any assessment tool must consider the following guiding principles [3, 7]:

- Students and teachers should be clear about not only what is being assessed but also how it is being assessed.

- All competencies should be assessed.

- The goal of assessment should be clarified as being either formative, that is, frequent, timely and for the purpose of further learning, or summative, and used to guide decisions about student progress.

- Assessment tools should consist of concrete, observable behaviours.

   The achievement of consistently valid and reliable assessment tools is easier to achieve when measuring discrete competencies, such as medical knowledge. On the other hand, some competencies, such as professionalism, have proven more difficult to measure using traditional psychometric tools [8]. In his recent review of competency assessments of the ACGME, Lurie concluded that competencies have proven to be more difficult to quantify than first thought [8]. As such, the use of qualitative assessments, as employed in the social sciences, may prove to be very useful in enriching the assessment armamentarium in medical education [9–11]. The future of assessment in medical education may indeed require new directions and incorporate more diverse methods of assessment.

   In this chapter, the various methods that have been used for assessing student competencies in psychiatry are described. In addition, the validity and reliability of these assessment methods will be presented and current recommendations for the assessment of individual competencies will be summarized.

17.2 Training

Selection criteria for entry into psychiatric training differ from country to country, varying from national examination to selection based on *curriculum vitae* (CV) alone; both a CV and an interview; CV, interview and six months psychiatric practice under supervision; waiting list or no selection at all. When selection does take place it can be as part of a national programme, be university based or be locally organized.

   In Europe the average length of psychiatric training is five years. Figure 17.1 illustrates the differences between European countries [12].

   An important part of quality insurance is inspection of training, highly recommended by the EFPT (European Federation of Psychiatric Trainees) and European Union of Medical Specialists (UEMS). Inspection of training should include all clinical and academic aspects as well as working conditions. The role of inspection teams is to insist on changes in training or – in the worst case – remove training status [13].

   Assessment of the workplace is important in understanding the real conditions of training and accessibility to clinical supervision, individual supervision and supervision in psychotherapy. The assessment of academic aspects includes the qualification of trainers, number of

Length of training in psychiatry in Europe

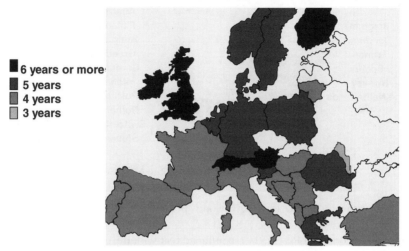

- ■ **6 years or more**
- ■ **5 years**
- ■ **4 years**
- □ **3 years**

Figure 17.1 Length of training in psychiatry in Europe.

trainees allocated to one supervisor, structure of theoretical courses, cases presentation and problem solving cases. Assessment of working conditions also includes workload, numbers of duty hours, number of patients examined by each trainee per day, presence of a trainees' room and a consultation room.

17.3 Knowledge Assessment

Postgraduate training in psychiatry is evolving and changing rapidly across the world [14]. The aim of training is to achieve the necessary knowledge and clinical experience required to work as a specialist in psychiatry.

Assessment of psychiatric education has been an issue for debate due to difficulties in checking knowledge, skills in diagnosis and treatment, decision making in real life conditions, leadership skills within therapeutic teams and research abilities. Different methods of evaluation have been discussed and criticised over time [15–17].

In Europe, national authorities are responsible for setting up programmes for quality assurance of training in psychiatry in accordance with national rules and European Union legislation, as well as according to the requirements of the European Board of Psychiatry [18].

The European Psychiatric Association (EPA) and World Psychiatric Association (WPA) have been preoccupied with standardizing education in psychiatry. To this end, the WPA established a core curriculum in psychiatry, which specifies the minimum knowledge required in psychiatry for specialists.

The evaluation of the structure of psychiatric training, made by the WPA, UEMS, EFPT and EPA in different European countries, showed significant differences, not only in the structure of training but also in types and levels of assessment in psychiatric education. These differences were underlined also by the trainees' research in an EFPT project to evaluate the quality of training in psychiatry across Europe [19]. The assessment of knowledge in a final

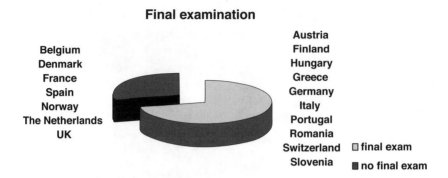

Figure 17.2 Assessment of knowledge in final examination.

examination at the end of the training period is present in some European countries but is not considered necessary in others (Figure 17.2).

The European Board of Psychiatry recommend that within national training programmes in psychiatry there should be a common core of fundamental knowledge and skills that is required of all candidates. This common core is compulsory and includes training in in-patient psychiatry, out-patient psychiatry, liaison psychiatry, emergency psychiatry and psychotherapy. Training should cover general adult psychiatry, old age psychiatry and psychiatric aspects of substance misuse. Training in developmental psychiatry and forensic psychiatry is highly recommended [13].

Training should include structured training (lectures, seminars etc.) over four years for, on average, four hours per week. van Diest *et al.* [20] have shown that knowledge of psychiatry and behavioural sciences increased significantly in the last decades. The subjects covered are as follows:

1. Scientific basis of psychiatry: biological, social and psychological aspects.

2. Psychopathology. Examination of the psychiatric patient. Diagnosis and classification. Psychological tests and laboratory investigations.

3. Specific disorders and syndromes.

4. Psychotherapies. Psychopharmacology and other biological treatments. Multidimensional clinical management. Community psychiatry.

5. Child and adolescent psychiatry. Mental handicap. Psychiatric aspects of substance misuse. Old age psychiatry. Women and psychiatry. Psychiatry of ethnic minorities. Legal and ethic issues in psychiatry.

6. Research methodology. Epidemiology of mental disorders. Psychiatric aspects of Public Health and prevention.

7. Medical informatics and telemedicine. Administration, management and economics.

National authorities should consider psychotherapy as an integral part of training in psychiatry, recognized as equal with the biological and social dimensions. The purpose of training in psychotherapy for a psychiatrist is to enhance their clinical skills in treating psychiatric patients. Psychotherapy should be understood as a psychological method of treatment based on a systematic theory, where efficacy should be scientifically proven. Psychotherapeutic training should include, as a minimum, psychodynamic and cognitive/behavioural approaches. Other theoretical models might be included [13].

Training in psychotherapy should include theoretical courses and compulsory supervision. The national authority should be responsible for the financing of the psychotherapy training, as it is for other kinds of training in psychiatry [19].

Despite the variance which existed, the majority of trainees considered nearly all the fields in question as essential for their training, with greatest priority given to psychopharmacology and biological psychiatry, by 91.7% and 91.4% of the trainees, respectively. It was notable that the stage of training, gender, training centre and medical school of graduation played an important role in the formation of the trainees' priorities [21].

Assessment of knowledge can be carried out at the end of the training period or after each module of training. This assessment could be by oral or by written examination. The type of evaluation differs from one training system to another and sometimes even from one centre to another. The methods of knowledge assessment vary between:

- a written or oral presentation of one or multiple specified topics from the core subjects selected by each examination commission,

- a written examination consisting of multiple choice questions,

- a dissertation on a psychotherapy case,

- an essay about a recommended theme from the speciality literature.

In recent years there have been significant changes in how knowledge is assessed, as the logistical and pedagogic flaws of examination methods have been scrutinised and questioned.

Whilst essays have theoretical advantages in assessing integrated knowledge they do pose logistical problems, as automated marking methods are not available and they are, therefore, labour intensive to mark. This is magnified when methods to improve reliability, such as double marking and additional marking/arbitration where there is disagreement over marks, are taken into account. On top of this, and arguably more important, are pedagogic issues. Formulating questions that are not open to a variety of reasonable interpretations (and therefore which permit a good candidate to diverge significantly from that which examiners intended) is difficult. Validity is further in doubt when it is considered that reliability of examiners in consistently marking work is poor. Even the same examiner remarking the same essay after a six month gap has been shown in one study to only have a correlation of 0.35.

Short answer questions (SAQs) are theoretically easier to focus but there remain issues as to how candidates interpret what is asked. That being said, improving reliability of marking in SAQs is easier than with essays but carries significant costs [22]. Some examination boards have therefore chosen to reject essays and SAQs in favour of other assessments of knowledge.

This is not without an impact on skills as, unless assessed in the workplace, the skill of writing, which is core to specialized psychiatric practice, can be missed out.

Multiple choice questions (MCQs) have been a core feature of medical assessments for many years but over recent years theories over their design have led to multiple changes and a variety of formats and marking schema have been implemented. One reason for this has been that question design has a marked influence on the validity of MCQs [23]. Recently, the shift has been to single item questions with an adjusted mark to take into account guessing. Previously, negative marking has been used to facilitate this but this carries a risk of rewarding examination technique as opposed to knowledge.

The move to MCQs at the expense of SAQs and essays has been viewed with some trepidation. The previous SAQ and other 'free response' formats are often said to test higher order skills than MCQs [24]. Additionally, MCQs can reward good guessing and thus reward 'recognition' rather than 'knowing' [25]. To address this extended matching items/questions (EMIs or EMQs) have been developed with the aim of better assessing knowledge application than with MCQs but with a higher reliability than can be had with SAQs and essays [26].

In EMIs candidates have less opportunity to guess answers successfully; 'recognition' cueing is less likely, too. The larger the list of options provided the more like a 'free response' question an EMI becomes [27]. Like any question format, design and adherence to theoretical models are important, so, for example, in EMIs there must be commonality between the items in the option list. Poorer ability candidates benefit from shorter option lists either because options are limited due to lack of commonality between the items available or simply because too few options are provided.

As an example, in Romania the assessment of psychiatric education is organized in examinations after each module (internal medicine, neurology, psychology, psychiatry) and a final national examination. The final examination is organized by the Ministry of Teaching and Education in different training centres and consists of a written examination, a clinical examination and a practical evaluation of para-clinical data.

The candidate is required to achieve a minimum mark of seven out of ten in the written examination before progressing to the clinical. In the United Kingdom, the latest format of the MRCPsych consists of three written papers taken over the first 12–24 months of speciality training. These assessments use single best answer from five MCQs and an extended matching item component. In Canada, many programmes administer standardized examinations, such as the PRITE[®] (Psychiatry Resident-In-Training Examination), on a yearly basis to monitor residents' level of theoretical knowledge. At the end of the residency, qualifying examinations are necessary to achieve Fellowship status and to practice as a specialist in psychiatry in Canada. These examinations are administered nationally by the Royal College of Physicians and Surgeons of Canada (RCPSC) and include both a written and an oral component. The written component in psychiatry consists of multiple choice and short answer questions, and while the oral examination comprises a number of OSCE stations.

The assessment of knowledge should correlate with that specified as core to the curriculum in each specific training system and reflects the structure of training. In Europe, the diversity and richness of training systems in psychiatry represent a continuous and challenging issue for international bodies like the EFPT, UEMS, EPA and WPA in their collaborative efforts to harmonise training in psychiatry.

The EFPT's efforts to identify this diversity and follow the changes over last 10 years showed significant differences in duration and structure, especially in Central and Eastern Europe [12].

Mihai *et al.* [28], in exploring psychotherapy training across Europe, found four categories of training system:

- Training in psychotherapy is compulsory. After completing training in psychiatry trainees are accredited as 'psychiatrist and psychotherapist' (Netherlands, Denmark, France, Germany and Italy).

- Basic training in psychotherapy is compulsory. After completing training in psychiatry trainees are not accredited as specialist psychotherapists. If a trainee wants to work as a psychotherapist he or she has to complete a specialist course in the chosen therapy (the United Kingdom, Denmark, Sweden, Estonia, Romania and Austria).

- Psychotherapy is a recommend but not a compulsory part of training (Bosnia, Herzegovina, Finland and Turkey).

- Training in psychotherapy is not recommended or compulsory. If trainees wish to become trained in psychotherapy then they have to pay for it and complete the training in their own time (Albania, Greece, Moldavia and Russia).

The assessment of psychotherapeutic knowledge depends on training requirements. In some countries this includes case presentation, in others only theoretical knowledge is assessed and in others knowledge in psychotherapy is not evaluated.

17.4   Skills Assessment

In the minds of regulatory bodies, clinicians and, perhaps most importantly, patients the key assessment of all doctors in training is the final clinical assessment. Traditionally this has taken the form of at least one 'long case', that is the assessment of a doctor in a setting as close to clinical practice as is possible. This mode of assessment is, unfortunately, not without its problems and over the last few decades considerable effort has gone into looking at alternatives.

17.4.1   The Long Case

The traditional form of clinical assessment has been to place a candidate in a room with a patient and require them to carry out an assessment from which they generate a diagnosis and management plan, which the candidate is then examined on. Typically, the candidate is not observed during the initial phase when the patient is assessed although they may be asked subsequently to demonstrate a portion of the assessment, usually examination, in front of the examiner(s). The actual assessment of their findings and conclusions has usually been carried out by a form of *viva voce* examination.

In Romania, as mentioned above, the clinical examination consists of two clinical cases in which the candidate interviews a patient in the presence of three examiners and then presents the case to them. Candidates are evaluated on the therapeutic relationship they establish with the patient, the conduct of the interview, the organization and presentation of data, phenomenology, differential diagnosis, prognosis and biopsychosocial treatment and particularities of the case.

This mode of assessment has apparent high face validity in that it simulates the clinical encounter, involves the assessment of real patients and requires 'higher order' clinical skills, such as the integration of clinical findings and knowledge. Unfortunately, it is not clear that it actually successfully tests the intended objectives. Key clinical skills are actually rarely observed and their assessment is largely by inferences drawn *post hoc* in the concluding viva. A solution to this has been to observe and mark the whole of the assessment carried out by the candidate [29] as a prelude to the final discussion, but this has significant resource implications and in itself does not resolve all of the problems associated with this form of examination.

As it has been traditional to use a single case, the reliability of this form of assessment is inadequate, as luck, either good or bad, has a significant role to play in candidates' experiences, as the case allocated may play to their strengths or weaknesses. The use of real patients introduces further variables, particularly in psychiatry, as their helpfulness or hostility can be independent of candidates' performances. The variability of cases in real patients will inevitably lead to variable signs and symptoms, some easier to elicit than others, and case selection will often be largely dependent on availability of patients at the examination centre, which in turn will be affected by the shape of the local clinical service. One further variable, perhaps the most difficult to control for, is the skill set and prejudices/preferences of the examiners. To address these problems would require assessment over a significant number of different cases with different examiners for each case. Work by Waas and Jolly [30] has indicated that reliability from a single long case of an hour is around 0.60, rising to 0.86 after four hours of testing and 0.90 after eight hours. This is a logistical impossibility for most examination boards and still wouldn't deal with the unreliability of the *viva voce* component, so alternative approaches have developed.

17.4.2 Modified Long Cases

Efforts to improve the reliability of the long case have, as already mentioned, included observation of the whole process but have not just been limited to this. Concerns about the reliability and validity of the *viva voce* component led to the development of the Objective Structured Long Examination Record (OSLER) [31], which structures the process in such a way that there is a focus on the candidate both carrying out observed clinical skills, whether history taking or examination, and presenting their conclusions and recommendations in response to a structured oral examination. This has not, however, eradicated all the concerns about reliability and validity.

17.4.3 The Objective Structured Clinical Examination

The Objective Structured Clinical Examination (OSCE) was developed out of a desire to focus on the objective assessment of clinical skills [32]. The candidate is required to move round a series of 'stations' in which a variety of clinical skills are assessed. The reliability of this form of examination is much higher than the long case, as each candidate can be given a similar experience through the use of simulated patients performing defined roles (Chapter 14). The candidates are also assessed against clear objectives, which can be designed to match an examination 'blueprint' that enables a sufficient breadth of skills to be assessed [33]. The OSCE didn't enter the psychiatric examination lexicon until relatively late [34] but has grown in use in both undergraduate and postgraduate settings. The UK Royal College of Psychiatrists (RCPsych) introduced the OSCE to what was the Part I examination in 2003 [35], and although the new RCPsych Membership examination now has only a final clinical examination the OSCE lives on, albeit in a modified format, in the new Clinical Assessment of Skills and Competencies (CASC).

A strength of the OSCE format is to allow the assessment of a depth and breadth of many skills in a structured way that cannot be readily done using real patients. This format is not without its detractors. Concerns about the verisimilitude of the clinical encounter and, in particular, empathic responses of candidates, but studies have suggested that this is not an issue [36] and that both the long case and OSCEs assess clinical competence 'no worse and no better' than each other [37]. Assessment of skills using OSCEs also appears to have reasonable correlation with assessment of skills in the workplace [38]. Additional evidence that OSCEs are focussed on the assessment of skills was obtained serendipitously in a paper by Wilkinson *et al.* [39], which showed that awareness of what was to be assessed did not appear to alter the assessed level of competence. Awareness of an assessment with a primary knowledge focus would have not shown a similar level of preservation of validity.

An area that has caused some concern in candidates attempting the previous Part I OSCE and current CASC of the RCPsych is the divergence of results between candidates with a UK primary medical qualification (PMQ) and those who have a non-UK PMQ. With both these examinations the overall pass result did not change significantly when compared with the previous assessment method, but there was a trend for candidates with a UK PMQ and in Postgraduate Medical Education and Training Board (PMETB) approved posts to do better. It is important to remember that the data available from the RCPsych compare the UK PMQ, PMETB approved post candidates with the whole cohort.

There are two main areas that contribute to this. Firstly, is the examination structure; secondly, is the candidate demographics. To deal with these in reverse order, since the introduction of Modernising Medical Careers in the United Kingdom there has been an opportunity for candidates who had previously failed the old examinations and who were no longer in training posts to sit the examination. As with any examination there is substantial evidence that when candidates attempt an examination after multiple attempts they have a diminishing chance of success. Additionally, these 're-sit' candidates are rarely in posts that provide significant training. Of course, there is an actual advantage for candidate with a UK PMQ in that their training in medical school is congruous with the roles they train for in speciality training. Finally, language, particularly in patient contact settings, plays a role independent of clinical knowledge. This feeds into the first area highlighted, that is, the examination structure.

Structured clinical examinations, in contrast to the older examinations, place an emphasis on clinical skills, not least of which is communication. As already highlighted, in the United Kingdom this may be an area of difficulty for those who are not primary English speakers; whilst they may well be able to communicate with fellow professionals this is qualitatively different from communication with patients, as the English in these encounters is not formal but colloquial. Cultural aspects of the examination, such as having patients who are challenging and sometimes in conflict with the doctor's views, add an extra layer of complexity for those candidates from outside the United Kingdom who may not be used to such 'robust' patient encounters. The use of simulated patients who are challenging and use colloquial English mirrors our patient population and is representative of real clinical encounters in the United Kingdom. It is also the case that the breadth of topics covered makes a more robust examination of breadth of skill. The longer spent out of training schemes that allow development of skills, the harder it is to hold onto the skills required for an examination such as the CASC. Finally, the benefit of having an undergraduate curriculum that emphasizes the importance of psychiatry and teaches core skills, as well as introducing the factual component of the speciality, should not be underestimated.

Whilst the above summarizes some of the issues that result in differential outcomes between UK PMQ, PMETB training candidates and the rest of the cohort, it is worth also noting that there are other variations in pass rate. For example, women in the whole cohort do better than men both in the knowledge and the clinical assessments. It is interesting, however, to note that in the CASC there is no significant difference between men and women in the reference group used (UK PMQ, PMETB approved post; first attempt). These issues are not specific to the United Kingdom experience. Similar patterns can be found in the Canadian speciality examinations, showing the universal importance of a good grounding in the culture of psychiatric practice and the local idiomatic language and culture for all specialist psychiatrists, for these examinations merely emulate every day clinical experience.

Ultimately, any examination stands or falls on its design. In OSCEs the key elements include numbers of stations and examiners, design and quality of each station and approach to marking. The original approach to OSCEs used checklists to mark operationalized skills. Hodges *et al.* [40] have highlighted that in testing more senior candidates and higher order clinical skills a more global schedule of marking has value in psychiatry. Again, length of testing is one of the most important variables, with reliabilities of 0.54 after one hour of assessment to 0.82 after four hours and 0.90 after eight hours of testing [41].

17.4.4 Workplace-Based Assessments

Much of assessment of clinical skills in psychiatry has been limited to what Miller [42] would have classified as the lower tiers of clinical assessment. In Miller's 'Pyramid' knowledge forms the base of clinical competence (Figure 17.3). Competence, knowing how to do something, is at the next level and where the traditional long case came in. The shift to the OSLER and other more complex long case variants and OSCEs shifted the emphasis to the second top level of Miller's hierarchy, as these methods seek to assess performance. Traditionally, higher speciality training in the United Kingdom, United States, Australia and New Zealand has been competency, but this has shifted in the United Kingdom to the assessment of the trainees ability to do their job, that is what Miller calls assessment of 'Action'. In the United Kingdom the tool to assess this is the workplace-based assessment (WPBA).

An issue of concern for many is that the quality of the assessment in these tools varies significantly between assessors. In the United Kingdom the WPBA is primarily used as a formative assessment. There is anecdotal evidence of significant variation in the quality of

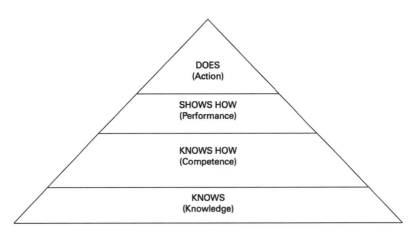

Figure 17.3 Framework for clinical assessment (adapted from Miller [42]).

assessors. It is undoubtedly the case that many find it difficult to be critical of their own trainees, as this requires a separation of the personal relationship and a transition to that of an impartial examiner.

The key to WPBAs is to ensure that there is suitable sampling of the clinical skills required by the trainee. Data on length of testing using tools, such as the Mini-Clinical Evaluation Exercise (mini-CEX) show reliability that is within a range that is at least comparable to other methods of clinical assessment, with reliability of 0.73 for one hour, increasing to 0.96 for eight hours of assessment [43]. Multiple assessments allow a spread of skills and multiple assessors assure a breadth of views is incorporated into a whole. This allows for the fact that mini-CEXs and other WPBA assessment tools are amongst the less structured and objective modes of assessment.

17.4.5 Summary

Many assessment bodies still use assessments around clinical encounters with real patients, either using long cases or short focussed tools such as the mini-CEX. This can be either in a formal examination or in the workplace (United Kingdom). In an ideal world the final conclusion as to whether a trainee has achieved a satisfactory level of clinical skills would use a combination of modes of assessment in a variety of settings, perhaps including a mix of the long case, mini-CEXs and their equivalents and OSCEs with workplace-based assessments.

17.5 Professionalism

In the past century, great strides occurred in the standardization of medical education, particularly with a focus on the acquisition of knowledge and specialized skills. In the last 15–20 years, however, the medical education literature has witnessed a resurgent interest in the concept of medical professionalism [1, 44]. Some authors proposed that a 'normative' definition of medical professionalism would enhance teaching and assessment of this very important quality of practising physicians [2, 45]. As a result, a number of psychiatric training programmes and national councils have joined their medical counterparts and included professionalism as a required competency for trainees and graduating specialists [3, 4, 46]. While there have been few studies on the assessment of professionalism specific to psychiatry, a recent review is available that summarizes the assessment of ACGME competencies in psychiatry [47–49]. The examination of the tools used to assess professionalism is complicated by the fact that it has been measured as both a global construct and as a number of individual qualities that are considered to contribute to the broader concept of professionalism, such as empathy, integrity, personal values and ethical principles [50, 51]. The studies and measures are extremely varied and, as a result, generalizations and recommendations based on these studies are difficult. These caveats aside, several reviews of the literature on this topic highlight the methods used to evaluate this construct in medicine and are useful to consider in the assessment of professionalism in psychiatry [2, 7, 49, 52–54].

The following methods have been used to measure various aspects of a student's degree of professionalism in medicine:

- **Portfolios**: Most portfolios include a collection of resident or medical student work and are useful in encouraging self-reflection in the educational process. Portfolios are, however, difficult to score reliably given their subjective and varied content.

- **Supervisor and peer assessments (generally involve global ratings)**: These can be useful in describing interpersonal skills but tend to be unreliable. Peer assessments may undermine relationships between learners.

- **Self-assessment (generally involve global ratings)**: This method has many inherent weaknesses that affect its reliability, including gender differences in self-assessment ratings. They tend to lack correlation with supervisor ratings and are influenced by the bias of social desirability. However, self-assessment tools may be useful when a student is asked to reflect on consistent discrepancies in self-ratings and external ratings of performance (see 360-degree feedback).

- **360-degree feedback**: These types of assessment were adopted from the business world and are useful for increasing self-awareness and driving efforts to change behaviour. These are especially useful if patient feedback is elicited.

- **Standardized written/oral examinations**: These have been shown to have good reliability and validity in the assessment of factual knowledge. Hence, their usefulness in the evaluation of professionalism may be restricted to the assessment of knowledge of ethical principles, for example.

- **Standardized patients and OSCES**: These are extensively used in summative assessments and may inform several aspects of students' professionalism, such as capacity for empathy or interpersonal skills. Drawbacks include cost and what some describe as an 'artificial' setting, as well as a lack of consistent reliability.

- **Direct observation**: Assessment forms such as the mini-CEX rely on direct observation of a specific clinical encounter. The effectiveness of such measures is dependent on effective and specific definitions of the rating criteria, as well as on the need to sample a range of clinical encounters in order to reduce sampling bias.

Bandiera *et al.* [55] recommended the following as the preferred tools to best assess resident competencies in professionalism:

- Portfolios

- Multisource feedback (360-degree feedback)

- Direct observations and In-Training Evaluation Reports (ITERs)

Some authors have proposed a developmental model in the teaching and assessment of professionalism [2]. Medical students could be taught the principles of ethics, humanism and responsibility, while doctors in speciality training would be expected to increasingly adopt these principles in their clinical work [56]. Initially, students would adopt these principles in order to avoid negative consequences from their peers, supervisors or other team members. By the time a doctor has achieved the competencies of a specialist psychiatrist, they would be expected to have internalized these principles and practice them spontaneously, incorporating them into their budding professional identity. With such a model, the methods used to assess professionalism in the medical student would be very different from those used to assess professionalism in a doctor about to achieve recognition as a specialist. Traditional psychometric methods may result in valid and reliable assessments of ethical knowledge in medical students, but they will be inadequate if applied to more complex and nuanced concepts, such as the evaluation of a senior trainee's management of boundary violations for example.

It is becoming clear to many in the field of educational health scholarship that qualities such as responsibility, altruism, integrity and the importance of placing patient interests above those of the physician cannot be measured in the same way that many aspects of medical knowledge are evaluated [10, 57]. Psychometric properties cannot take into account the contextual and relationship-specific factors unique to professionalism [9, 52]. Hence, the tools to assess professionalism will need to be broadened and take into account the stage of training of the person being evaluated [9].

Cruess *et al.* [1] state that professionalism is '. . .an ideal to be sustained' and it will be crucial to ensure that medical students, residents and practising physicians live up to that ideal. Consequently, psychiatry, and medicine as a whole, needs to encourage the ongoing development of sound and accurate assessment methods that will maintain the integrity of the profession.

17.6 Who Passes

In any assessment process the decision about who passes can be a significant bone of contention. This is a particular issue for those candidates who perform around the borderline and it is here, therefore, that educationalists have focussed their efforts to try and assist in this decision making process.

In establishing any examination this issue needs to be resolved at an early stage, as it will affect approaches to marking, standard setting and examiner training. It is, of course, only fair that this is transparent and candidates understand the principles upon which the final decision is going to be made. Issues of test quality have already been touched upon above. The two main factors are reliability and validity.

Validity is a measure of whether a test assesses what it purports to and reliability is whether what it measures does so in a consistent and reproducible manner. Validity is divisible into three main types:

- Content validity, sometimes called face validity, is whether the examination actually tests the objectives chosen.

- Construct validity is whether the test shows correlation with what might be considered a 'gold standard'.

- Criterion validity is whether the test result has predictive value. An example might be whether a final medical examination can predict competence as a first year doctor.

Some also include whether the assessment process imposes constraints on learning in that it changes what candidates learn in preparation for the examination in the list of types of validity.

Reliability is a statistical method that aims to provide data on how consistent and generalizable an examination is. Types of reliability include:

- Test–retest reliability

- Inter-rater reliability

- Intra-rater reliability

- Internal consistency

- Equivalent test forms.

Literature on reliability typically considers measures of reliability with values above 0.8 as being acceptable, whilst if the value is below 0.7 there is a need to improve the assessment methodology.

Standard setting requires that prior to an examination being delivered an assessment is made by an 'expert' group which has insight into the what is expected of a passing, or minimally competent, candidate. They review the examination with the aim of deciding which questions are of 'easy', 'moderate' or 'hard' difficulty. From this the individual 'expert' ratings are combined, for example using the Angoff method [58], to quantify the threshold at which a minimally competent candidate would pass the examination. This also allows the examination board to try and ensure that from diet to diet examinations remain of a consistent and appropriate difficulty. This can be aided by the use of 'anchor' questions where cohorts of candidates can be compared over time, allowing conclusions to be drawn about whether differences in performance between cohorts reflect differences between them or the examination.

Once the examination has taken place questions which are statistical outliers can be reviewed and those that are particularly discrepant and do not appear to discriminate (either between those who are or are not competent, or between the 'excellent' and 'minimally competent' candidates) can be excluded from the final consideration of results. Here, two main methods of defining a pass mark are often used. The borderline groups method and the contrasting groups method.

In the borderline groups method (as used in the UK General Medical Council's Professional and Linguistics Assessment Board) each candidate obtains two marks. One is a percentage mark; the other is a decision as to whether they have achieved an overall 'Pass', a 'Fail' or whether their performance is 'Borderline'. The scores for all those marked 'Borderline' are reviewed and the mean of those candidates graded at the 'Borderline' is used to determine the pass mark for that examination item.

In the contrasting groups method the examiner again makes a global judgement as well as giving a percentage mark. This time the decision is dichotomous, either 'Pass' or 'Fail'. The marks for each group are then plotted separately on the same graph and the point where the two curves intersect becomes the pass mark for that item.

From here, in both the above methods, the results can be handled in a variety of ways. The individual item pass marks could be summated, giving a pass mark for the whole examination, or a threshold can be chosen where candidates have to pass an agreed number of items. The potential problem with the former is that it is possible for a candidate to pass a minority of items but still pass the examination, whilst the latter method can be seen as arbitrary.

17.7 Summary

Most, if not all, of those involved in teaching medicine have probably encountered a variant on the question, 'Will this be in the examination?' There can be no more accurate truism in medicine than 'Assessment drives learning.' With this in mind, it is evident that, whatever the focus of a training programme, if assessment is not at the centre of planning the curriculum, efforts to direct trainee learning will fail.

It is easy to become nihilistic when faced with an awareness that trainees will choose to focus on that which is examined but if we see this not as an impediment but an opportunity, trainees can be directed down a chosen learning path and appropriate attributes developed. Assessment then becomes central to any curriculum, not as an end in itself but as a signpost and driver to excellence.

It is therefore encouraging to see the beginning of adoption of worldwide standards in the teaching and assessment of psychiatric knowledge and skills. That being said, it is clear that there's still a need for more work to be done to ensure that assessment methods are driven by the current and future evidence base and focussed appropriately to drive trainees learning. In the forefront of all of our minds should be that the objective is to deliver high quality specialist psychiatrists, individuals to whom we would feel comfortable entrusting the care of those we care about.

References

1. Cruess, R.L., Cruess, S.R. and Johnston, S.E. (2000) Professionalism: an ideal to be sustained. *The Lancet*, **356**, 156–159.
2. Arnold, L. and Stern, D.T. (2006) What is Medical Professionalism? in *Measuring Medical Professionalism* (ed. D.T. Stern), Oxford University Press, Oxford, pp. 15–37.
3. European Board of Psychiatry (2009) European Framework for Competencies in Psychiatry. Draft. http://www.acgme.org/outcome/implement/Profm_resource.pdf (accessed 4 August 2010).
4. Frank, J.R. (2005) The CanMEDS 2005 Physician Competency Framework. Better Standards. Better Physicians. Better Care, The Royal College of Physicians and Surgeons of Canada, Ottawa.
5. Zaretsky, A. (2009) Evaluation of resident competency in psychiatry: a Canadian perspective, in *Approaches to Postgraduate Education in Canada: What Educators and Residents Need to Know* (eds J.S. Leverette, G.S. Hnatko and E. Persad), Canadian Psychiatric Association, pp. 241–257.
6. Leverette, J.S., Hnatko, G.S. and Persad, E. (2009) *Approaches to Postgraduate Education in Canada: What Educators and Residents Need to Know*, Canadian Psychiatric Association.
7. Arnold, L. (2002) Assessing professional behaviour: yesterday, today and tomorrow. *Academic Medicine*, **77**, 502–515.
8. Lurie, S.J., Mooney, C.J. and Lyness, J.M. (2009) Measurement of the general competencies of the Accreditation Council for Graduate Medical Education: a systematic review. *Academic Medicine*, **84**, 301–309.
9. Kuper, A., Reeves, S., Albert, M. *et al.* (2007) Assessment: do we need to broaden our methodological horizons? *Medical Education*, **41**, 1121–1123.
10. Ginsburg, S., McIlroy, J., Oulanova, O. *et al.* (in press) Towards authentic clinical evaluation: pitfalls in the pursuit of competency. *Academic Medicine*, **85** (5), 780–786
11. Regher, G., Bogo, M., Regher, C. *et al.* (2007) Can we build a better mousetrap? Improving the measures of practice performance in the field practicum. *Journal of Social Work Education*, **43**, 327–343.
12. Mihai, A. (2006) European Federation of Psychiatric Trainees (EFPT) and harmonisation in training programs, in *New tools for clinical practice*, 28th Nordic Congress of Psychiatry abstracts, pp. 28–29.
13. UEMS (2002) Report of the European Board of Psychiatry – Quality assurance in specialist training in psychiatry.
14. Langsley, D.G. (1981) Changing patterns of psychiatry specialty certification in the English-speaking countries. *American Journal of Psychiatry*, **138**, 493–497.
15. Morgenstern, A.L. (1970) A criticism of psychiatry's board examinations. *American Journal of Psychiatry*, **127**, 33–42.
16. Druss, R.G. (2002) Board exams. *American Journal of Psychiatry*, **159**, 1827–1828.
17. Quick, S.K. and Robinowitz, C.B. (1981) Examination success and opinions on American Board of Psychiatry and Neurology certification. *American Journal of Psychiatry*, **138**, 340–344.
18. Hohagen, F. (1996) Training in psychiatry in Europe – recommendations of the European Board of Psychiatry. *European Psychiatry*, **11**, 248s–248s.
19. Mihai, A. (2002) EFPT Statements, in *EFPT: Education in Psychiatry across Europe* (ed. U.M.F. Mures), Sinaia, pp. 13–32.
20. van Diest, R., van Dalen, J., Bak, M. *et al.* (2004) Growth of knowledge in psychiatry and behavioural sciences in a problem-based learning curriculum. *Medical Education*, **38**, 1295–1301.

21. Margariti, M.M., Kontaxakis, V.P., Madianos, M. *et al.* (2002) Psychiatric education: a survey of Greek trainee psychiatrists. *Medical Education*, **36**, 622–625.

22. Milton, O. (1979) Improving achievement via essay exams. *Journal of Veterinary Medical Education*, **6**, 108–112.

23. Shively, M.J. (1978) Improving the quality of multiple-choice examinations. *Journal of Veterinary Medical Education*, **5**, 76–76.

24. McGuire, C. (1987) Written methods for assessing clinical competence, in *Further Developments in Assessing Clinical Competence* (eds I. Hart and R. Harden), Can-Heal Publications, Montreal, pp. 46–58.

25. Newble, D., Baxter, A. and Elmslie, R. (1979) A comparison of multiple-choice and free-response tests in examinations of clinical competence. *Medical Education*, **13**, 263–268.

26. Case, S.M. and Swanson, D.B. (1993) Extended matching items: a practical alternative to free-response questions. *Teaching and Learning in Medicine*, **5**, 107–115.

27. Veloski, J., Robinowitz, H. and Robeson, M. (1988) Cuing in multiple-choice questions: a reliable, valid and economical solution, in *Research in Medical Education*, Association of Medical Colleges, Washington, DC, pp. 195–200.

28. Mihai, A., Weiss, E., Beezhold, J. *et al.* (2009) Psychotherapy training across Europe: Status quo. *Die psychiatrie*, **6**, 84–88.

29. Newble, D.I. (1991) The observed long case in clinical assessment. *Medical Education*, **25**, 369–373.

30. Wass, V. and Jolly, B. (2001) Does observation add to the validity of the long case? *Medical Education*, **35**, 729–734.

31. Gleeson, F. (1997) AMEE Medical Education Guide No 9: assessment of clinical competence using the Objective Structured Long Examination Record (OSLER). *Medical Teacher*, **19**, 7–14.

32. Harden, R.M. and Gleeson, F.A. (1979) Assessment of clinical competencies using an objective structured clinical examination (OSCE). *Medical Education*, **13**, 39–45.

33. Lunn, B. (2005) The OSCE blueprint and station development, in *OSCEs in Psychiatry* (ed. R. Rao), Gaskell, London, pp. 24–32.

34. Famuyiwa, O.O., Zachariah, M.P. and Ilechukwu, S.T. (1991) The objective structured clinical examination in undergraduate psychiatry. *Medical Education*, **25**, 45–50.

35. Tyrer, S. and Oyebode, F. (2004) Why does the MRCPsych examination need to change? *The British Journal of Psychiatry*, **184**, 197–199.

36. Sanson-Fisher, R.W. and Poole, A.D. (1980) Simulated patients and the assessment of medical students' interpersonal skills. *Medical Education*, **14**, 249–253.

37. Wass, V., Jones, R. and Van Der Vleuten, C. (2001) Stadardized or real patients to test clinical competence? The long case revisited. *Medical Education*, **35**, 321–325.

38. Melding, P., Coverdale, J. and Robinson, E. (2002) A 'fair play'? Comparison of an objective structured clinical examination of final year medical students training in psychiatry and their supervisors' appraisals. *Australian Psychiatry*, **10**, 344–347.

39. Wilkinson, T., Fontaine, S. and Egan, T. (2003) Was a breach of examination security unfair in an objective structured clinical examination? A critical incident. *Medical Teacher*, **25**, 42–46.

40. Hodges, B., Regeher, G., McNaughton, N. *et al.* (1999) OSCE checklists do not capture increasing levels of expertise. *Academic Medicine*, **74**, 1129–1134.

41. Van Der Vleuten, C.P.M., van Luyk, S.J. and Swanson, D.B. (1988) Reliability (generalizability) of the Maastricht Skills Test. *Research in Medical Education*, **27**, 228–33.

42. Miller, G.E. (1990) The assessment of clinical skills/competence/performance. *Academic Medicine*, **6** (suppl.) S63–S67.

43. Norcini, J.J., Blank, L.L., Duffy, D. *et al.* (2003) The mini-CEX: method for assessing clinical skills. *Annals of Internal Medicine*, **138**, 476–481.

44. Medical Professionalism Project (2002) Medical professionalism in the new millennium: a physicians' charter. *The Lancet*, **359**, 520–522.

45. Swick, H.M. (2000) Toward a normative definition of medical professionalism. *Academic Medicine*, **75**, 612–616.

46. Royal College of Psychiatrists (2007) A Competency Based Curriculum for Specialist Training in Psychiatry: Core and General Module. Royal College of Psychiatrists, London.

47. Bienenfeld, D., Klykylo, W. and Lehrer, D. (2003) Closing the loop: assessing the effectiveness of psychiatric competency measures. *Academic Psychiatry*, **27**, 131–135.

48. Bennett, A.J., Roman, B., Arnold, L.M. *et al.* (2005) Professionalism deficits among medical students: models of identification and intervention. *Academic Psychiatry*, **29**, 426–432.

49. Swick, S., Hall, S. and Beresin, E. (2006) Assessing the ACGME competencies in psychiatry training programs. *Academic Psychiatry*, **30**, 330–351.

50. Arnold, E.L., Blank, L.L., Race, K.E.H. *et al.* (1998) Can professionalism be measured? The development of a scale for use in the medical environment. *Academic Medicine*, **73**, 1119–1121.

51. Veloski, J.J., Fields, S.K., Boex, J.R. *et al.* (2005) Measuring professionalism: a review of studies with instruments reported in the literature between 1982 and 2002. *Academic Medicine*, **80**, 366–370.

52. Ginsburg, S., Regher, G., Hatala, R. *et al.* (2000) Context, conflict and resolution: a new conceptual framework for evaluating professionalism. *Academic Medicine*, **75**, S6–S10.

53. Larkin, G.L., Binder, L., Houry, D. *et al.* (2002) Defining and evaluating professionalism: a core competency for graduating emergency rotation. *Academic Emergency Medicine*, **11**, 1249–1256.

54. Lynch, D.C., Surdyck, P.M. and Eiser, A.R. (2004) Assessing professionalism: a review of the literature. *Medical Teacher*, **26**, 366–373.

55. Bandiera, G., Sherbino, J. and Frank, J.R. (2006) *The CanMEDS Assessment Tools Handbook. An Introductory Guide to Assessment Methods for the CanMEDS Competencies*, The Royal College of Physicians and Surgeons of Canada, Ottawa.

56. Roberts, L.W., Green Hammond, K.A., Geppert, C.M.A. *et al.* (2004) The positive role of professionalism and ethics training in medical education: a comparison of medical student and resident perspectives. *Academic Psychiatry*, **28**, 170–182.

57. Ginsburg, S., Regher, G. and Mylopoulos, M. (2009) From behaviours to attributions: further concerns regarding the evaluation of professionalism. *Medical Education*, **43**, 414–425.

58. Zieky, M.J. (2001). So much has changed: how the setting of cutscores has evolved since the 1980s, in *Setting Performance Standards* (eds G.J. Cizek and N.J. Mahwah), Lawrence Erlbaum Associates, pp. 19–52.

18

The Support and Welfare of the Student

Michael F. Myers

Department of Psychiatry & Behavioural Sciences, SUNY Downstate Medical Center, NY, USA

18.1 Introduction

> The future is today
>
> —(Sir William Osler) [1]

One of the exciting dimensions of teaching psychiatry in the twenty first century is the increasing attention being paid to the health and well-being of medical students and residents. Accompanying, or embedded in, the burgeoning literature on the subject of physician health and illness are many evidence-based and anecdotal studies of trainees. Sadly, this has not always been so. Prior to the recognition and treatment of 'the impaired physician' in the 1970s (mainly substance abuse), troubled medical students and residents generally buried their distress in overwork, struggled academically and under-performed, fell by the wayside or were simply dismissed. Some killed themselves and although their deaths were seen as tragic, many of these individuals were judged as unfit for medicine and not up for the task. Deemed flawed, they alone were responsible for their demise. Not only were they under-diagnosed and under-treated, there was no understanding of context then. The 'culture of medicine' with its toxic and protective factors did not exist.

Discussed in this chapter are some of the more common psychiatric illnesses in students, common stressors in the lives of students today, unique issues for ethnic minority and IMG trainees and, most important, how it is possible to assist both at an individual and systems level of intervention. But firstly, a review of what is happening around the world.

Teaching Psychiatry: Putting Theory into Practice Edited by Linda Gask, Bulent Coskun and David Baron
© 2011 John Wiley & Sons, Ltd

18.2   An International Perspective

At least two studies from the United Kingdom have noted poor mental health in medical students, worsening as the years of school go on [2, 3]. In Norway, Tyssen *et al.* [4] have found a significant amount of suicidal thinking in medical students, some of which included a suicidal plan. A study of Turkish medical students uncovered significant depression and anxiety [5]. Swedish medical students reported significant symptoms of depression and suicidal ideation [6]. Over a six year course of training, Finnish medical students reported increasing levels of fatigue, sleeping problems, anxiety, irritability and depression – without gender differences [7]. And at least three Canadian studies have documented high levels of stress and depression in medical students and residents [8–10].

18.3   Psychiatric Illnesses

18.3.1   Burnout

Although this is not a diagnosis in DSM-IV, there have been a number of recent papers on burnout in both medical students and residents. Most have employed the Maslach Burnout Inventory (BMI), a 22 item instrument that is considered the gold standard for measuring burnout [11]. Emotional exhaustion, depersonalization and low personal accomplishment are its three domains. Burnout was found in 45% of medical students in one study [12] and 50% of medical students in a larger study [11]. Burnout increased with each year of schooling and was felt due to both personal life events in students (divorce, major illness in self or family member, death of family member) and curricular factors (academic failure, deaths of patients, increasing educational debts). In the 2008 study, 10% of the students also experienced suicidal ideation. Not surprisingly, these same researchers [13] found an inverse relationship between degree of burnout and empathy for others.

What about burnout in residents? Martini *et al.* [14] found burnout in 50% of residents, ranging from 75% in obstetrics and gynaecology to 27% in family medicine. An Argentinian study of cardiology residents found high levels of burnout, perceived stress and depressive symptoms [15]. Although it did not use the Maslach Burnout Inventory, a large Canadian study by Cohen and Patten [10] found the following: 34% reported their life as stressful (40% in females, 27% in males) and up to 55% reported experiencing intimidation and harassment (12% of males and 38% of females). Of concern is that 17% rated their mental health as fair or poor. Finally, a study of family medicine and psychiatric residents reported significant depersonalization and emotional exhaustion scales on the MBI but less so in psychiatry residents [16]. Residents who were parents had lower depersonalization and emotional exhaustion scores.

What are the implications of these findings for psychiatric educators? Firstly, teachers must accept that a medical student or resident who seems disinterested, apathetic and lacking in compassion – and is under-functioning – may be burnt out. Secondly, it is imperative to reach out to the trainee and express one's concern. Thirdly, one must suggest a number of options (see later).

18.3.2   Depression

A systematic review of studies by Dyrbye *et al.* [17] found a high prevalence of depression and anxiety amongst medical students. Levels of overall psychological distress were consistently higher than in the general population and age-matched peers by the later years of training. Distress was generally reported to be higher in female students. Levine *et al.* [18], using the Beck Depression Inventory (BDI), found that the percentage of medical students who experienced a depressed mood (in the moderately to severely depressed range) increased from the beginning of year one to the end of second year medicine but the rates were not as high as in two previous studies [19, 20], that is less than 12%. This is in contrast with a 2002 study reporting depression in up to 25% of medical students [21].

What about depression in residents? Older data [8, 22] indicate that one quarter to one third of residents develop clinical symptoms of depression during their training. Most studies of residents are not speciality specific. There is no research on the prevalence of bipolar mood disorder in trainees. In one unpublished look back study of 110 psychiatrists presenting for treatment (Myers, private practice, 1974–2004), the most common diagnoses were mood disorders, substance use disorders and dual diagnoses; two of the residents were diagnosed with bipolar illness. In this review, one third were residents and the gender mix was 39 females and 61males. The referral patterns were: self, primary care physician, programme director, employer, spouse or partner, medical colleague, physician friend, licensing body, attorney or one of their patients. Some of the resident patients confused being a patient (that is, being in treatment) with being a trainee. In other words, although they were symptomatic and presented for help, they had a lot of difficulty accepting being a patient. They preferred to see this more as part of their education and development toward becoming a psychiatrist. Many of the patients had procrastinated for some time about seeking treatment. A number of the patients lived with significant internalized stigma (that is, despite being in training or working in the mental health field, they felt ashamed about their need for treatment). Some felt fraudulent because they were prescribed psychotropic medications; for example, they felt duplicitous as a doctor treating patients when they were in treatment themselves. International Medical Graduates had higher levels of internalized stigma.

It has long been felt that there is significant self-selection into psychiatry as a career choice. In other words, an unknown percentage of applicants to psychiatry residency have a previous history of at least one episode of depression. Many have a family history of mood disorders in first degree relatives. An unknown percentage of medical students recovering from a bout of depression become interested in psychiatry residency. They may become attracted to the field because of their personal experience of illness, first hand empathy for those who suffer from a psychiatric illness and a desire to make a difference. Others, considering the importance of self-care and life style considerations in maintaining mood stability, select psychiatry because of a perception of more humane faculty, more reasonable work hours, less demanding on call schedules and the potential for more autonomy and control in setting limits on how much one works after training. A fundamental belief is that should the trainee have a relapse of their illness he/she would receive a more understanding, informed and compassionate response by the training office and clinical supervisors.

Teachers of psychiatry must accept and respect that an unknown number of their medical students and residents may have had a previous personal experience with a mental illness. When lecturing whole classes, when conducting seminars and when facilitating case conferences, it behoves the psychiatrist teacher to refrain from an 'us and them' duality in explaining the symptoms and behaviours of a particular mental illness. Historically, too many trainees have been hurt and offended when the teacher talks about patients as 'other', using highly intellectualized and psychopathological jargon that is distancing and disrespectful. 'Mr Brown is a man suffering with mania' is more humanistic than 'Mr Brown is a manic'. When describing the symptoms of depression, instead of reciting a checklist, a teaching point will be made much more empathically by saying something like 'Those of you who have suffered from depression yourself will know first hand how profound the fatigue is, how terrible the absence of feeling or the loss of self-worth and the despair of hopelessness. It's a very, very painful illness'.

18.3.3   Substance Use Disorders

Good data on the incidence of substance use disorders in medical students are not generally available. What has been known for decades is that many medical students have alcoholism or other drug abuse in one or more first degree relatives. This places them at risk for developing the disease themselves. A recent study of first year military medical students revealed at least one episode of binge drinking within two weeks of the survey in one fifth of the women students and one third of the male students [23]. In a recent study of Irish business and medical students, 14.4% of the medical students had an alcohol use disorder that is CAGE[1] score = 2 [24]. Rates of alcohol abuse were higher in Turkish medical students (20.0–22.4%) [25]. A questionnaire study of Swedish medical students' alcohol and drug habits in 1995 found that 12% of the male and 4% of the female students were deemed at risk for alcohol problems. About 7% of the medical students reported having used illegal drugs, such as hashish, marijuana and cocaine, during the past 12-month period and about 9% to have used sedative and/or hypnotic drugs [26].

The prevalence of substance use disorders amongst physicians in general is 10–15% [27]. What is relevant for our purposes as psychiatric educators is the following: 'Specialities such as anaesthesia, emergency medicine and psychiatry have higher rates of drug abuse, probably related to the high-risk environment associated with these specialities, the baseline personalities of these health care providers and easy access to drugs in these areas. Drugs and alcohol are mostly used for recreational purposes by medical students. Residents and attending physicians use drugs of abuse for performance enhancement and as self-treatment for various reasons, such as pain, anxiety or depression' [28].

Case Example

> Paul, a fourth year medical student, came for assessment after being charged with impaired driving and having his driver's licence suspended. His wife Clair had been trying unsuccessfully to get him to seek treatment for alcoholism for at least two years. He often drank too much, especially on weekends. During these times he was boisterous, touchy and sarcastic,

---

[1]CAGE – Have you ever felt you should *cut* down on your drinking? Have people *annoyed* you by criticising your drinking? Have you ever felt bad or *guilty* about your drinking? Have you ever had a drink first thing in the morning to steady your nerves or get rid of a hang-over (*eye-opener*)?

not only with Clair, but with her friends as well. He had 'blackouts' during these episodes, but because he never struck Clair and never drank when on call, he considered his drinking 'no different than that of any other medical student'. His father, one brother, two paternal uncles and two maternal aunts were severely alcoholic. He dismissed this as 'unimportant'.

Although addiction is diagnosed in some medical students and residents, the vast majority of physicians who come to attention and begin treatment are in their early to middle career years. However, a longitudinal and detailed history of increasing abuse and dependence commonly denotes problem or excessive use that began during the training years. And because obvious signs of addiction like intoxication at work and suicidal thinking are end-stage signs, it is critical to watch students for early signs, like tardiness for rounds, not responding to beepers, mysterious absences while on duty, frequent 'sick days', diminished attention to grooming, forgetfulness, irritability with peers and colleagues, faulty record keeping and lapsed clinical skills. It is necessary to take seriously any and all concerns expressed by the student's classmates, allied health professionals, family or patients. This is especially relevant when what is being reported is clearly a decline in the trainee's performance baseline from which he/she normally functions [29].

18.3.4 Anxiety Disorders

There is little research on the anxiety disorders in medical students. However, there is plenty of anecdotal evidence gleaned from the practices of psychiatrists and psychologists who look after trainees that the entire spectrum of anxiety disorders (generalized anxiety disorder, panic disorder, simple phobias, social anxiety disorder, obsessive compulsive disorder and post traumatic stress disorder) exist in mild to severe forms. Heru [30] found that 73% of third and fourth year medical students reported witnessing or experiencing mistreatment 'suggesting symptoms of post traumatic stress, with no differences in scores across the intended field of study, age or gender'. With regard to residents, Klamen et al. [31] studied 212 residents with a standardized questionnaire. 13% met diagnostic criteria for post traumatic stress disorder (PTSD) (20% of the women and 9% of the men).

Case Example

Dr Brown, a 29 year old resident in psychiatry was referred to a psychiatrist for the following symptoms: unrelenting fluctuating anxiety, broken sleep, nightmares, intrusive imagery of a pistol being held to someone's head, emotional lability, crying and numbness. Her symptoms began 10 days earlier when she was seeing patients in the out-patient department of a teaching hospital. Suddenly she heard a loud angry voice coming from the waiting room. She excused herself and went into the hall where she witnessed a large man with a pistol in his hand yelling 'Where is he? Where's my doctor? I'm going to kill him! He's been fucking with my mind!' Terrified she ran back into her room, rang the help alert buzzer and called hospital security. There was no lock on the door but she and her patient barricaded the door with the desk and waited. Minutes felt like hours. The man kept yelling as he ran from office to office but no shots were heard. He did not attempt to enter her office. Soon she heard sirens and heard the voices of police officers. The patient was subdued and no one was hurt. Dr Brown was diagnosed with post traumatic stress disorder and she responded nicely to medication and cognitive behavioural therapy.

Although exposure to this type of trauma is not common in students, they are, though, subject to other clinical situations that they may find disturbing, especially when they are new to a service or feel unprepared. Examples might include: treating patients with mutilating injuries from high speed motor vehicle accidents, falls or burns; assessing and treating battered infants; watching an amputation of a limb in the operating room; first exposure to an intensive care unit; assisting at an unsuccessful cardiac arrest, especially in a young or previously healthy patient; listening to the painful story of someone who has been brutally raped; witnessing the laboured breathing of someone who is in pulmonary oedema and who is fully conscious and terrified.

Some students suffer from obsessive compulsive disorder (OCD) and this is not only disabling but can seriously impair their ability to function effectively at school or work.

Case Example

> Mr Baxter's chief complaint was 'I need help, I think I've got OCD'. He was a third year medical student. When asked why he thought he had obsessive compulsive disorder, here was his response: 'Well I looked up my symptoms in DSM-IV and I think that I meet criteria – I've got both obsessions and compulsions – I get this – it's really embarrassing to talk about but I know I have to – I get this thought over and over again, like maybe 10 times a day, that really scares me – it's a thought and a fear – that I'm going to suddenly mount a female patient up in stirrups – it all started when I was on OBGYN two months ago – I was fine at first but sometime during the third week of the rotation I awoke early one morning from a dream, I was terrified, I had just thrown myself on a patient that I was doing a bimanual pelvic exam on – it all happened so fast, that's when I woke up – I was sweating like mad. Anyway, from then on I was nervous being around female patients, I could still do my physical and pelvic exams but only if I said the Lord's Prayer under my breath. That worked. But this doesn't make sense to me. I really like OBGYN, I might even specialize in it but if I told anyone they'd think I was a pervert, a sicko, depraved. What's weird – but reassuring – is that I'm not turned on at all, like I'm not thinking sexual thoughts, I don't get erections when I'm examining women. I'm really professional. So why would I have this thought, this idea or impulse that I'm going to jump her. And this stuff is nothing like my relationship with my girlfriend, we have a wonderful sex life together, still do, even with this sick shit going on in my head. The praying seems to help, both at work and when the thoughts come back to me. But now I have to say the Lord's Prayer 16 times over. Then I can move on. I have no idea why the number 16 but it works'. This medical student was treated with a high dose of a selective serotonin reuptake inhibitor and a course of CBT. He became asymptomatic within six weeks and remained symptom free after the medication was stopped nine months later.

18.3.5 Attention Deficit Disorder (With or Without Hyperactivity)

This is a disorder that is being uncovered in students much more often than 10–15 years ago. Some are adults who were diagnosed as children and who have already been treated with medication like methylphenidate. Some are students who begin to encounter academic difficulties that they've never encountered before; assessment by educational psychologists in the student learning centre point to ADD or ADHD. Some begin to learn about the disorder in paediatrics or child psychiatry blocks and wonder about their long standing disorganization, distractibility, short attention span, restlessness, forgetfulness, impulsiveness or other deficits; they may seek the assistance of a specialist in the area. And others recognize that they have been self-medicating with alcohol and really see their symptoms clearly when they stop drinking. Most respond nicely to appropriate medication and academic accommodations on examinations or other procedures that simply take them more time to complete.

18.3.6   Eating Disorders

These exist in both female and male students but are more common in women. Both types – anorexia nervosa and bulimia nervosa – are seen. Most cases are mild in students but some are severe and cause impairment, requiring the student to take time out from their studies or residency to receive appropriate treatment. One of the risk factors for anorexia is perfectionism, which is not uncommon in medical students and residents. Men with eating disorders share the same preoccupation with body image and thinness as do women; some of these men may be gay but not always. Excessive exercise is seen in both men and women students who are striving to be thin.

18.3.7   Personality Disorders

Although personality disorders in physicians do exist, they are usually not diagnosed until after the training years are completed. However, retrospective analysis illustrates many examples of traits or deficits during the phases of medical school or residency. All three clusters of personality disorders may be seen. Cluster A personality disorders are seen in those students who are loners, somewhat eccentric, excessively shy or suspicious and mistrustful. Not uncommonly, their professors or clinical supervisors have noticed that they are not part of the 'group' and may seem odd in their verbal behaviour or written work. Cluster B personality disorders are more obvious by their high emotion, 'in your face' behaviour, cheating on examinations or lying about on call schedules, dramatic actions, self-injurious behaviour and so forth. Cluster C personality disorders describe some of the more anxious, obsessional, immature, dependent and unsocialised medical students and residents. Without inappropriately labelling students with personality traits or disorders, clinical teachers in psychiatry might be better able than their colleagues to recognize these students and ensure that they receive a far-reaching assessment (and treatment) should they come to their attention.

18.4   Common Stressors in the Lives of Students Today

The four years of medical school constitute a time of massive transition from undergraduate life (or a first career in non-traditional students) that involves many different challenges and goals. Some of these are: learning a new language and acquiring a new role of young professional [32]; coming to terms with the limits on how much one can be expected to know and master; often for the first time, accepting academic decline (and failure in some students); adjusting to a new programme and course of study; leaving friends and family support if one has moved to begin medical school; consolidating one's sexuality and intimacy in a significant relationship, including marriage in some students and separation or divorce in others [33]; confronting developmental tasks – increasing maturity, responsibility, commitment and autonomy; living with enormous debt; confronting ethical dilemmas and challenges in clinical medicine, including abusive behaviour in some residents, faculty or patients toward medical students [34, 35]; and, for some, facing serious illness and death in grandparents or parents.

What follows is an example of a marital crisis in a resident:

> Dr Ramsey called a therapist asking if he could be seen as soon as possible, that he was afraid that 'I'm coming unglued'. His voice was quivering and he sounded very down. He told the therapist that he was on call that evening and he didn't know if he should be working or not. He arranged to see him that afternoon. His story was that he had begun to spend 'lots and lots' of time with Dr Lori, an ObGyn resident since starting his rotation at the Women's Hospital. This began as coffee together, talks in the residents' lounge when they were on call together, and a few walks together on the university campus. Three days earlier, when he and Dr Lori were post-call, they slept together back at her apartment. He immediately felt awful – and by his report, so did she. Dr Ramsey was married and his wife was home full time with their six month daughter. Dr Lori was married too – her husband was a resident in Neurosurgery. He was given a diagnosis of adjustment disorder with mixed anxiety and depressive symptoms; he was not clinically depressed, did not use or abuse substances and his overall health was good. Dr Ramsey agreed to see the therapist for individual treatment until he felt better and more fully appreciated the underlying dynamics contributing to the single episode of extramarital behaviour.

As residents embark on a four to six year period of training, they too must face challenges. In addition to similar stressors listed above for medical students, the top ten stressors are shown in Table 18.1.

There are additional stressors: ambivalence about the speciality and self-doubts about career choice; relationship strain given the huge numbers of hours worked and the ascendancy of training over the demands of an intimate relationship; difficulty finding a partner for some female residents and some gay and lesbian doctors; continuing financial worries; for residents

Table 18.1 The top ten stressors.

- Insufficient sleep (less than 3 hrs)
- Frequent night calls (every third night or more)
- Uncompromising attending physicians
- Large patient load
- Too much 'scut' work (tedious, unrewarding, trivial)
- Too much medical records work
- High rates of death among patients
- Little or no contact with fellow residents
- Inadequate sexual activity
- High peer competition to impress staff

Source: Peterkin, personal communication

who are parents, role strain in trying to balance work and family wishes and demands; studying for board examinations; and finding a fellowship or job at the completion of residency.

18.5   Unique Issues for Ethnic Minority and International Medical Graduate (IMG) Trainees

Like the population that doctors serve, medical students and residents are a mosaic of race, ethnicity and culture. In the United States, the cultural studies of African Americans, Hispanics and Asian Americans give us some context for the diversity and multiculturalism of our students. To appreciate some of the special challenges of minority students, the reader is advised to consult the following publications: African Americans [36–39]; Hispanics [40,41]; and Asian Americans [42,43]. Many of the principles outlined by these authors are unifying, despite the recognition that an Hispanic student from New Mexico comes from a different cultural context than one from Chile or Spain, as does a trainee from Harlem versus someone from Nigeria. Each will bring a unique story to their medical studies. The following vignette of a resident is illustrative.

Case Example

Dr Thomas was a 33 year old black physician who was a junior resident in cardiology when he came to see a psychiatrist. He was quite depressed. Given the history of a previous illness in medical school and a significant family history of mood disorders (and suicide), he was diagnosed as having Major Depressive Disorder – recurrent type. He was restarted on the same antidepressant that had been helpful for his earlier depression. Within 10 days, he was beginning to feel better. With improvement of his mood and cognition, his psychiatrist was able to obtain valuable history, and the psychosocial factors at work in the precipitation of his clinical symptoms.

Firstly, Dr Thomas felt very isolated in his department. He was the only black resident and there were no faculty – academic or clinical – who were black. 'In fact, I'm it. There are minority nurses, aides, laboratory technicians, clerical staff and housekeeping personnel – but not one is black. I've had a couple of black patients and that's been refreshing. I think I'm a bit of an oddity in this city'. Having attended a mostly minority student medical school, Dr Thomas' work setting was very foreign to him. Secondly, he was single and good looking. 'I get a lot of attention from the nurses and others at work. I've done a lot of dating. It's great for the ego. Most of the women ask me out. Easy sex too. But there's no intimacy. It's very empty. And very lonely'. Thirdly, Dr Thomas felt dismissed for what he called his humanistic side. 'I've always been interested in story telling. It's part of my black heritage, going back so many generations. This is what attracted me to medicine. I would have pursued psychiatry but I'm in cardiology because heart disease is rampant in my family and I want to contribute to research into this killer. But my attendings are not interested in the nuts and bolts of my patients' lives. They've been very critical of the time I spend at the bedside and my presentations at rounds (getting teary... 'that hurts...').

—Myers and Gabbard [29, page 19]

It is important to delineate some of the common challenges for international medical graduates (IMGs), challenges that exist on top of the 'normal' trials that all residents have as they pursue graduate medical education (Table 18.2).

Table 18.2 Challenges for international medical graduates.

- Becoming acculturated to North America
- Learning English, especially idioms and slang (if they are from non-English speaking countries)
- Facing temporary periods of isolation from their peers
- Coping with a sense of longing for family and friends
- Preparing for one or more examinations
- Coming to terms with examination failure on first attempts
- Facing financial hurdles
- Confronting a myriad of medical licensing board regulations
- Facing discrimination
- Dealing with the stigma associated with emotional strain or psychiatric illness
- Balancing the adoption of the values of North America with the preservation and abandonment of some of their home customs.

Each of these challenges is no easy feat and, in the aggregate, the journey can become overwhelming [29].

Case Example

Dr Mirwan, a fellow in endocrinology, called with this chief complaint: 'I think I'm starting to behave a little weird at work'. He was 33 years old, unmarried and the only member of his family living abroad. Born in the Middle East, he came to North America to do residency training. Struggling with early morning wakening, crying outbursts, lowered self-esteem, poor appetite and a 10 pound weight loss, he wondered if he was depressed. Then he added, 'Or I wonder if I have a histrionic personality disorder'. His psychiatrist confirmed the former and challenged the latter.

Statements from several interviews with Dr Mirwan illustrated many of the strains contributing to his mood disorder. 'Three members of my family are very ill – one is my brother – he's been diagnosed with multiple sclerosis – he doesn't deserve it'. 'I feel like I have failed them, if I were there I could oversee their care'. 'I am very closed, I don't talk about my feelings, I don't want to show my insecurities – and my culture is macho'. 'I have become too focused into myself, very self-absorbed – this is not good, not normal where I come from. That's why I worry that I have developed histrionic personality disorder since coming here'. 'I miss the intimacy of the Middle East – you people are different – cool, busy, no time to talk about things outside of medicine'.

There was a family history of depression and suicide. The fact that Dr Mirwan acknowledged this history was instrumental in his accepting the notion of antidepressant medication. He responded nicely to a SSRI drug and was compliant in taking it. Stigma was ever present, both at the beginning and during the entire time that he was in treatment. 'I accept the biomedical part of depression, that I am genetically predisposed – as I am for diabetes – and that my neurotransmitters are off. But I am ashamed that I have depression. I feel deficient, not just chemically, but in strength and resistance to stress. As an IMG I must be very guarded that no one learns of this. I am almost paranoid that if anyone in authority finds out, I will be asked to leave the residency and be deported home. I am made to feel 'lucky' to have this residency position. I must be very careful. Even though I know that mental illness exists globally, I believe also that I have shamed my home country by getting sick here. That geopolitically I have let her down. That as a visitor here, I must be a good ambassador'.

—Myers and Gabbard [29, page 29]

18.6   How We Can Assist

18.6.1   Promote Self-Care

Stuber has written, '*Medical school is the best time to set up habits that can help you to be a better doctor and a happier, healthier person for the rest of your life*' [32]. Her recommendations include: prioritizing one's time, making and maintaining friendships, getting regular exercise, taking the time for relaxation and respecting good sleep hygiene. One of the best venues to introduce these basic notions of self-care is during orientation to medical school and residency training [44]. However, these principles will not be followed or accepted by trainees if their role models have a different philosophy. All too often medical students and residents complain that their chiefs or attending physicians over-work, eat poorly, are sleep-deprived, rarely exercise and lead lives that are desperately out of balance. And worse, trainees may quickly get the message that the rigours of study and clinical work eclipse all notions of self-care. The goal, of course, is some blend or harmony of competing forces but this takes commitment and effort on everyone's part.

18.6.2   Overcoming Barriers to Getting Help

The stigma associated with recognizing and accepting that one's symptoms require attention needs to be addressed on day one of medical school or residency. Lectures and small group peer discussions help a lot. Voluntary self-disclosures of previous illness and treatment by students, residents and faculty have great appeal and deliver a clear message that stress and vulnerability are human conditions that do not escape physicians. In many medical centres or at national meetings, physicians who are in recovery from alcoholism or other substance abuse disorders or non-chemical illnesses like mood or anxiety disorders are often willing to share their stories at orientation [45].

18.6.3   Establishing Resources for Students

In the United States, the Liaison Committee on Medical Education (LCME) has established standards for medical schools to establish systems for psychological and psychiatric coun-selling. This includes the development of programmes to promote medical student wellness [46]. Examples of interventions include lectures and seminars on stress management, cogni-tive restructuring and relaxation techniques, mindful-based stress reduction (MBSR) tech-niques and simple reflection. Many programmes today have a student counselling service for symptomatic individuals, staffed with masters or doctoral level psychologists or clinical social workers. These professionals provide assessment and short term treatment that is available quickly (same day or within days) and at no cost (or minimal expense). Their services are invaluable and may even be life-saving for students in crisis. Most on site services have rapid access to psychiatrists who make themselves available on an urgent basis to assess and treat those students who are severely ill, at risk of self-harm or harm to others or perhaps psychotic.

In 2001, the Joint Commission on Accreditation of Healthcare Organizations (JCAHO) required that identification and education of impaired physicians be mandated but separate from disciplinary action [47]. Further, it ordered that all staff and resident physicians be educated on physician impairment and offered resources for psychiatric or substance abuse concerns [48, 49]. Confidentiality is essential.

All students need to be told at orientation – and repeatedly over their training – that services are available, that they are on site or nearby, that the care is confidential and totally separate from the dean's office (and their academic file) and that it works! Very few students – whether medical students or residents – are actually diagnosed with impairment (meaning that their illness or use of drugs has adversely affected their ability to study, attend classes or practice medicine safely and competently). Individuals who are (or who may be) impaired are usually assessed and followed by the state physician health programme over time; this fact is known to the medical school or residency programme, but only by key individuals in authority and personal health details are never shared.

18.6.4 Training Experts in Medical Student and Physician Health

Most mental health professionals would argue that medical students and residents are really no different than other people in postgraduate training and one can apply the same skill set when assessing and treating these individuals. This is largely true. However, there are findings over 30 years of study that can enlighten professionals who treat this population. Some of these are:

- There is a significant risk of burnout in students.

- Perfectionism is a common trait that is a risk factor for anxiety, depression, burnout and suicide.

- There are family pressures to succeed at all costs in some ethnic minority trainees.

- Students admit to a high level of felt or perceived stigma in acknowledging psychological or psychiatric vulnerability.

- Today's medical culture can be overly rigorous and unforgiving.

- Trainees are prone to over function, including over studying or over working.

- There are significant rates of alcohol and/or other substance abuse in medical students and residents.

Continuing medical education on this subject includes many publications, web sites, courses and international conferences [50, 51].

18.6.5 Changing the Culture of Medicine

Despite the fact that our students continue to face major educational and psychological challenges through their training years and beyond, gains have been made from a few decades ago. Directors of medical student education and residency programme directors are not just focused on pedagogical matters and clinical excellence in their students and residents. They are universally aware that a variable number of students completing psychiatry clerkships and electives – and residents and fellows – are struggling with a myriad of issues that may affect their well-being. There is increasing interest in medical student and physician health by academic psychiatrists [52].

Most educators in today's medical centres would agree that the culture of medicine is changing. There is more evidence-based research on medical students and physicians. This helps to identify at-risk medical students and residents – and to strive for earlier intervention and treatment. This diminishes morbidity, suffering, impairment, medical error, physicians on disability insurance and premature death.

As an example of how seriously one country has confronted the subject of physician health, the Canadian Medical Association launched the Centre for Physician Health and Well-Being in 2003. It is housed in Ottawa, Ontario, and is a clearing house and coordinating setting for information resources for medical students, physicians and their families. Its four key areas are: health promotion and disease prevention, awareness and education, advocacy and leadership and research and data collection [53].

Finally, most psychiatric educators today are committed to the notion of balance in their own lives and those of their students. There are many challenges [54]. There is a long history of overwork in medicine, a high commitment to one's patients (and teaching, research and administration) and, despite being in the mental health field, a tendency to not always recognize marital strain and/or problems with one's children [55]. Medical students and residents will confront these competing commitments throughout their lives. Hopefully, this journey will be eased by their teachers and clinical supervisors modelling some modicum of balance in their own professional and personal lives.

18.7 Key Points

- It is well known that being a medical student or resident is a time of transition. Not uncommonly, trainees develop symptoms of burnout, anxiety disorder, mood disorder, chemical dependency and more.

- Even without a DSM-IV diagnosis – or contributing to a specific diagnosis – there may be significant stressors in the lives of students, such as financial worries, sleep deprivation from being on call, adjustment to training, harassment or abuse in the medical setting, relationship strain at home and so forth.

- Minority trainees and international medical graduates often face additional challenges that can complicate their work or put them at greater risk of illness.

- Medical institutions must have free (or affordable) resources available for their symptomatic students to receive timely and state-of-the-art care.

- Deans of medical schools, programme directors and psychiatric educators must recognize the stigma that students feel regarding accepting psychiatric help. This calls for a collective effort to fight this.

- The culture of medicine must continue to change and evolve so that all students safely progress through their training and thrive as young professionals.

References

1. William Osler Quotes. BrainyQuote. www.brainyquote.com (accessed 30 July 2010).
2. Guthrie, E., Black, D., Bagalkote, H. *et al.* (1998) Psychological stress and burnout in medical students: a five year prospective longitudinal study. *J R Soc Med*, **91**, 237–243.
3. Moffat, K.J., McConnachie, A., Ross, S. *et al.* (2004) First-year medical student stress and coping in a problem-based learning medical curriculum. *Med Educ*, **38**, 482–491.
4. Tyssen, R., Vaglum, P., Gronvold, N.T. *et al.* (2001) Suicidal ideation among medical students and young physicians: a nationwide and prospective study of prevalence and predictors. *J Affect Disord*, **64**, 69–79.
5. Aktekin, M., Karaman, T., Senol, Y.Y. *et al.* (2001) Anxiety, depression and stressful life events among medical students: a prospective study in Antalya, Turkey. *Med Educ*, **35**, 12–17.
6. Dahlin, M., Joneborg, N. and Runeson, B. (2005) Stress and depression among medical students: a cross-sectional study. *Med Educ*, **39**, 594–604.
7. Niemi, P.M. and Vainiomaki, P.T. (2006) Medical students' distress – quality, continuity and gender differences during a six year medical programme. *Medical Teacher*, **28**, 136–141.
8. Hsu, K. and Marshall, V. (1987) Prevalence of depression and distress in a large sample of Canadian residents, interns and fellows. *Am J Psychiatry*, **144**, 1561–1566.
9. Toews, J.A., Lockyer, J.M., Dobson, D.J. *et al.* (1997) Analysis of stress levels among medical students, residents and graduate students at four Canadian schools of medicine. *Acad Med*, **72**, 997–1002.
10. Cohen, J.S. and Patten, S. (2005) Well-being in residency training: a survey examining resident physician satisfaction both within and outside of residency training and mental health in Alberta. *BMC Medical Education*, **5** (21), 1–11.
11. Dyrbye, L.N., Thomas, M.R., Massie, F.S. *et al.* (2008) Burnout and suicidal ideation among US medical students. *Ann Intern Med.*, **149**, 334–341.
12. Dyrbye, L.N., Thomas, M.R., Huntingdon, J.L. *et al.* (2006) Personal life events and medical student burnout: a multicenter study. *Acad Med*, **81**, 374–384.
13. Thomas, M.R., Dyrbye, L.N., Huntingdon, J.L. *et al.* (2007) How do distress and well-being relate to medical student empathy? A multicenter study. *J Gen Intern Med*, **22**, 177–183.
14. Martini, S., Arfken, C.L., Churchill A. and Balon, S. (2004) Burnout comparison among residents in different specialities. *Acad Psychiatry*, **28**, 240–242.
15. Waldman, S.V., Diez, J.C.L., Arazi, H.C. *et al.* (2009) Burnout, perceived stress and depression among cardiology residents in Argentina. *Acad Psychiatry*, **33**, 296–301.
16. Woodside, J.R., Miller, M.N., Floyd, M.R. *et al.* (2008) Observations on burnout in family medicine and psychiatry residents. *Acad Psychiatry*, **32**, 13–19.

17. Dyrbye, L.N., Thomas, M.R. and Shanafelt, T.D. (2006) Systematic review of depression, anxiety and other indicators of psychological distress among US and Canadian medical students. *Acad Med*, **81**, 354–373.

18. Levine, R.E., Litwins, S.D. and Frye, A.W. (2006) An evaluation of depressed mood in two classes of medical students. *Acad Psychiatry*, **30**, 235–237.

19. Clark, D.C. and Zeldow, P.B. (1988) Vicissitudes of depressed mood during four years of medical school. *JAMA*, **260**, 2521–2528.

20. Zoccolillo, M., Murphy, G.E. and Wetzel, R.D. (1986) Depression among medical students. *J Affect Disorders*, **11**, 91–96.

21. Givens, J.L. and Tija, J. (2002) Depressed medical students use of mental health services and barriers to care. *Acad Med*, **77**, 918–921.

22. Hendrie, H.C., Clair, D.K., Brittain, H.M. *et al.* (1990) A study of anxiety/depressive symptoms of medical students, house staff and their spouses/partners. *J Nerv Ment Dis*, **178**, 204–207.

23. Lande, R.G., Marin, B.A., Chang, A.S. *et al.* (2007) A survey of alcohol consumption among first-year military medical students. *Am J Drug and Alc Abuse*, **33**, 605–610.

24. Curran, T.A., Gawley, E., Casey, P. *et al.* (2009) Depression, suicidality and alcohol abuse among medical and business students. *Irish Med J*, Online version.

25. Akvardar, Y., Demiral, Y., Ergor, G. *et al.* (2004) Substance use among medical students and physicians in a medical school in Turkey. *Soc Psychiatry and Psychiatric Epidemiology*, **39**, 502–506.

26. Borschos, B., Kuhlhorn, E. and Rydberg, U. (1999) Alcohol and drug use among medical students 1995: more than every tenth male student had hazardous alcohol drinking habits. *Lakartidningen*, **96**, 3253–3258.

27. Hughes, P.H., Brandenburg, N., Baldwin, D.C. *et al.* (1992) Prevalence of substance use among US physicians. *JAMA*, **267**, 2333–2339.

28. Baldisseri, M. (2007) Impaired health care professional. *Critical Care Medicine*, **35**, 106–116.

29. Myers, M.F. and Gabbard, G.O. (2008) *The Physician As Patient: A Clinical Handbook for Mental Health Professionals*, American Psychiatric Publishing, Inc., Washington, DC, p. 84.

30. Heru, A., Gagne, G. and Strong, D. (2009) Medical student mistreatment results in symptoms of posttraumatic stress. *Acad Psychiatry*, **33**, 302–306.

31. Klamen, D.L., Grossman, L.S. and Kopacz, D. (1995) Posttraumatic stress disorder symptoms in resident physicians related to their internship. *Acad Psychiatry*, **19**, 142–149.

32. Stuber, M.L. (2006) Medical student and physician well-being, in *Behavior and Medicine*, 4th edn (eds D. Wedding and M.L. Stuber), Hogrefe and Huber, Cambridge, MA, pp. 167–174.

33. Myers, M.F. (2000) *Intimate Relationships in Medical School: How to Make Them Work*, Sage, Thousand Oaks, CA.

34. Coverdale, J.H., Louie, A.K. and Roberts, L.W. (2005) Protecting the safety of medical students and residents. *Acad Psychiatry*, **29**, 329–331.

35. Coverdale, J.H., Balon, R. and Roberts, L.W. (2009) Mistreatment of trainees: verbal abuse and other bullying behaviors. *Acad Psychiatry*, **33**, 269–273.

36. Anderson, L.P. (1991) Acculturative stress: a theory of relevance to Black Americans. *Clin Psychol Rev*, **11**, 685–702.

37. Pyskoty, C.E., Richman, J.A. and Faherty, J.A. (1990) Psychosocial aspects and mental health of minority medical students. *Acad Med*, **65**, 581–585.

38. Post, D. and Weddington, W. (1997) The impact of culture on physician stress and coping. *J Nat Med Assoc*, **89**, 585–590.

39. Webb, C., Smith, S., Hawkins, M. *et al.* (2000). Focus on African American medical students, in *Taking My Place in Medicine* (ed. C. Webb), Sage, Thousand Oaks, CA, pp. 139–155.

40. Glymour, M.M., Saha, S. and Bigby, J.A. (2004) Physician race and ethnicity, professional satisfaction, and work-related stress: results from the physician worklife study. *J Nat Med Assoc*, **96**, 1283–1294.

41. Canive, J.M., Castillo, D.T. and Tuason, V.B. (2001) The Hispanic veteran, in *Culture and Psychotherapy: A Guide to Clinical Practice* (eds W.-S. Tseng and J. Streltzer), American Psychiatric Publishing, Inc, Washington, DC, pp. 157–172.

42. Du, N. (2006) Asian American patients, in *Clinical Manual of Cultural Psychiatry* (ed. R.F. Lim), American Psychiatric Publishing, Inc, Washington, DC, pp. 69–117.

43. Comas-Diaz, L. and Jacobsen, F.M. (1991) Ethnocultural transference and countertransference in the therapeutic dyad. *Am J Orthopsychiatry*, **61**, 392–402.

44. Dickstein, L.J. (1998) *Health Awareness Workshop Reference Manual*, Proactive Press, Louisville, KY.

45. Myers, M.F. and Dickstein, L.J. (1997–2010) Psychiatrists Living with a Mental Illness. Workshop "Treating Medical Students and Physicians". Syllabus and Proceedings Summary, American Psychiatric Association Annual Meeting, American Psychiatric Association, Washington, DC.

46. Liaison Committee on Medical Education (2009). AAMC. Washington, DC (http://www.aamc.org/meetings/annual/2009, accessed 30 July 2010).

47. Joint Commission on Accreditation of Healthcare Organizations Selected Medical Staff Standard (2001). Physician Health: MS 2.6. (http://www.jointcommission.org, accessed 30 July 2010).

48. Greenup, R.A. (2008) The other side of the stethoscope. *Acad Psychiatry*, **32**, 1–2.

49. Broquet, K.E. and Rockey, P.H. (2004) Teaching residents and program directors about physician impairment. *Acad Psychiatry*, **28**, 221–225.

50. Myers, M.F., Dickstein, L.J. and Zigler, P. (2008) Treating Medical Students and Physicians (Workshop). Syllabus and Proceedings Summary, American Psychiatric Association Annual Meeting, American Psychiatric Association, Washington, DC.

51. Faculty and Physician Wellness Program (2009). Vanderbilt University Medical Center, Nashville, TN (http://healthandwellness.vanderbilt.edu, accessed 30 July 2010).

52. Myers, M.F. (2008) Physician impairment: is it relevant to academic psychiatry? *Acad Psychiatry*, **32**, 39–43.

53. Center for Physician Health and Well-Being (2009). Canadian Medical Association, Ottawa, ON, Canada (http://www.cma.ca, accessed 30 July 2010).

54. Louie, A., Coverdale, J. and Roberts, L.W. (2007) Balancing the personal and the professional: should and can we teach this? *Acad Psychiatry*, **31**, 129–132.

55. Sotile, W.M. and Sotile, M.O. (2000) *The Medical Marriage: Sustaining Healthy Relationships for Physicians and Their Families*, American Medical Association, Chicago, IL.

19

Psychiatrist Educators

David Baron[1] and Bulent Coskun[2]

[1]Department of Psychiatry, Keck School of Medicine, University of Southern California, Los Angeles, CA, USA
[2]Department of Psychiatry, Kocaeli University Medical School, Kocaeli, Turkey

19.1 Introduction

The word 'doctor' comes from the ancient term 'docere'. The translation of this word is not 'to diagnose' or 'to treat', but rather 'to teach'. When we stop and think about what we do as physicians, and particularly psychiatrists, to help our patients maintain health or treat disease, *teaching* them how to maintain emotional homoeostasis and better deal with life stress is an important component of every treatment strategy and clinical intervention. While medical education has focused on the acquisition of knowledge in understanding how the body functions, and our skills in diagnosing and treating dysfunction, precious little time is devoted to instructing doctors how to teach. The model of see one, do one, teach one continues to dominate clinical medical education worldwide. How will the next generation of psychiatric educators be trained?

In this chapter, methods to train psychiatric educators are discussed, relevant target groups identified, examples of effective teacher training programmes provided and teacher training programmes for psychiatric residents recommended.

19.2 Examples of Teacher Training Programmes

The concept of instructing psychiatric residents and faculty how to be better teachers is increasingly being recognized as an important component of formal training and career development. Creative programmes devoted to 'teaching the teacher' are being recognized and rewarded by national psychiatric professional organizations in most developed countries worldwide. In the United States, for example, the American College of Psychiatrists gives

Teaching Psychiatry: Putting Theory into Practice   Edited by Linda Gask, Bulent Coskun and David Baron
© 2011 John Wiley & Sons, Ltd

an annual award to residency programmes from all over the world that have developed and implemented creative teaching programmes. Most of the programmes focus on creative ways of teaching psychiatry residents how to better teach medical students. An important outcome of this friendly competition has been a significant increase in the number of residents choosing to pursue careers in psychiatric education.

Effective teaching, like conducting psychotherapy, is a skill that requires the acquisition of core competencies along with a supervised clinical experience. Observing a good teacher is necessary, but not sufficient to becoming an effective teacher. Like psychotherapy training, learning to be a competent teacher has both content and process components. Content issues include topics such as the development of specific goals and objectives, the proper use of action verbs, development of effective slides and educational aides, and maintaining relevancies for the learners (amongst other issues). Process issues include effective communication styles, knowing your audience and sharing a positive affect with the learners. Virtually all students can differentiate a good lecture from a bad one.

The role of instructing how to become a good teacher involves dissecting what components are necessary to provide a meaningful learning experience. Education includes a cognitive and affective component. The facts (cognitive) are the basis of education. The teacher must know his/her student. How those facts are presented will determine how much the learner is able to absorb. A boring lecture with no affect from the teacher, or one not sensitive to the learning style and abilities of the learners, will not result in a quality educational experience. This underscores the need to abandon the see one, do one and teach one mentality and move towards formal education in how to teach. Credentialing organizations can promote this concept by adding requirements for core didactics in how to teach for all psychiatric residents. Their target learners should be medical students, patients, the public, peers, faculty and non-psychiatric colleagues.

19.3   Methods for Teaching Psychiatric Educators

The methods used to train psychiatric educators are as varied as any in the educational field. Competent educators require both content and process knowledge in psychiatry, as well as in adult learning theory.

The rapid advances in educational technology have altered the expectation of medical students and residents. The days of 35 mm slides have given way to PowerPoint and Blackboard. Students now expect to receive material before the lecture is even given, and many choose to not even attend formal lectures at all. It is a new generation of students who have grown up with the Internet and advanced IT. Despite these technical advances, a good lecturer must still have a passion to teach, be organized, demonstrate relevance of the material to the students and know the subject.

The current instructional technologies available are not reviewed in this chapter. This is not meant to diminish their importance, but the topic is too broad and levels of core competence and availability vary widely across the globe. What does not vary is the basic characteristics of a good teacher and what goes into presenting a lecture that teaches the students what they need to know.

Medical students, residents and postgraduate physicians are all professional students. They would not have gotten into medical school if they did not succeed academically. They also tend to be excellent critics of teachers. They may not know the specific subject matter, but they know a good lecture when they hear one.

The most important component of teaching psychiatric educators is to identify those that want to be educators in the first place. People who do not want to teach, should not. Many individuals will want to teach, but feel inadequate and fearful they will do it poorly. Instilling confidence is essential in training educators of all types, especially in psychiatry. A good way to identify potential psychiatric educators is to allow them to self-identify while still in medical training. Once identified, these students should be offered additional training in educational techniques. The 'see one, do one, teach one' mentality of pre-Flexner medical education and the mentorship model of many residency programmes is no longer sufficient. Future psychiatric educators need formal instruction on how to organize a lecture or course, prepare educational materials and, most importantly, how to engage their students (whatever their level). Books are available on instructional design, but require mentorship from experienced educators. Would we ever consider teaching a student how to conduct psychotherapy by merely reading a book? Like becoming a better athlete, practice makes perfect. More accurately, perfect practice makes perfect. Novice teachers need to get in front of a class and receive feedback from their mentors.

Training to become an educator should ideally start during the undergraduate years, but this is not often possible with the rigours of premedical education or the intensity of the ever-expanding medical curriculum. A few programmes worldwide offer advanced postgraduate training in medical education, but these are too few in number. There needs to be a greater focus placed on training psychiatric educators at all levels (premedical, medical, residency, postgraduate and community education). Some universities with schools of education offer advanced training for physicians wanting to become educators, but these are limited. National psychiatric organizations, like the American Psychiatric Association (APA) and UK Royal College of Psychiatrists (RCP), offer courses at their scientific symposia, as does the World Psychiatric Association (WPA) (the editors of this text all met through their involvement with the WPA Education Section). Quality teaching provides more than just well educated students who can appreciate the vital role of mental health in physical health. It is our best recruiting tool and the most effective way to address the stigma towards psychiatric patients by our non-psychiatric colleagues and society at large. We need to continue to emphasize the need to train the next generation of psychiatric educators and provide resources and incentives to maintain interest. The future of our field and the ability to provide quality patient care depends on it.

19.4 Target Groups for Psychiatrist Educators

The important role of the physician as an educator can be traced back to the origin of the word 'doctor' meaning 'teacher'. To be an effective educator, one must be cognisant of the students' background and abilities, and be able to articulate specific goals and objectives. There are numerous variables which will effect the style and content of material being presented. These include the availability of resources, the amount of time available to present the material, the experience and knowledge of the teacher and the motivation of the students. This is particularly important for psychiatric educators. Medical students around the world often do not regard psychiatry as their most important subject and do not see themselves as ever caring for patients with mental illness. Psychiatric educators must be aware of this potential issue and establish relevance of the subject for the students at the beginning of the course. Each target group of students will have a different core understanding of basic principles and varying expectations of what they want from the instruction. The skilled educator will alter the instruction to better fit the needs of the students, given the limitation of time and resources, and the requirement to achieve specific goals and objectives (Box 19.1).

Box 19.1   Target Groups for Psychiatrist Educators

1. **Medical students, psychiatry residents, other physicians and medical staff:**

   (a) medical students

   (b) psychiatry residents

   (c) non-psychiatric physicians.

2. **Professionals from other sectors and opinion leaders:**

   (a) non-physicians (professionals from other sectors and opinion leaders)

   (b) decision makers and opinion leaders.

3. **The community in general, including patients, family members and people at risk:**

   (a) patients and their family members

   (b) people at risk of developing mental problems

   (c) the general population/lay people.

Psychiatrist educators need to customise curricular content for medical students according to their specific needs. Most medical students are concerned with passing required examinations so they can progress in their medical training. A small number will choose to become psychiatrists. Their motivation is very different than that of a psychiatric resident. For the residents, an additional aim should be to demonstrate their future role as psychiatrist educators themselves, in addition to the needs and expectations of the residency programme. For non-psychiatric physicians and other medical staff, sharing psychiatric knowledge and skills should be presented in a way that emphasizes the role of psychiatry in the practice of medicine. It is important to use medical models to emphasize key clinical points. The use of psychiatric jargon is not effective and should be avoided.

For other non-physician professionals, including teachers, social workers, coaches, government officials, business men and women, the content and delivery style must be adapted to the audience. A detailed description of psychopharmacology is likely not appropriate. However, a description and overview of key issues might be very effective and help achieve the desired goals. For decision makers and opinion leaders, the content should be evidenced based whenever possible and the take home message must be clear and well articulated. An underlying agenda will often be to advocate for mental health promotion and proper prevention, treatment and rehabilitation programmes for patients with mental illness, in addition to any other didactic objective.

When teaching patient groups, their families, at-risk groups and the general public, different approaches may be required. The psychiatrist educator is not only providing information but also representing the entire field of psychiatry. The stigma associated with mental illness and addictive disorders must be kept in mind. Cardiologists lecturing on heart disease need not be concerned about stigma, but psychiatrists must always address this issue when speaking to the public. No opportunity to address stigma should ever be lost. Topics such as dealing with stress and the role of emotional stress on physical health are particularly relevant for the general public. The message that there is no health without mental health is valuable for this group of learners. Liberal use of medical analogies may also help diminish stigma. The fact that psychiatrists are medical doctors with a special expertise in understanding how people think, feel and behave cannot be overstated. Our patients have treatable diseases, just like the rest of medicine. Psychiatric educators need to share the advances taking place in the field, while keeping them in proper context. An example would be discussing exciting work taking place in understanding the role of psychogenomics, while not having the public becoming vulnerable to claims that psychopathology can be predicted by a single genetic test. Valid and reliable data should be the basis for all education.

The education of specific groups will now be considered. These sections are summarized in Boxes 19.2, 19.3 and 19.4, along with recommendations for how to evaluate these activities.

19.4.1   Psychiatrist Educators for Medical Students

It is a challenging task for all clinician teachers to act as a clinician and an educator. But since medicine is an applied science, it is inevitable to have two roles synchronized [1]. Clinicians working at hospitals or Academic Medical Centres are usually expected to be equipped with teaching skills, yet most of them have not received any formal training on teaching [2]. Recently this problem has been recognized; training is now provided and special departments have been established on medical education at medical schools to draw the attention of the faculty members to teaching principles.

Other than the various approaches and tools medical educators use during teaching, the decision about the focus of the education is vital. In daily practice it may be the medical content, the vision or the interested area of the instructor or the learner. The main focus is strongly suggested to be the learner. The content has to be structured and executed in a manner that facilitates learning instead of inhibiting it [3]. The educator should also realize that learners have different learning styles, and teaching methods should be designed accordingly [4]. Amongst all the target groups, medical students may be the youngest and with less knowledge and skills when compared to other groups, but still they would benefit from adult learning techniques. Even at this level, they have achieved the success in getting into this challenging training.

Box 19.2   Recommendations Regarding Medical Students, Psychiatry Residents, Other Specialists, GPs and Medical Staff

	What to do and how	In collaboration with	Outcome measures
Medical students	Start teaching to be an educator at an early level. Teach to be advocates of mental health promotion and prevention of mental disorders Encourage involvement in social responsibility projects	Committees on undergraduate education National and local psychiatry organizations Residents NGOs	Following up of attitudes and behaviour on physician patient relations Following up recruitment into psychiatry Involvement with voluntary mental health related projects
Psychiatry residents	Teach to be 'educators' for different groups Give responsibility in teaching and evaluation of medical students Encourage involvement in community projects	Psychiatry residents and their national, local organizations NGOs	Feedback from students Following up graduated residents' career development
Medical staff at hospitals and Academic Medical Centres	Organize liaison activities with other departments ('learning together' projects) Work on common education projects with different disciplines Encourage collaborative symposia, workshops, research Organize educational activities on stigma, stress management, communication skills	Other departments, education committees Interested individuals or organizations of nurses, psychologists, social workers, hospital administrators etc.	Following up patient satisfaction Following up job satisfaction, burnout and stress levels in the hospital personnel
Medical staff at Primary Care Centres	Organize 'learning together' projects with primary care workers Organize coordinated patient and public education programmes on health issues (behaviour changing regarding healthy lifestyles)	National and local health administrations Organizations of family physicians / GPs / Nurses	Following up patient satisfaction comparatively Following up job satisfaction, burnout and stress levels in the hospital personnel

Psychiatrist educators may very well be role models for medical students, amongst whom new psychiatrists will develop. However, the 'educator role' can also be modelled. In a study for fourth year medical students, to teach them how to teach during their internship, Haber *et al.* [5] found that students who had participated in this programme were highly in favour of the inclusion of the programme into the medical education. 97% of respondents 'agreed' or 'strongly agreed' with the statement: 'Formal instruction in teaching should be a required part of medical education'. Participants of this course were surveyed during the last month of their internship and then 84% 'agreed' or strongly agreed' with the statement: 'The teaching to teach course helped prepare me for my role as a teacher during internship'.

Education of medical students in psychiatry and the roles of psychiatrists in this process have been discussed extensively in other chapters of this book.

19.4.2 Psychiatrist Educators for Psychiatry Residents

An important component of every residency training programme should be formal instruction on how to be an effective teacher. Residents need to learn how to teach to different learners, including peers, medical students, non-psychiatrist physicians, patient groups and the general public. Residents should receive instruction on both the process and content of how to teach. Process issues relate to the effective component of learning and include delivery style, use of instructional aides, engaging the audience and other factors. Content issues include the material being presented, using recent data and having a command of the subject. Residents often feel unqualified to be lecturing despite having an adequate knowledge base. They need to gain confidence and be reassured they do not have to be the world expert on a topic to give a good lecture. They should be counselled on how to organize and prepare a lecture, then practice giving it in front of a mirror before getting up to the podium. Public speaking is a common social phobia even for many physicians. Preparation and practice are the most effective strategies to bind this form of performance anxiety. If time permits, giving the lecture to a supervisor before presenting to a larger group will allow for constructive feedback and valuable experience for the resident. The supervisor should also assist the resident by providing suggestions on how to bind their anxiety prior to giving lecture or conducting an educational activity.

Residents must also be taught how to present to different groups of learners at a level that is appropriate to their knowledge base. Physicians sometimes forget the language routinely used with colleagues may not be fully understood by non-physicians, even well educated individuals. The resident must be instructed how to adapt the material to maximize its effectiveness and impact for the audience. A key concept is 'translational education'. This is the process of taking complex material not familiar to the learner and presenting it in a fashion which makes sense and is understandable to the learner. An important rule to follow is to avoid 'psychobabble' or the use of terms unique to psychiatry but not generally used as a component of the general lexicon. When these terms are used, for example 'transference' or 'splitting', the educator defines the term and offers examples to better clarify the use of the word. Presenting a lecture that sounds scholarly but is not understood by the learner is not good teaching. The goal of teaching is not to impress but to educate.

19.4.3   Educating Non-Psychiatric Physicians

The need to educate non-psychiatric physicians cannot be overstated. It is imperative that our non-psychiatric colleagues understand and appreciate the role of mental health in the practice of medicine. Although the core content is similar, the delivery should be customized to best match the work environment and experience of the learner. The different groups are broadly divided into those working in Academic Medical Centres and those in Primary Care settings or General Hospitals/Out-patient Clinics. A key issue is to ensure that the material being taught is relevant to the audience and not merely viewed as something only a psychiatrist would treat. For example, when lecturing to internists on depression, discuss the increased mortality from virtually every physical illness in depressed patients versus illness matched controls and the robust extant data demonstrating poorer response to somatic interventions in depressed physically ill patients. To enhance credibility, providing an overview of the mechanism of action, by reviewing research demonstrating alterations in immune functioning in depressed and anxious patient, will enhance relevance for the learner (Chapter 13).

Recently, there has been an increasing interest in effective treatment of medically un-explained symptoms and psychosomatic disorders. It is said that the treatment for these is often ineffective and there may be costly investigations which may be 'unnecessary, un-pleasant and not without risk'. The solution is stated to be the continuous improvement of communication skills and patient centred practice. The inclusion of practical assessment of communication skills into the examination in the United Kingdom seems to be an encour-aging factor for General Practioner (GP) training. GPs have to pass the college examination to enter general practice [6]. In this process there is responsibility for psychiatrist educators to share their experiences.

19.4.4   Educating Non-Physicians (Professionals from Other Sectors and Opinion Leaders)

The general lack of public mental health literacy is a global problem, but more pronounced in developing countries. This plays a major role in the stigma of mentally ill patients, which continues to exist in all areas of the world. An effective strategy is for psychiatrists in all clinical settings to engage in public education programmes at every level. Presenting to local civic groups, schools and, especially, politicians and public servants, can make a significant contribution towards better public understanding of mental health and mental illness. These must be viewed as illnesses with a biopsychosocial diathesis, just like the rest of medicine. It should not be assumed that just because someone is educated they understand even the basic principles of psychiatry. As noted above, presentations should avoid psychiatric jargon and focus on the use of analogies that are familiar to the learner. Special efforts should be made to engage political leaders. As the world's economy has become stressed, often the first cuts are made to mental health and drug and alcohol treatment programmes. The most effective strategy to combat this problem is to educate the decision makers and stay actively involved with a strong voice. Not taking time to educate this important group will very likely result in even greater reductions in services and funding.

Box 19.3   Recommendations Regarding Professionals Working at Schools, Workplaces and the Decision Makers and the Opinion Leaders

	What to do and how	In collaboration with	Outcome measures
Schools, work-places, social institutions	Organize research (needs assessment and follow up after implementations) and educational projects (aiming to empower professionals from other disciplines and sectors)	Teachers, psychologists, counsellors, social workers, lawyers, parent organizations, NGOs	Following up attitudes and behaviour on stigma
	Try to be aware of and to contribute to projects on all sectors related to educational activities on psychosocial well-being	Administrators of schools, workplaces, armed forces, prisons, social institutions Involvement of residents and voluntary medical students in the projects	Following up satisfaction levels of the service users Following up absenteeism, job satisfaction, burnout and stress levels in the relevant personnel
Decision makers and opinion leaders	Be an advocate of mental health promotion, disease prevention	International, national, local governmental organizations and NGOs	Increase in budget for projects related with mental health
	Try to see the needs and motivations behind the needs	Work together with opinion leaders who have experience on people with mental problems	Following up of the news on media
	Contribute to producing evidence regarding crucial role of awareness and education in overall development of nations		
	Contribute to positive mental health in media		

The number of professionals is almost never sufficient for the need, even in developed countries or in developed parts of less developed countries. But as would be expected in developing areas the conditions are much worse. It is possible to find institutions with no physician, no psychologist, sometimes only very few when compared with the demand. In such conditions psychiatrist educators may organize supportive visits for institutions where the human resources are limited. Those supportive visits and consultations would help to reduce burnout in the mental health professionals working in hard situations. Other than the supportive visits, mental health professionals working at different institutions may be invited to periodic case discussion meetings to enrich their knowledge and skills. Monthly meetings have been held for about two years in Kocaeli, Turkey, for the mental health professionals working at crisis centres and at two regional prisons. Sometimes psychiatry residents also attend the meetings, where 'difficult situations' are discussed and solutions are sometimes searched for by various techniques, including role plays.

19.4.5   Educating Decision Makers and Opinion Leaders

The decision makers are the key people who need to learn evidence-based scientific facts applicable to their realities. They have their own motivations, priorities and responsibilities [7]. Psychiatrist educators should be able to focus on the needs behind the needs, to persuade the decision makers, for the promotion of mental health.

It may be helpful to mention a practical note on 'knowledge and skills sharing': psychiatrist educators should avoid the paternalistic attitude of some instructors. It should be kept in mind that all other specialists – GPs or professionals of different disciplines or sectors – have their own areas of expertise and will expect respect for their previous knowledge and implementation styles, though some of those may be in contradiction to what the psychiatric educator will believe or practice. So as not to cause resistance to what is being suggested, the psychiatrist educator should be able to use their general knowledge and skills in convincing, in a respectful manner. If some kind of change in the attitude or the behaviour of the other professionals is going to be suggested, some time should be spent to understand the rationale behind those attitudes or behaviours. Psychiatrist educators should be ready to learn, ready to compromise or, where necessary, ready to strongly disagree and insist, but always with an understanding and egalitarian attitude.

19.4.6   Educating Patients and Their Family Members

Acceptance of psychopathology as a 'real disease' has increased over the past 20 years. As a result, families have played a more active role in caring for loved ones experiencing psychiatric disease and are requesting more information from psychiatrists. In addition, advocacy groups continue to grow in developed and, to a lesser extent, developing countries around the world. Psychiatrists need to engage these groups in meaningful dialogue to educate them about advances in the field, including new research in the aetiology and treatment of psychopathology. As mentioned earlier in this chapter, teaching this audience needs to be sensitive to the educational background of the learners. Given the availability of the internet globally, this can be a valuable resource. It is important for the psychiatrist educator to screen Internet educational material for the quality of the content. The internet is not peer reviewed and information should be screened by a professional. Patients and their families need to be alerted to fraudulent and grossly biased information they may encounter.

19.4.7   Educating People at Risk of Developing Mental Problems

Individual survivors of severe psychological and/or physical trauma (violence and/or sexual assault), people with fatal or severely disabling diseases, their family members or masses of people as victims of natural or man-made disasters or poverty are a few examples in a list of people under risk of mental problems.

Usually it is not easy to access people under risk; some may not comprehend the risks, if they are informed about the risks some may not accept that their conditions are risky, many may have rational reasons for continuing their risky behaviour, some may not have any choice to change their situation, others who may be offered the chance may not have the courage or motivation to move. Some of these people, if not most of them, may have lost many things in their lives and may not have much more to lose, so almost all may be hopeless and aimless. They may not be willing to be advised or educated.

Box 19.4   Recommendations Regarding Patients, Family Members and the General Population

	What to do and how	In collaboration with	Outcome measures
Patients and their family members	Encourage participation to patient and family organizations Organize or contribute to education programmes for awareness Be part of educational activities to reduce stigma (contribute to media – through newspapers, radio, TV)	Patient and family organizations Opinion leaders, mainly people from media	Patient and family member satisfaction on the services Products of rehabilitation activities Employment of former users of mental health services
People at risk of developing mental problems	Provide advice to governmental organizations and NGOs Develop and contribute to educational projects on rehabilitation, fight against dependency, violence, suicide etc.	Other professionals (teachers, psychologists, social workers, counsellors), Governmental organizations and NGOs	Statistics on dependency, crime, violence and suicide Some research on the situation of people representing those at risk
The general population/lay people	Organize or contribute to projects on public awareness in psychosocial well-being and healthy lifestyles Develop and contribute to projects on stress management Be part of educational activities to reduce stigma	Work together with other professionals, former users of mental health services or voluntary people	Statistics on dependency, crime, violence and suicide

---

The psychiatrists may meet some of those people at prisons, some at hospitals, others in some special institutions. If they are referred to the psychiatrist because of their symptoms, the attempt at psychoeducation may be together with proper treatment. If these people are recognized through any kind of scanning they should be informed and encouraged about possible alternatives to their risky behaviours.

As has been emphasized above, the psychiatrist can only be a part of a team of mental health professionals and some volunteers. One of the best groups of volunteers may come out of former users of mental health services, for whom helping others would have valuable therapeutic effect as well [8]. A radio broadcast for mental health promotion in Australia, presented by people who themselves had mental problems, not only gave members of the public a better understanding of the mental health issues but also appeared to give consumers of mental health services empowerment, confidence and self-esteem, and allow them to lead productive lives again [9].

19.4.8   Educating the General Population/Lay People

The educator role of the psychiatrist for the general population should be part of a general mental health programme. It should be in line with the overall health policy and the mental health policy, if there is one. There may be innovative activities in response to local needs, but to have a sustainable and effective public education, psychiatrists must be aware of the national and local programmes. If there are problems with the existence of such policies or programmes, the very first task should be to work for raising awareness to advocate for such programmes.

Psychiatrist educators, through their instructor role for medical students and residents, advocate public education on mental health issues at different levels and on different occasions. In addition to sharing knowledge and skills, they may encourage students and residents to take part in community mental health projects where they themselves may be the models.

Education programmes for the general public may be classified in several ways, according to the method, the topics and, finally, the media through which the education is conducted.

Although details are beyond the scope of this chapter, it would be fair to say that before going into any kind of education process the first step should be to assess the needs, priorities and learning styles of the target population. Assessments for the effectiveness of the education should be used for monitoring the level, the depth, the periodicity and the length of the education. For the various media to be used, it must be kept in mind that the messages should complement each other, in line with the main theme of the education. Some psychiatrist educators may prefer to focus on training of other professionals or volunteers, others may prefer to reach directly the population [10], either in small groups or through books, brochures or channels like radio [9], video [11] or internet-connected graphic environments [12].

A compendium of public education projects can be found in a book published by the World Health Organization and the World Federation for Mental Health [13].

19.5   Recommendations

As has been highlighted in other chapters in this book, teaching psychiatry is a complex, albeit highly rewarding, task. As the field continues to evolve with significant advances being made in the neurosciences, the core concepts of biopsychosocial factors interacting to influence phenotypic presentation remains the keystone of understanding mental health and psychopathology. A well educated medical student needs to understand and appreciate this complex interaction of salient factors. All clinicians, not just psychiatrists, need to be advocates for their patients overall well-being. Psychiatric educators must demonstrate the importance of eliciting clinical information, beyond merely documenting physical symptoms, and must be a role model for how to effectively engage the patient to elicit this data.

In this chapter, specific examples of topics to be covered at various stages of training, from medical students through post graduate courses, have been offered. The need to present this information from a public health perspective, rather than just a mental health perspective, will assist the educator in decreasing the inherent stigma that continues to negatively affect attitudes and opinions of the field.

References

1. Taylor, E.W., Tisdell, E.J. and Gusic, M.E. (2007) Teaching beliefs of medical educators: perspectives on clinical teaching in pediatrics. *Med Teach*, **29**, 371–376.
2. Wilkerson, L. and Irby, D.M. (1998) Strategies for improving teaching practices: a comprehensive approach to faculty development. *Academ Med*, **73**, 387–396.
3. Stahl, S.M. and Davis, R.L. (2009) Applying the principles of adult learning to the teaching of psychopharmacology: overview and finding the focus. *CNS Spectr*, **14**, 179–182.
4. Dobbing, K.R. (2001) Applying learning theories to develop teaching strategies for the critical care nurse. Don't limit yourself to the formal classroom lecture. *Crit Care Nurse Clin North Am*, **13**, 1–11.
5. Haber, R.J., Bardach, N.S., Vedanthan, R. *et al.* (2006) Preparing fourth-year medical students to teach during internship. *J Gen Intern Med*, **21**, 518–520
6. Walton, I. (2008) Mental health education and resources for general practitioners in the UK. *Mental Health in Family Medicine*, **5**, 121–123.
7. Jenkins, R. (2003) Supporting governments to adopt mental health poicies. *World Psychiatry*, **2**, 14–19.
8. Ikkos, G. (2005) Mental health service user involvement: teaching doctors successfully. *Primary Care Mental Health*, **3**, 139–144.
9. Ormsby, N. (2004) Radio beyondblue: Radio broadcast in South Australia, in *Mental Health Promotion Case studies from Countries* (eds S. Saxena and P.J. Garrison), World Health Organization and World Federation for Mental Health, France, pp. 8–9.
10. Vassiliadou, M.S. (2004) Athens mental health promotion programme: Raising the awareness of health professionals and the public in Greece, in *Mental Health Promotion Case Studies from Countries* (eds S. Saxena and P.J. Garrison), World Health Organization and World Federation for Mental Health, France, pp. 41–43.
11. Coskun, B. (2006) Utilization of Video Recorded Experiences after a Natural Disaster as a Tool for Disaster Preparedness Education. *Slice of Life 2006 Abstract Book, 18th International Meeting for Medical Multimedia Developers and Educators, Lausanne, Switzerland*, pp. 28.
12. Yellowless, P.M. and Cook, J.N. (2006) Education about halucinations using an internet virtual reality system: a qualitative survey. *Acad Psychiatry*, **30**, 534–539.
13. Saxena, S. and Garrison, P.J. (eds) (2004) *Mental Health Promotion Case studies from Countries*, World Health Organization and World Federation for Mental Health, France.

Index

Teaching Psychiatry: Putting Theory into Practice   Edited by Linda Gask, Bulent Coskun and David Baron
© 2011 John Wiley & Sons, Ltd

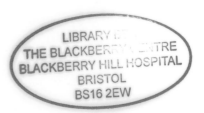

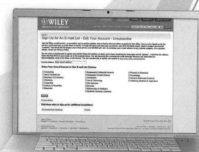